Ashok Muzumdar (Editor)

Powered Upper Limb Prostheses

Control, Implementation
and Clinical Application

Springer

Berlin
Heidelberg
New York
Hong Kong
London
Milan
Paris
Tokyo

Ashok Muzumdar (Editor)

MB, BS, FRCPC, FACP, AFCASI, DAAPM, LM

Powered Upper Limb Prostheses

Control, Implementation and Clinical Application

With 154 Figures and 11 Tables

Springer

ISBN 3-540-40406-6
Springer-Verlag Berlin Heidelberg New York

Ashok Muzumdar
Ottawa, Canada

Library of Congress Cataloging-in-Publication Data
Muzumdar, Ashok, 1940– . Powered upper limb prostheses/
Ashok Muzumdar. p.; cm. Includes bibliographical references
and index. ISBN 3-540-40406-6 (hard cover: alk. paper) 1. Artificial limbs. 2. Myoelectric prosthesis. 3. Prosthesis. 4. Human
engineering. 5. Amputees–Rehabilitation. I. Title. [DNLM: 1.
Artificial Limbs. 2. Arm. 3. Prosthesis Design. WE 172 M994p
2004] RD756.M89 2004 617.5'7403–dc22

Springer-Verlag is a part of Springer Science + Business Media

springeronline.com

© Springer-Verlag Berlin Heidelberg 2004
Printed in Germany

Cover design: E. Kirchner, Heidelberg
Product management and layout: B. Wieland, Heidelberg
Reproduction and typesetting: AM-production, Wiesloch
Printing and bookbinding: Appl, Wemding

21/3150 – 5 4 3 2 1 0
Printed on acid-free paper

Preface

Powered Upper Limb Prostheses represents, in my view, a concise yet comprehensive book on the subject of myoelectrically controlled externally powered prostheses for both child and adult upper limb amputees. It is a natural successor to the series of monographs on myoelectric prostheses produced by the Institute of Biomedical Engineering and published by the University of New Brunswick in Canada. The UNB monographs have been out of print for some years now. Therefore, this body of work on powered upper limb prostheses not only fills that void but, in addition, provides new and updated information on the many facets of powered prostheses for patients with upper limb loss or absence.

There are various factors that determine the success of the application, fit and function of a powered upper limb prosthesis. Selecting the appropriate prescription for any patient, client or user requires the knowledge, experience and skills of a multidisciplinary team of professionals. Expertise for such a specialized amputee clinic team comes from a wide variety of specialities and sub-specialities of health care and engineering.

The flow pattern of the book follows the philosophy of informing the reader of the past, present and future of powered upper limb prostheses. The text begins with a historical perspective followed by basic muscle anatomy and electrophysiology as well as the origins, acquisition and processing of the myoelectric signal. With the intention of remaining unbiased, analysis is made of the commercially available components for upper extremity prostheses for young children, adolescents and adults. The clinical chapters deal with the prevalence, psychosocial issues and outcomes pertaining to upper limb deficiencies along with assessment and prosthetic fitting of paediatric and adult amputees. This is followed by training which includes the pre- and post-prosthetic phases and subsequent rehabilitative care. The book reviews the current research on the subject and examines the future of myoelectric upper extremity prosthetics. It concludes with a bibliography which is in addition to the suggested reading and references provided at the end of the chapters.

While there is general consensus among academics and practitioners on the many aspects of powered upper limb prostheses in children and adults, in some centres prevailing philosophy and practices may differ from those outlined in this book by various authors. In order to present a broad spectrum of viewpoints in a balanced manner, this book brings together authors who are experienced practitioners, academics and researchers in the field from Canada, Great Britain and the United States. The bibliography allows the reader to pursue their own ideas and further their search on specific topics of interest to them.

This book should serve as a foundation for students as well as a resource for professionals in related disciplines of engineering and medicine. It is my hope that the confluence of information presented by the contributing authors of this book will provide the knowledge for those involved in the field of powered upper limb prosthetics to progress well into the twenty-first century.

Ashok Muzumdar

Disclaimer

While the advice and information in this book are believed to be true and accurate at the time of submission for publication, neither the authors nor the editor and publisher can accept any legal responsibility for any errors or omissions made in any part of this book. The material presented in this volume is not intended to represent the only method or application appropriate for the medical situations discussed, but rather is intended to present an approach, viewpoint, statement or opinion of the author or authors, which may be helpful to others who encounter similar clinical situations.

The opinions expressed, suggestions made and advice given in this book are those of the respective author or authors and not necessarily those of the editor or the publisher. The publisher and the editor make no warranty, express or implied, with respect to any material contained herein.

Table of Contents

Contributing Authors

Randall D. Alley BSc, CP, FAAOP
Clinical Research and Business Development
Upper Extremity Prosthetic Program, HPO, Inc
Thousand Oakes, California, USA

Robert R. Caldwell Dip E Eng, CET
Manager, Institute of Bio-Medical Engineering
University of New Brunswick
Fredericton, New Brunswick, Canada

Paul H. Chappell BSc, PhD, CEng, MIEE,
MIPEM, ILTM
Lecturer, Medical Engineering, Electronics
and Computer Science
University of Southampton
Southampton, UK

Shane Glasford CP(c)
Prosthetic and Myoelectric Services
Bloorview MacMillan Children's Centre
Toronto, Ontario, Canada

David Gow BSc Hons, CEng, SRCS
Director, Rehabilitation Engineering Services,
Lothian Primary Care NHS Trust
Eastern General Hospital
Edinburgh, Scotland, UK

Hanna Heger BA, OT Reg(Ont)
St. John's Rehabilitation Hospital and
Sunnybrook Centre for Independent Living
Toronto, Ontario, Canada

Winfried Heim CP(c)
Prosthetic and Myoelectric Services
Bloorview MacMillan Children's Centre
Toronto, Ontario, Canada

Sheila A. Hubbard BSc PT, OT Reg(Ont)
Manager, Amputee Team
Bloorview MacMillan Children's Centre
Toronto, Ontario, Canada

Peter J. Kyberd BSc, MSc, PhD
Lecturer, Cybernetics Department
University of Reading
Whiteknights, Reading, Berkshire, UK

Dennis F. Lovely BSc, PhD, PEng
Professor, Dept. of Electrical
and Computing Engineering
University of New Brunswick
Fredericton, New Brunswick, Canada

Linda McLean BSc(PT), MScE, PhD
Assistant Professor, Physical Therapy
School of Rehabilitation Therapy
Queen's University
Kingston, Ontario, Canada

Gert Montgomery BScN, MSW, RSW
Social Worker & Professional Advisor
for Social Work,
Chaplaincy & Creative Arts Service
Bloorview MacMillan Children's Centre
Toronto, Ontario, Canada

Stephen Naumann PhD, PEng
Director, Rehabilitation Engineering Department
Bloorview MacMillan Children's Centre
Toronto, Ontario, Canada

Sandra Ramdial CP(c)
Manager, Custom Silicone Services,
Otto Bock
Oakville, Ontario, Canada

Robert N. Scott BSc, DSc, PEng
Professor Emeritus
Department of Electrical Engineering
University of New Brunswick
Fredericton, New Brunswick, Canada

Harold H. Sears BS, MS, PhD
General Manager
Motion Control Inc
Salt Lake City, Utah, USA

Heather Smart BA, Dip Lib, MIInfSc
Information Officer, RECAL Information Services
National Centre for Training and Education
in Prosthetics and Orthotics
University of Strathclyde
Glasgow, Scotland, UK

Dinah Stocker MEd, BSc OT
Institute of Bio-Medical Engineering
University of New Brunswick
Fredericton, New Brunswick, Canada

The Early History of Myoelectric Control of Prosthetic Limbs (1945–1970)

L. McLean · R. N. Scott

Contents

Summary

This chapter traces the development of myoelectric control of prosthetic arms from its conception in post-war Germany through its popular acclaim in "bionic arms" toward its acceptance as a routine and valid option for many arm amputees. Separate and apparently unrelated conceptions of myoelectric control in Germany, the United Kingdom, the USSR, the USA and Canada are followed with particular attention to the gradual achievement of collaborative ties research and the even slower development of commercial products for clinical application. The impact of wars, epidemics and world political climate upon this activity is noted. The chapter is written from the perspective of one of the authors (RNS), who directed a program of myoelectric controls research at the Institute of Biomedical Engineering at the University of New Brunswick, Fredericton, NB, Canada through this period and is based on a careful review of the extensive collection of relevant literature held at the Institute, much of which is unpublished or has had only a very restricted circulation.

1.1 Introduction

The concept of a myoelectric prosthesis is simple. The electrical activity naturally generated by contracting muscle in a residual limb is amplified, processed and used to control the flow of electricity from a battery to a motor, which operates an artificial limb.

However the design of a clinically useful myoelectric prosthesis is extremely difficult. The prosthesis must be comfortable, must work reliably and must have a natural appearance both at rest and during functional activities. In addition, as noted by Weiner

[69], the prosthesis ideally should replace not only mechanical function but also cutaneous and kinaesthetic sensation. The challenge of achieving a comfortable fitting becomes greater as the weight of the prosthesis increases; thus minimizing weight becomes an important design objective. To achieve clinical acceptance, ease of fitting, adjustment and training are essential. The challenge of achieving a natural (anthropomorphic) appearance creates size constraints. A natural appearance during function, what Tucker called "dynamic cosmesis", is equally important [58] and contributes to the complexity of design both in terms of segmental trajectories and in terms of mechanical noise. Versatility, typically achieved through modular design, is important if the needs of a variety of individuals are to be met.

It is these aspects of myoelectric prosthesis design which have challenged designers since myoelectric control was conceived and it is the failure to meet these design criteria which continues to challenge users, clinicians, engineers and researchers alike. Finally, despite all of the above design constraints, the cost of the device should be controlled. Like most technological products, mass production of myoelectric prostheses would contribute to affordability. However, the market is both small in numbers and complex in its diversity and research and development costs are high, leaving little scope for cost reduction

As with many medical technologies, developments in myoelectric prosthetics have tended to follow major political, economic or epidemiological world events. After a war, the demand for technological development is enhanced by the presence of victims of the war. Funding tends to increase due to a feeling of accountability by governments. Sometimes technological developments driven by military requirements can be applied to prosthetics. Of all victims, however, the "Thalidomide Children" – children born to mothers who had taken the drug Thalidomide during pregnancy – provided the most touching appeal as single and multiple limb amelia or phocomelia were common, leaving clinicians and researchers desperate for improved limb prostheses. The political response was to provide public funds for research and development into improved prostheses for these children.

1.2 The Beginnings of Myoelectric Control

Myoelectric control was first implemented by Reinhold Reiter, a physics student at Munich University. The first written evidence of Reiter's research was a May 1945 patent application [51].

The only published report of Reiter's work, in a German medical newspaper, [53], described a myoelectric prosthetic arm designed for the amputee factory worker. A prototype was demonstrated at the Hannover Export Fair in that year. The research leading to this device was supported by the Bavarian Red Cross and private sources [53]. Pudlusky, who was Reiter's business manager for the project, noted that development of the system was terminated due to the lack of funds after the German currency reform in 1948 [51].

The prototype prosthesis, intended for concept testing, was not portable: its control system employed vacuum tubes which required considerable power* and the electric hand was quite inefficient, so the prosthesis was dependent on energy from the building wiring. It could be used at a factory work station, where the amputee would don the limb once seated, use it for gross motor tasks as required and remove it at the end of his shift. But in this form the prosthesis would be of little use in general activities of daily living.

The idea behind the control system was to amplify the myoelectric signal from a contracting muscle in order to control a wooden hand, which was modified to be actuated by an electric solenoid. Reiter used a single muscle site in the residual limb. Control of opening and closing motions was derived from using "two different rhythms of contraction". This scheme of using the signal from a single muscle to control two motions (plus an "off" state) was later to be known as "three state control" [15]. Reiter's version of this control was a rate-controlled system, in which a short duration, large burst of signal (identified by its rapid rate of rise) would send power to the solenoid, opening the prosthetic hand. In the absence of any

---

* The transistor was not invented until 1948 [2]

signal, after a certain prescribed period of time the hand would close. While the hand was open, a lower amplitude pulse of myoelectric signal (identified by its lower rate of rise) would reduce the current in the solenoid, causing the hand to be nudged closed before the prescribed delay. This combination of voluntary opening with automatic closing of a terminal device was later to become known as a "cookie crusher" control [56].

It is clear now that Reiter's work was doomed, in terms of clinical use, by the limitations of available technology. But beyond that, it appears that Reiter's invention was not known to the researchers who were responsible for pioneering work in this field in Europe and elsewhere – or, at least, this knowledge was not admitted. Certainly the work was not well known until the oversight was reported in a widely read engineering journal in 1969 [51].

Reiter's work was not alone in being overlooked in the early development of myoelectric control. The myoelectric signal had been used to monitor lookout alertness as early as 1947 [63], and by 1957 to control respirators for polio victims [3]. Indeed, it had been investigated as a possible control source for prostheses as early as 1949, with encouraging results [5].

Perhaps publication in different journals would have made a difference, particularly as there was no computer-based literature search capability in this era. Reiter's report was published in a medical newspaper, Travis and Kennedy's in a journal of physiology and psychiatry [63], Batson's in the journal "Science" [3] and Berger and Huppert's in The American Journal of Occupational Therapy [5]. Hence the pioneers of this work likely did not benefit from idea sharing with their contemporaries in other disciplines.

In any event, through the late 1950s and early 1960s researchers began re-inventing parts of Reiter's myoelectric control system. This work occurred independently and almost simultaneously in the USSR, the United Kingdom, the USA, Europe and Canada. It was aided greatly by the availability of transistors, without which a truly portable myoelectric prosthesis was not practical.

1.3 National Beginnings of Myoelectric Prosthetics

1.3.1 The United Kingdom

Research on myoelectric control in the United Kingdom was initiated in an effort to provide control to polio patients requiring orthotic devices and was extended to include the control of prosthetic limbs. Much of this research was funded by the British National Fund for Research into Poliomyelitis and other Crippling Diseases [7]. The primary researchers in this field were A. H. Bottomley, C. Battye, A. B. Kinnier Wilson and A. Nightingale.

Battye and Nightingale were the first British researchers to describe a myoelectric control system for an artificial hand (M. Näder, O. Bock Orthopädische Industrie, Duderstadt, personal communication with R. N. Scott, 1986 [9]) and published their first work regarding a functional myoelectric control system in 1955 [4]. Their initial work was based on the premise that the signals used to control a prosthesis should be derived from remnants of the muscles that would have produced these movements in the normal limb [8]. This led to the conclusion that two muscles are needed to control hand opening and closing. This work does not seem to have progressed beyond the laboratory prototype stage.

1.3.2 The USSR

Research in myoelectric control at the USSR Academy of Sciences and the Central Prosthetics Research Institute, Moscow, had begun by 1957 [37]. This group was aware of prior research in the area of myoelectric control of prostheses, referencing specifically the work of Battye et al. in the UK [10, 35, 36]. However the Russian group considered that work quite elementary and credited themselves with the first formulation of bioelectric control principles [35, 36]. It is interesting that this group, in selecting the myoelectric signal power as the information carrier for control purposes, noted the probability that other parameters of the myoelectric signal, including parameters related to its frequency characteristic would prove useful in the future [37].

Kobrinski's group shared Bottomley's view that two independent sources of bioelectric signals were required to control an artificial hand [37]. Accordingly their prosthetic limb used separate muscle sites for pickup of myoelectric signals, one to control hand opening and the other to control hand closing. They developed the first myoelectrically controlled prosthesis to be manufactured for clinical use. It was battery operated, designed for an adult male with a below elbow amputation. After reports of clinical success in the USSR, the fitting rights were sold to groups in the UK, Canada and other countries, where clinical trials began amidst a flurry of highly exaggerated media reports of "Bionic Arms" [56]. The engineers responsible for the technical aspects of these trials were frustrated by design limitations and by the use of inferior quality components in the USSR systems, the latter problem being attributed by the USSR personnel to funding limitations (A. Lippay 1964, Trip report – Roehampton and Manchester, England, 13–20 Dec 1964, unpublished work). (This suggests that the project may have had a rather low priority for USSR government funding). Clinical response, of which McKenzie's report [43] is typical, likewise was rather subdued.

1.3.3 The United States

The first research in the United States involving myoelectric control of prostheses had been conducted some years before by Berger and Huppert at New York University [5]. Their research, begun in 1949, involved feasibility studies on muscle bulging and on myoelectric signals as possible sources of prosthesis control. As noted above, this work was overlooked in the USA for some time along with that of Batson and Montgomery.

By 1959, a group headed by Lyman of the University of California at Los Angeles (UCLA) was involved in research into myoelectric control for applications in prosthetics and orthotics. These researchers were aware of the work of Travis and Kennedy, as well as Battye's work and that in Moscow. Their first techni-

cal report [70], provides a remarkably accurate analysis of the challenges in myoelectric control systems development, identifying problems and forecasting likely solutions. This academic research was not translated into devices or systems for clinical use, however.

Interestingly, members of Lyman's group apparently did not rebut the negative reports on USSR myoelectric controls research given at the Lake Arrowhead Conference by Reswick of Case Western Reserve University [48]. Reswick had been in Moscow at the First International Congress on Automatic Controls earlier that year and had witnessed a demonstration of the Russian arm. He reported that the Russians had "hinted" at myoelectric control but would not divulge any details, and suggested that myoelectric control would not be feasible.

1.3.4 Austria

Zemann of Austria began working on a myoelectric control system as a result of publicity given to the U.S.S.R. system. By 1966 he had contacted Otto Bock Orthopädische Industrie, of Duderstadt, which had a strong foundation in related rehabilitation technology, in order to obtain a suitable hand (M. Näder, O. Bock 1986, Orthopädische Industrie, Duderstadt, personal communication with R. N. Scott). The Hüffner Hand was adapted by Otto Bock for this purpose, however it was not satisfactory due to the lack of space available to incorporate the control circuitry and to its low efficiency and thus Otto Bock developed a new electric hand, Model Z1, intended for use with myoelectric controls. Zemann's work was continued by Viennatone, a hearing aid manufacturing company in Austria and eventually marketed as the Viennatone Hand system, incorporating a hand nearly identical to the Otto Bock Z1 hand.

1.3.5 Germany

Otto Bock, meanwhile, under the leadership of Dr. Max Näder, began development of a myoelectric prosthesis and introduced its first system for clinical use in 1967, incorporating an improved electric hand, Model Z6 (M. Näder, O. Bock 1986, Orthopädische Industrie, Duderstadt, personal communication with R. N. Scott). As well, Otto Bock was the supplier of electric hands to Schmidl in Italy.

1.3.6 Italy

Two apparently separate research efforts in the area of myoelectric control began in Italy. Professor G. W. Horn, aware of the work in Russia and Britain, used some of the same principles to construct a myoelectric prosthesis [24]. His prosthesis included a position servo, which, in the absence of any myoelectric signal, would allow voluntary positioning of the fingers as determined by a potentiometer controlled by active rotation of the residual limb within the socket. There seems to have been no clinical follow-up.

The most important contribution in Italy however was by an Austrian, Hannes Schmidl, of the I.N.A.I.L. (the Instituto Nazionale per l'Assicurazione contro gli Infortuni sul Lavoro) in Budrio, who began myoelectric controls research in the early 1960s. Schmidl was motivated by the large numbers of children born with severe congenital limb deficiencies due to their mothers' use of Thalidomide. His first below-elbow prosthesis used relays to control the electric hand, one set of electrodes over the wrist flexors to close the hand and a set over the wrist extensors to open it. The control mechanism provided a degree of proportional control by using the duration of a contraction to create proportional power in the output [54]. Schmidl worked closely with Otto Bock in Germany, who provided a hand that would house the necessary circuitry in order to enable the system to be used clinically (M. Näder, O. Bock 1986, Orthopädische Industrie, Duderstadt, personal communication with R. N. Scott). Schmidl was to become well respected internationally for his innovative fitting of complex powered prostheses to persons with multiple limb loss.

1.3.7 Sweden

Researchers in Sweden began to look at myoelectric control of prostheses later than some others, essentially beginning their work in the mid 1960s. The emphasis in Sweden was on collaboration between various specialized groups in order to produce the best end product. The Swedish Council for Applied Research, the Swedish Medical Council and the Medical Society of Göteborg started joint research in 1963. They began concentrating on myoelectric control in 1964 and began looking at signal processing techniques as being the key to improved control at that time. In 1965, the division of Applied Electronics at Chalmers University of Technology in Göteborg began research in the area of myoelectric prostheses. As well, one of the key Swedish researchers, Roland Kadefors, was granted a scholarship to the US to study with the Case Western Reserve group [26]. Kadefors provided an invaluable link between myoelectric controls research in the US and Sweden.

1.3.8 Japan

The Japanese also joined late in the development of myoelectrically controlled prostheses. It seems surprising that a nation so devoted to technological advances and manufacturing would not be at the forefront of research in this area. However, upon further reflection, the Japanese are known for their marketing of technology and the demand for limb prostheses would not likely have proven to be lucrative. One researcher stands out among the Japanese. Kato, a professor of engineering at Waseda University, led the Waseda hand project, which was begun in 1964 in response to suggestions by Tomovic to design a feedback control system for use with myoelectric system hands [29]. This project was initiated in 1964, with the goal of incorporating an element of pressure feedback into the system. In the first prototype hand, a pressure sensitive resistor in the finger would initiate grasp automatically. Later on, this system progressed to the incorporation of independent movement of each of the five fingers, all triggered by pressure sensors [29]. By 1967, myoelectric control was incorporated into the system using two channel ago-nist-antagonist myoelectric signals to provide ampli-tude-modulated control. The project continued and by 1969 a multi-function hand with pressure feed-back (Waseda hand 4P) was being evaluated [29].

A second group in Japan was that headed by Su-zuki, then professor of bio-electronics at Tokyo Med-ical and Dental University. He actually became in-volved in research in upper limb prosthesis control before Kato. Beginning in 1962, Suzuki produced a servo motor control system by 1964, and by 1965, he too was working on myoelectric control strategies, including a backlash circuit (as done by Bottomley) to overcome fluctuations in the myoelectric signal amplitude without degrading the response of the sys-tem. This amplitude information was used to control both velocity and force of hand movements [60]. Su-zuki went on to concentrate on the development of small implantable electrodes for use with multifunc-tion control systems.

Although the research done by these two, seeming-ly independent, Japanese groups was timely and of clinical importance, apparently none of their re-search led to a clinically fitted, manufacturable and marketable limb prosthesis.

1.3.9 Canada

The first myoelectric controls research in Canada was initiated by Scott, of the University of New Brunswick (UNB) in Fredericton [55, 57]. The initial goal was to provide wheelchair control and/or control of a feeder appliance for a high level quadriplegic patient, using myoelectric signals. This project was initiated in 1961, and very shortly was re-directed toward myo-electric control of prostheses, in response to the "Thalidomide crisis".

Influenced greatly by the clinical advice of re-search prosthetist Bill Sauter, of the Ontario Crippled Children's Centre in Toronto (OCCC), the UNB group concentrated on eliciting the maximum possible in-formation from a single muscle site, developing three-state control systems intended particularly for children with short below elbow amputations [15]. The first clinical fitting of a Canadian myoelectric

prosthesis, in 1965, was a collaborative effort between these two centres, using a system developed at UNB to control an electric prosthesis developed at OCCC. Interestingly, this prosthesis used a cable-powered, voluntary opening hook with a motor-driven wrist rotator– a marvelous prosthesis for pouring tea! [56]

1.4 Collaboration in Myoelectric Controls Research

Overall, myoelectric controls research has been aided significantly by formal and informal interactions among researchers in various countries. Information sharing began slowly, often impeded by individual, institutional or national desire for recognition. Be-cause the most important factors limiting the early clinical use of myoelectric prostheses were problems of hardware implementation, the natural tendency of potential manufacturers of these systems to work in secrecy was very important in limiting overall progress. When information was published, mem-bers of the various disciplines involved tended to publish in their own disciplinary journals, further impeding communication. Thus, many of the basic concepts of myoelectric control were re-invented in-dependently at several centers. After some time, how-ever, the political climate seemed to become more conducive to collaborative efforts both within and among countries. With encouragement from health organizations worldwide, conferences that empha-sized the importance of information transfer made a significant contribution to the evolution of a collabo-rative endeavour.

The Committee for Prosthetic Research and De-velopment (CPRD) of the US National Academy of Sciences/National Research Council played a major role in facilitating collaboration in prosthetics re-search, including myoelectric prosthetics. Interna-tional conferences such as those at Lake Arrowhead, California, in 1960 [48] and at Warrenton, Virginia, in 1965 [49], as well as many more specialized meetings, were organized and funded by CPRD, with the prima-ry mandate of bringing together the world leaders in prosthetics research to promote the sharing of knowledge and ideas and ultimately to promote global advancement in the field of prosthetics. Canadian centres participated fully in CPRD activities, with Colin McLaurin of Toronto, Canada, serving as CPRD chairman from 1969–1975, at a time when as many as three other members of the Committee were from Canada. As well, through its economic aid program the USA sponsored an important series of international research conferences in Yugoslavia, in the 1960s and 1970s.

In 1963, the Canadian government was faced with a public outcry due to its approval of clinical trials of the drug Thalidomide, which had resulted in some thirty infants being born in Canada with significant limb abnormalities. The number of victims in Canada was very low compared to the hundreds affected in Europe but this did nothing to reduce public criticism of the government, especially since the drug had not been approved by the US Food and Drug Administration. In response, promising to "solve the Thalidomide problem", Canada's Department of Health allocated funds to establish and operate new "prosthetics research and training centres" in Montréal, Toronto and Winnipeg and to support the existing group at UNB in Fredericton. A condition of this funding was that the research groups were to collaborate with one another, meeting together at least once per year. In retrospect, this research did little to help the Thalidomide victims but it did provide a foundation on which developments beneficial to many amputees were based.

1.5 Developments in Myoelectric Control

While the national beginnings of myoelectric controls research were independent and highly redundant re-inventions of Reiter's ideas, the activities of the next decade or so were quite collaborative. Research groups pursued different objectives but with increasing knowledge of work in other centres. There was even discussion about design standards to facilitate interconnection of components from various centres. What redundancy remained in the research programs, generally was intentional and useful.

1.5.1 The United Kingdom

Bottomley became the central investigator in many studies following his initial review of myoelectric control [7]. He tended to favor the idea of proportional control, wherein the power of the myoelectric signal would determine the degree of opening or closing of a prosthetic hook or hand [7, 9]. This type of control used more of the information embedded in the myoelectric signal to provide the user with a more graded and natural form of prosthetic function. One of Bottomley's contributions was his "autogenic backlash" circuit, which allowed for small fluctuations in the myoelectric signal amplitude to occur without disrupting the smooth control of the motor. Many groups involved in subsequent myoelectric controls systems research incorporated some form of backlash into their design.

By 1964, the Hanger Limb Factory was delivering the Russian Arm, the first functional myoelectric prosthesis to be manufactured in bulk, to orders from the British Limb Fitting Centres of the Ministry of Health throughout the UK. The company was modifying the design of the arm somewhat and upgrading the electronics using British components (A. Lippay 1964, Trip report – Roehampton and Manchester, England, 13–20 Dec 1964, unpublished work). At this time, while the Russian Arm was being distributed with some success throughout the UK, Bottomley's myoelectric arm was in the hands of the British Atomic Energy Research Institute, for miniaturization and development (A. Lippay 1964, Trip report – Roehampton and Manchester, England, 13–20 Dec 1964, unpublished work). To the authors' knowledge, it never emerged from that Institute.

1.5.2 The United States

Weltman and Lyman at UCLA continued research intended to achieve more accurate control in myoelectric systems [71]. Later on, Lyman and Freedy at the Biotechnology Laboratory of UCLA approached prosthesis control as an information transfer problem. They began to draw on techniques of pattern recognition, information theory and adaptive systems in order to develop the concept of limb tracking and adaptive aiding [18]. They described an "Autonomous Control System" capable of supplementing the operator's own conscious control by generating future end-point positions using the Maximum Likelihood decision rule to accept or reject a predicted position based on past movements performed by the system.

The UCLA group and others used military advances as precursors to myoelectric control research. Lyman contributed to the work done by Spacelabs Inc., which was interested in the servo control of spacecraft [59]. In 1961, Ellis and Schneidermeyer worked on a myoelectric control system for Litton Systems [17], in which myoelectric data would be used to control robots, aircraft at high G-forces and, as an afterthought, prosthetic and orthotic devices. The urgency of this research was primarily for military purposes due to the US involvement in Vietnam [14]. This war, however, did provide casualties who would then benefit from further prosthetics developments and thus in the post-war period, the medical use of myoelectric controls was a priority as well.

Others were also enticed by military funding to look at the properties of the myoelectric signal. Philco Laboratories were interested in using the myoelectric signal to provide performance capabilities beyond what would normally be possible under, for example, extreme G-forces in military aircraft. They offered a grant to Finley and Wirta in order to follow through with this research (F.R. Finley and R.W. Wirta 1965, A correlational study of myopotential response and force of muscle contraction during varying activity demands, (unpublished) interim report on contract no. Nonr 4292(00) for the Office of Naval Research, Washington; Bio-Cybernetics Laboratory, Philco Corporation, Willow Grove Pennsylvania). Later, as precision and accuracy became more important, pattern recognition techniques were developed in order to provide myoelectric control systems with multifunction control [72]. This research, as with most myoelectric controls research, was beginning to take on more of a civilian orientation, with applications to amputees and paralyzed individuals.

By the early 1960s, research into myoelectric control had finally begun to form some roots in the US other than at military funded laboratories. The advances made to this point had, for the most part, been derived from investigations which were intended for other purposes but which could be extrapolated for use in the prosthetics and orthotics field. Michael and Crawford at Oregon State University looked at the possibility of developing a "myoelectric language". Their intent was to employ fine control techniques to emulate the natural muscle movement patterns of a normal arm [47]. This theory did not go far, however it is the same type of theory that continues to dominate much of the research done even today. Engineers and health care professionals alike became involved in the advances in prosthetic limb research, with many centers across the United States working to develop a marketable myoelectrically controlled limb.

In 1961, Melvin Glimcher, Associate Medical Director of the Medical Services Center, Liberty Mutual Insurance Company, traveled to Russia in order to witness the most recent developments in myoelectric prosthesis control. Obviously Glimcher was more impressed by the Russian work than Reswick had been just one year earlier. Upon his return, he urged his colleagues at the Massachusetts Institute of Technology (MIT) to become involved. Then doctoral candidate Altman, through the assistance of his supervising professor, Bose, and with funding from Liberty Mutual Insurance Company, introduced prosthetic limb research as a specialty at MIT [1]. The group eventually developed the "Boston Arm", a high performance electric elbow with myoelectric control, which was and still is marketed internationally. This led to a strong academic research program in myoelectric control at MIT. Liberty Mutual provided the financial security necessary to promote high quality research and development at Liberty's Research Centre in Hopkinton Massachusetts, where fabrication of prosthetic limb systems for clinical use was undertaken on a commercial scale. The "ball-screw" mechanism of the original elbow being very inefficient, a new mechanism with a harmonic drive was developed by Gerard. As well, force feedback was removed from the system, permitting the use of a self-locking clutch that further reduced energy consumption. This mechanism was still in production, with only minor changes, as of the year 2000 (T.W. Williams

2000, Liberty Research, Hopkinston MA, personal communication).

Jacobsen, a graduate student working under Mann at MIT became well known in the field of prosthetics control [42] after leaving MIT in the late 1960s and going to the University of Utah. The "Utah Arm", developed by Jacobsen and others in the early 1970s was sold to a private bidder, becoming property of Motion Control Inc., which then began production for clinical use [25]. Those at MIT eventually began to collaborate with researchers at the University of Utah through Jacobsen and his colleagues. A more sophisticated system was designed to provide fine trajectory control. The collaboration between MIT and Utah continued in development of the "MIT/Utah dexterous hand" [56].

A large research group in Cleveland was formed by the combined efforts of Case Western Reserve University, Highland View Hospital and the Case Institute of Technology. By the mid 1960s, this group, headed by Reswick, was investigating the possibility of multiple control sites for myoelectric control. One interesting project studied the possibility of using small muscles behind the ear (the auricularis superior and posterior) in order to provide fine motor control of prostheses. Reswick (whose initial opinions of myoelectric control must have changed by this point) and Taba had been involved in this study previously, with funding by Northrop Aircraft [6]. This research was eventually discontinued due to the practical difficulties of accessing the muscles [46]. At this same center, collaboration with Vodovnik (from Yugoslavia) was aimed at the development of implanted telemetry devices with miniaturized circuit technologies [34, 41]. Vodovnik, Lippay and Starbuck developed the Case Research Arm Aid, a laboratory system for evaluating control systems for a variety of prosthetics or orthotics applications [34]. Continued investigation into telemetry was pursued by Ko and his associates, whose work developed radio transducers for telemetry control of prosthetic limbs [31–33].

Another myoelectric controls research group was formed by Snelson at Rancho Los Amigos Hospital in California. Unlike the groups at MIT and Philco Laboratories, the primary concern at this center was orthotics as opposed to prosthetics [68]. As with most groups, this one began with an on/off control strategy and then worked on proportional control. By the mid to late 1960s they had developed the Rancho Electric Arm, which had seven degrees of freedom [67]. In the case of orthotics, general problems of electrodes, noise, crosstalk etc. applied, as had been the case for prosthetics. An advantage in working with orthotics was that the target group for the devices was predominantly wheelchair bound and thus the size and weight of power supplies and batteries was less of a concern [11].

One last group in the US doing research in the area of prosthetic limbs was that headed by Dudley Childress at Northwestern University. This group began myoelectric controls research slightly later than some of the other American centers (i.e. in the late 1960s). The clinical focus of this center was exemplified in its advocacy for a self suspended, self contained myoelectric below elbow prosthesis, which the centre did achieve. This research incorporated much of the work done previously by other groups in order to produce the desired fitting characteristics. Bottomley's "autogenic backlash" for the production of a steady control signal, as well as the appropriate electrode configurations to maximize signal to noise ratios and to minimize crosstalk were of the utmost importance [13].

A three-state controller developed at Northwestern University used the rate of change of myoelectric signal amplitude as a control signal. This system was approved by the Veteran's Administration Prosthetics Center (VAPC) and contracted to Fidelity Electronics for production [12]. This three state control strategy used the absence of myoelectric signal to indicate that the motor should be off, thus the hand remained in whatever position it happened to be in. A large rate of change of signal amplitude would cause the motor to open the hand and a smaller rate of change of signal amplitude would close the hand. The final prosthesis offered a high speed prehension movement until a resistance was encountered and then a lower speed prehensile grip would ensue, offering more precise control to the user. This strategy, called "synergistic prehension" was later imitated by others. By 1970, Childress and others at Northwestern University were experimenting with immediate post-surgical fittings of their self contained, self suspended below elbow prosthesis. Initial trials were successful technically, but the logistical problems of having the interdisciplinary team and all necessary components available on short notice precluded clinical adoption of the procedure.

1.5.3 Yugoslavia

Key researchers in Yugoslavia at the time when myoelectric control was becoming a broad area of research across the United States were Vodovnik, Tomovic and Rakic, all of whom were involved with Reswick's group at the Case Institute in Cleveland. Vodovnik was involved in myoelectric control by 1964, beginning with the development of an automobile brake for severely disabled persons. This brake was activated by contraction of the muscles above the eyebrow [65]. He was in Cleveland working with McLeod and Reswick in 1964, returning to Yugoslavia in 1965 [66]. Vodovnik was interested in the use of implanted transmitters for myoelectric control and in the information content of the myoelectric signal for control parameter development. He continued to collaborate with the Case Institute group long after leaving Cleveland.

An important contribution to the development of powered prostheses was made by Tomovic's group in Belgrade. Tomovic was convinced that mathematics and control theory were applicable to this field [61] and that it would be helpful to provide prostheses that required minimal supervision by their wearers. This led to the "Belgrade Hand" project [52, 62], which yielded a hand capable of varied grasping patterns dictated by details of its contact with an object. Clinical success of that project was limited [30], primarily because of the mechanical complexity of the prosthesis: the principle was sound and was to be implemented in later years in a variety of applications. One of the primary objectives was movement patterns which appeared natural, an important objective aptly termed by Tucker "dynamic cosmesis" [58].

Gavrilovic and Maric were similarly concerned with providing coordinated control of prostheses having several functions. Their work was mostly in-volved with determining rules to govern multi-joint movement. By using proximal joint movements as the control input to a co-ordination algorithm, tangential or translational movements would be output as basic pre-programmed coordinated actions [19].

1.5.4 Canada**

Canada's Department of Health provided funds for the establishment and operation of new research and training centres in Montréal (at l'Institute de réadptation de Montréal), Toronto (at the Ontario Crippled Children's Centre) and Winnipeg (in the Manitoba Rehabilitation Centre). The Fredericton group (later to become the Institute of Biomedical Engineering at the University of New Brunswick) was invited to share in this "Thalidomide program" by redirecting its research from orthotics to prosthetics, in collaboration with the three new centres. In the period 1961–1970, this was the only research group working exclusively on myoelectric control systems for applications in prosthetics. The group used prosthetics components designed elsewhere to conduct clinical trials of the control systems. Myoelectric controls research remains a primary activity at the UNB Institute of Biomedical Engineering to this day.

The Montréal group, under the direction of Gustav Gingras, began myoelectric controls research once the Thalidomide grant was approved. The engineer in that group, Andy Lippay, had been involved with myoelectric control systems researchers in the US (Case Institute) and had visited Britain (Hanger) and Yugoslavia (Tomovic) in an attempt to collaborate with these groups in the determination of design changes required to improve upon the USSR limb commercially available at the time (A. Lippay 1964, Trip report – Roehampton and Manchester, England, 13–20 Dec 1964, unpublished work). By 1964 this group had purchased the right to import the Russian Arm for evaluation [20, 39, 50]. Modifications were made to

---

** In preparing this section, use was made of the (unpublished) minutes of annual meetings of the Canadian Prosthetics Research Groups for the years 1964 through 1972.

the wrist unit to improve hand position and all wiring was placed inside the device [44]. By 1965, the Montréal group had contracted with the Northern Electric Company to work on the miniaturization of their myoelectric prosthesis and by 1967 Northern Electric had produced a child size electric hand made for use with a four function hydraulic arm [45].

The Toronto group, with John Hall as medical director and Colin McLaurin as engineering director, focused on the development of powered prosthetic components and had developed an electric hook and a powered wrist rotation unit by 1965 [56]. The group's prosthetist, Bill Sauter was responsible for significant advances in fitting techniques, especially for the more challenging cases. Excellent collaboration existed between this group and researchers in Fredericton, and as a result of this collaboration patients from Toronto would, by 1965, be fitted with the first fully Canadian-made myoelectric prostheses [45].

The Fredericton group, under the direction of Bob Scott, reported the completion of the design of a current limiter device and supplied a prototype unit to Toronto for testing (the original "cookie crusher") by 1968. They were then working on the possibility of implanted myotelemetry devices [16, 64] (while Scott was spending a sabbatical leave with the Winnipeg group) and on redesigning the three state controller. By 1969 the Fredericton group was producing myoelectric control systems that provided one site, two state ("cookie crusher") control; one site, three state control and one site, three state proportional closing control. Emphasis was on the one site, three state systems, because of clinical demand in the Toronto group for such systems for below elbow amputees with very short residual limbs [56]. As well, through the leadership of Phil Parker, the Fredericton group did considerable research on modeling the myoelectric signal generation process and on optimum signal processing for myoelectric control.

The Toronto group went on to develop an electric elbow unit by 1969. The need for a production center was evident, and with the assistance of the local Variety Club the "Variety Village Electro-Limb Production Centre" was established in Toronto in 1971 in order to provide Canadian made prosthetic and orthotic components. (This centre is still in operation at the time of writing, as Variety Ability Systems Inc.)

In Winnipeg, where the medical director was Bob Tucker and the technical director Jim Foort, the main research interest initially was lower extremity prostheses. In upper extremity applications, they worked with the Fredericton group on development of implantable myotelemetry systems [64], this initiative being facilitated by the presence in Winnipeg of Scott and three of his graduate students from UNB during a sabbatical leave. This work progressed to a single clinical trial in a human amputee, which was successful initially. Early failure of the device encapsulation and inadequate access to appropriate encapsulation technology, led to the abandonment of this project in the mid-1970s.

1.5.5 Sweden

In 1965, the SVEN-group for research in technical rehabilitation had been formed in Stockholm [21] and through collaborative efforts, the "SVEN Hand" design was completed in 1973 [23]. Among those involved in this area in Sweden were Kadefors, Herberts, Hirsch, Kaiser, Alstrom and Petersén. While Kadefors directed most areas of design, Herberts was concerned with signal processing and pattern recognition [22], Kaiser and Petersén with electrode characteristics [26, 28, 38] and Hirsch with telemetry devices [27]. The unified goal of these separate projects was the development of a statistical pattern recognition algorithm for the myoelectric control of a three degree of freedom below elbow prosthesis. They hoped to do this by isolating a sufficient number of hand movement signals to avoid time consuming multiplexing and signal processing. The end product of this research was the "SVEN Hand", a three degree of freedom below elbow prosthesis controlled by six pairs of electrodes placed on the residual limb. Later developments eventually evolved a hand with six degrees of freedom [22]. Kadefors eventually concluded that myoelectric control was still impractical. Collaborative efforts were continued between the SVEN group and Reswick's group in the US and eventually began with the British groups as well. Kadefors, after leaving the field of prosthetics, became the director of a research center studying ergonomics in the workplace [67], although he was destined to re-enter the field of prosthetics toward the end of the century.

1.6 Discussion

The initial research on myoelectric control was entirely empirical: reasonably adequate models of the process by which myoelectric signals are generated were developed only gradually, long after these signals were being used to control prostheses. Advanced signal processing techniques that could simplify use and lead to greater functionality did not begin to be applied until the late 1970s. This was not inappropriate – the most critical limitations of early systems arose from inherent problems of available technology and demanded ingenious packaging of components rather than more efficient signal processing. Indeed the most critical factors in the rapid development of myoelectric prostheses in the 1960s and 1970s were advances in battery technology and in magnet technology that resulted in significant reductions in motor size and weight.

Despite the great advances in myoelectric prosthesis technology, it has remained a challenge to address the functional needs of the users. Rarely in the early work on myoelectric prostheses was clinical evaluation at the forefront of research concerns and many of the original prostheses were never used clinically. It is apparent that the lack of clinical trials was a major limitation. Perhaps had these first limbs been evaluated in the clinical setting, especially if this had been done on a broad scale, the needs of the intended users would have been understood more clearly, deficiencies recognized and technical limitations overcome more effectively.

The development of a marketable commercial product has also remained elusive. In fact, only one supplier, Otto Bock, continues to carry a really broad product line of components for myoelectric prostheses and that product line was, at least until recently, being subsidized by some of the Company's high volume products. Nevertheless, myoelectric prostheses are accepted in most modern rehabilitation centres as one of the standard options for upper extremity amputees.

Some nations, such as Sweden and to a more limited extent the UK, routinely provide myoelectric prostheses within a national health service program. In others, such as the USA, funding generally must be obtained from private sources (including workers' compensation and other insurance carriers). In Canada, the situation varies among provinces, but with a mix of government, insurance and charitable agency funding most amputees for whom myoelectric prostheses are prescribed can obtain them without personal cost. The provision of these limbs remains an expensive endeavor. Generally, individual fittings are devised using available components from a wide variety of sources among which there is little or no standardization. Neither the clinical fitting of myoelectric prostheses nor the manufacture of the components of these prostheses is a profitable commercial activity. This is due to the great variety of components and systems needed to meet the widely varied needs of amputees, the relatively limited market size and the rapid development of the technology.

The thrust towards multifunction control systems has, since the mid 1970s, remained a key area of research at most myoelectric controls research centres. Techniques developed for robotics, such as end-point control and pattern recognition via neural networks, have been investigated. Advanced signal processing and computing techniques have been an integral part of this research, with strategies being modeled to provide "cybernetic" movement patterns. Most of this work remains unsuccessful, partially due to limitations in the control systems and also due to limitations in the mechanical design. The research continues, but thus far offers only limited benefit compared to the simpler control systems of the past. Again, much is lost due to the lack of clinical trials and other techniques of conveying to the researchers the real needs of the intended users.

Acknowledgements. The development of myoelectric prostheses has been dominated by contributions of a relatively small number of individuals who, in solo research or more often as team leaders, had the vision and tenacity to pursue what was often a very frustrating objective. Unfortunately, when these individuals are identified as they are in this essay, it is easy to forget the hundreds of their colleagues, staff and students who made their successes possible. Further, the contribution of thousands of amputees who tested experimental and often woefully unsatisfactory prostheses is often overlooked. To all of these persons, some known and many unknown, the authors extend most sincere thanks.

References

1. Alter R (1966) Bioelectric control of prostheses. Massachusetts Institute of Technology, Research Laboratory of Electronics (Tech report no 446)
2. Bardeen J, Brattain WH (1948) The transistor, a semiconductor triode. Phys Rev 74:230–231
3. Batson RL et al (1957) Electronically controlled respirator. Science 26:819–821
4. Battye CK, Nightingale A, Whillis J (1955) The use of myoelectric currents in the operation of prostheses. J Bone Joint Surg 37B:506–510
5. Berger N, Huppert C (1952) The use of electrical and mechanical muscle forces for the control of and electrical prosthesis. Am J Occup Ther VI:110–114
6. Bontrager EL (1965) The application of muscle education techniques in the investigation of electromyographic control. Case Western Reserve Univ Rep no 4-65-13
7. Bottomley AH (1959) The control of muscles. Prog Cybernet 1:124–131
8. Bottomley AH (1962) Working model of myoelectric control. Proceedings of the international symposium on the application of automatic control in prosthetic design, Belgrade, Yugoslavia, pp 37–45
9. Bottomley AH (1965) Myoelectric control of powered prostheses. J Bone Joint Surg 47B:411–415
10. Breido MG et al (1961) A bioelectric control system. Prob Cybernet 2:556–566 (MS received 1957)
11. Childress D (1969) Design of a myoelectric signal conditioner. J Audio Eng Soc 17
12. Childress D (1971) Progress report – prosthetic research laboratory. Northwestern University Medical School, Chicago, Illinois
13. Childress DS, Billock JN (1970) Self-containment and self suspension of externally powered prostheses for the forearm. Bull Prosthet Res BPR 10 (14):4–21
14. Dodge C (1966) Bioelectrically controlled upper extremity prosthesis – review article. Aerospace Technology Division Report, Library of Congress
15. Dorcas DS, Scott RN (1966) A three-state myoelectric control. Med Biol Eng 4:367–370
16. Dunfield VA, Scott RN (1970) A surgically implanted myotelemetry unit. Proceedings of the 3rd Canadian Medical and Biological Engineering Conference, Halifax, pp 32–32
17. Ellis DO, Schneidermeyer F (1961) EMG control system, publ no 1688. Medical Electronics and Bionics Department, Advanced Development Laboratory, Litton Systems, Woodland Hills, CA
18. Freedy A, Lyman J (1969) Adaptive aiding. Proceedings of the 3rd international symposium on external control of human movement, Dubrovnik, pp 155–170
19. Gavrilovic MM, Maric MR (1969) An approach to the organization of artificial arm control. Proceedings of the 3rd international symposium on external control of human extremities, Dubrovnik, Yugoslavia, pp 307–322
20. Gingras G et al (1966) Bioelectric upper extremity prosthesis developed in Soviet Union: preliminary report. Arch Phys Med Rehabil 47:232–267
21. Herberts P (1969) Myoelectric signals in control of prostheses. ACTA Orthop Scand [Suppl] 124
22. Herberts P, Petersén I (1970) Possibilities for control of powered devices by myoelectric signals. Scand J Rehabil Med 2:164–170
23. Herberts P et al (1973) Hand prosthesis control via myoelectric patterns. ACTA Orthop Scand 44:389–409
24. Horn GW (1963) Muscle potentials control artificial arm movements. Electronics 11:213–227
25. Jacobsen SC et al (1982) Development of the Utah Arm. IEEE Trans Biomed Eng BME-29:249–269
26. Kadefors R (1969) The voluntary EMG in prosthetics – contributions to the theory and application of myo-electric control. Final Report of a Scholarship in Prosthetics. Chalmers University of Technology, Göteborg, Sweden (The Swedish Board for Technical Development, Basic Grant no 4442)
27. Kadefors R, Taylor CM (1973) On the feasibility of myoelectric control of multifunctional orthoses. Scand J Rehabil Med 5:134–146
28. Kadefors R et al (1968) Electrodes for myoelectric control of prostheses. Medicoteknik 1:43–59
29. Kato I et al (1970) Multifunctional myoelectric hand prosthesis with pressure sensory feedback system – Waseda Hand 4P. Advances in external control of human extremities. Proceedings of the 3rd international symposium on the control of human extremities, Dubrovnik, Aug 1969, pp 155–170
30. Kay HW, Kajganic M, Ivancevic N (1970) Medical evaluation of the belgrade electronic hand. In: Gavrilovic MM, Wilson AB (eds) Advances in external control of human extremities. Proceedings of the 3rd international symposium on external control of human extremities, Dubrovnik, pp 128–137

31. Ko WH (1965) Progress in miniaturized biotelemetry. Bioscience 15:118–120

32. Ko WH, Reswick J (1965) Miniature FM implant bio-telemetering transmitters. Digest of the 6th international conference on medical electronics and biological engineering, pp 213–214

33. Ko WH, Yon E (1965) RF induction power supply for implant circuits. Digest of the 6th international conference on medical electronics and biological engineering, pp 206–207

34. Ko WH et al (1964) Implantable radio transducers for physiological information and implant techniques. Proceedings of the 2nd national biomedical sciences instrumentation symposium, Albuquerque, New Mexico, vol 2

35. Kobrinski AY (1959) Utilization of biocurrents for control purposes. Report of the USSR Academy of Science, Department of Technical Sciences, Energetics and Automation, no 3 (translation by P Barta, UNB, 1966)

36. Kobrinski AY (1960) Bioelectrical control of prosthetic devices. Herald of the Academy of Sciences USSR, Moscow, vol 30, no 7, pp 58–61 (translation by US Office of Technical Services, Washington DC, 1960)

37. Kobrinski AY et al (1960) Problems of bioelectric control. Transactions of the 1st international congress on automatic controls, vol 2. Butterworths, London, pp 619–620

38. Lawrence P, Herberts P, Kadefors R (1973) Experiences with a multifunctional hand prosthesis controlled by myoelectric patterns. In: Gavrilovic MM, Wilson AB (eds) Advances in external control of human extremities. Etan, Belgrade, pp 47–65

39. Lippay AL, Corriveau C, Lozac'h Y (1965) A practical exercise in bioelectric control – the Soviet myoelectric arm. Proceedings of the 18th annual conference on engineering in medicine and biology, p 149

40. Long C, Ebskov B (1965) Research applications of myoelectric control. Paper presented at the 43rd annual session of the American Congress of Physical Medicine and Rehabilitation, Philadelphia, USA

41. Lorig R, Greene L, Vodovnik L (1967) Some topics on myoelectric control of orthotic/prosthetic systems. Report no EDC 4-67-17. Case Western Reserve University, Cleveland, Ohio

42. Mann RW, Reemers SD (1970) Kinesthetic sensing for the EMG controlled 'Boston Arm'. In: Gavrilovic MM, Wilson AB (eds) Proceedings of the 3rd international symposium on advances in external control of human extremities, Belgrade

43. McKenzie DS (1965) The Russian Myo-electric Arm. J Bone Joint Surg 47B:418–420

44. McLaurin CA (1965) On the use of electricity in upper extremity prostheses. J Bone Joint Surg 47B:448–452

45. McLeod W (1965) Ampersand report, Highlandview Hospital

46. McLeod W (1967) Ampersand report, Highlandview Hospital

47. Michael RR, Crawford FR (1963) Myoelectric surface potentials for machine control. Electr Eng 689

48. National Academy of Sciences (1961) The application of external power in prosthetics and orthotics. Proceedings of the 1960 Lake Arrowhead Conference, publ 874. National Academy of Sciences – National Research Council, Washington DC

49. National Academy of Sciences (1965) Proceedings of the conference on the control of external power in upper extremity rehabilitation. Warrenton, VA, National Academy of Sciences – National Research Council, Washington DC

50. Ontario Crippled Children's Center, Toronto, Ontario, Canada (1965) Prosthetic Research Training Unit, annual report

51. Pudulski (1969) The Boston Arm. Forum IEEE Spectrum 6

52. Rakic M, Jaksic D, Ivancevic N (1970) Technical evaluation of the belgrade hand prosthesis. In: Gavrilovic MM, Wilson AB (eds) Advances in external control of human extremities. Proceedings of the 3rd international symposium on external control of human extremities, Dubrovnik, pp 139–143

53. Reiter R (1948) Eine neue Elektrokunsthand. Grenzgeb Med 4:133–135

54. Schmidl H (1965) The INAIL Myoelectric B/E prosthesis. Orthop Prosth Appl J 298–303

55. Scott RN (1962) Orthotics systems research. Prog Rep 1. Research Lab Rep 62–5. Department of Electrical Engineering, University of Brunswick, Fredericton NB, Canada

56. Scott RN (2001) Institute of Biomedical Engineering, University of New Brunswick, Fredericton NB, Canada, personal recollection

57. Scott RN, Thompson GB (1963) Orthotics systems research. Prog Rep 2. Res Lab Rep 63–5. Department of Electrical Engineering, University of Brunswick, Fredericton NB, Canada

58. Scott RN, Tucker FR (1968) Surgical implications of myoelectric control. Clin Orthop Relat Res 61:248–260

59. Sullivan GH (1963) Myoelectric servo control. Technical documentary report no ASD-TDR-63-70. Wright-Patterson Air Force Base, Ohio

60. Suzuki R (1969) Myoelectric control of a multifunction system. Proceedings of the 8th international conference on medical and biological engineering, Chicago, session 5.2

61. Tomovic R (1966) Control theory and signal processing in prosthetic systems. The control of external power in upper extremity rehabilitation. A report on a conference at Warrenton, Virginia. National Academy of Sciences – National Research Council, Washington DC, pp 221–226

62. Tomovic R (1970) A new model of the Belgrade hand. In: Gavrilovic MM, Wilson AB (eds) Advances in external control of human extremities. Proceedings of the 3rd international symposium on external control of human extremities, Dubrovnik, pp 151–154

63. Travis RC, Kennedy JL (1949) Prediction and automatic control of alertness III – calibration of the alertness indicator and further results. J Comp Physiol Psychiatry 42:45–57

64. Tucker FR, Scott RN (1968) Development of a surgically implanted Myo-telemetry control system. J Bone Joint Surg 50B:771–779

65. Vodovnik L (1964) An electromagnetic brake activated by eyebrow muscles. Electr Eng 694–695

66. Vodovnik L, Kreifeld F (1967) The information content of myoelectric signals. Cybernetics Systems Group, report no RDC 4–67–17. Case Western Reserve University, Cleveland, Ohio, pp 30–46

67. Waring W (1968) Investigation of myoelectric control of functional braces. Attending Staff Association, Rancho Los Amigos Hospital, Downey, California

68. Waring W, Antonelli DJ (1967) Myoelectric control systems. Orthop Prosthet J 27–32

69. Weiner N (1948) Cybernetics, or control and communication in the animal and the machine. Wiley, New York

70. Weltman G, Groth H, Lyman J (1959) An analysis of bioelectrical prostheses control. Department of Engineering, UCLA (Biotechnology laboratory technical report no 1)

71. Weltman G, Lyman J (1960) The effects of electronic transformation on the patterns of myoelectric activity during arm movement. Department of Engineering, UCLA (Biotechnology laboratory technical report no 6)

72. Wirta RW, Taylor DR (1969) Development of a multi-axis myoelectrically controlled prosthetic arm. Advances in external control of human extremities. Proceedings of the 3rd international symposium on external control of human extremities, Dubrovnik, pp 245–253

The Origins and Nature of the Myoelectric Signal

D. F. Lovely

Contents

Summary

This chapter explains the origin and nature of the myoelectric signal (MES) as used in the control of powered prostheses. The first part of the chapter covers basic muscle anatomy and explains the contraction mechanism. This is followed by the electrophysiology associated with the contraction process and the resultant generation of the MES. Finally, the appearance of the MES, as obtained using surface electrodes from the wrist flexors of the author, is presented. These examples illustrate many of the points made throughout the chapter.

2.1 Introduction

The roots of "myoelectric" involve two words, namely "myo" from the Greek *mys* meaning muscle and *electric* pertaining to electricity. From this we can define a myoelectric signal (MES) as the "*electrical activity produced by a contracting muscle*". This is a simple definition, however, in this chapter we will delve deeper into the origins and nature of the myoelectric signal that are far from simple.

Knowing more about any subject usually improves both our understanding and application skills and with the MES this is not an exception. We will show that when a muscle contracts, ionic currents are generated deep within the muscle structure that can be detected using electrodes. The amplitude and appearance of this signal is a function of many variables including the depth of the muscle, size of the muscle, strength of the contraction, the overlying tissue, type of electrodes used for detection, their location and their orientation.

The MES can be detected beneath the skin surface using needle electrodes. As its origin lies deep within the structure of the muscle, moving closer to the source will increase the magnitude of the signal. However, as the application to which this book is targeted is the myo-electric control of powered prosthesis, the signal is typically detected using a pair of surface electrodes.

There are three basic muscle types within the body, *smooth*, *cardiac* and *skeletal*. Smooth muscle lines the gut and is generally under autonomic control. Cardiac muscle is the non-fatiguing contractile mechanism of the heart. Skeletal muscle is under voluntary control and effects the movement of limbs. The functions of these three types of muscle are radically different and so it is not unexpected that the electrical properties of the corresponding MES differ accordingly. As the focus of this book is that of myoelectric control, which by its very definition involves voluntary control by the user, attention has been concentrated on the MES from skeletal muscle.

2.2 Anatomy

In the anatomy of any structure in the body, there is always a question of the level of detail. One can look at the structure with the un-aided eye or delve deeper using a microscope until we arrive at the cellular level and beyond. What we can see with the naked eye is generally termed gross anatomy (Fig. 2.1). This is where we will start with the anatomy of skeletal muscle. Our first observation is that skeletal muscle is very red. This is because muscle requires a good blood supply not only to provide the necessary energy for contraction but also to remove the large amounts of metabolic waste products that are built up during the contraction process. In addition, the blood vessels in skeletal muscle tend to be long and winding. This feature permits them to accommodate changes in muscle length – by straightening when the muscle is stretched and contorting when the muscle contracts.

To allow skeletal muscle to move bones, there must be an attachment so that when the muscle contracts movement is produced. In general, there are two types of attachment mechanisms; namely direct and indirect.

In direct attachments, the outside covering of the muscle, the *epimysium*, is fused to the outer layer or *periosteum* of a bone or *perichondrium* of a cartilage. In indirect attachments, the connective tissue of the muscle extends beyond the muscle as a ropelike *tendon* or a flat, broad *aponeurosis*. The tendon or aponeurosis anchors the muscle to the connective tissue covering of the skeletal element or to the *fascia* of other muscles. Of the two methods the indirect attachments are much more common in the body be-

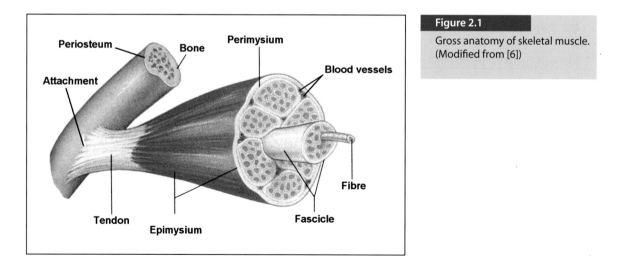

Figure 2.1

Gross anatomy of skeletal muscle. (Modified from [6])

Figure 2.2

Fine anatomy of skeletal muscle. (Modified from [6])

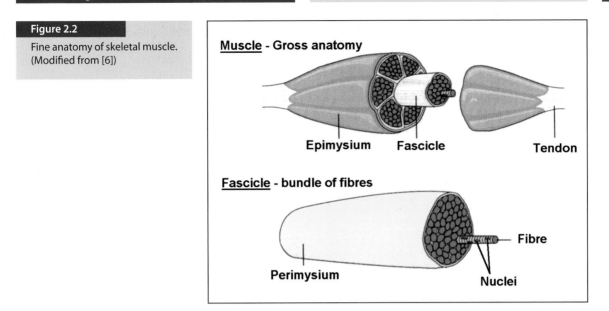

cause of their durability and small size. As tendons are mostly tough *collagenic* fibres, they can cross rough bony projections that would tear apart the more delicate muscle tissues.

If we delve deeper into the microscopic or fine anatomy of the muscle, its structure resembles a bundle of spaghetti. The bulk of the muscle is composed of muscle *fibres* that are arranged in bundles called *fascicles*. The fascicles are covered with a membrane called the *perimysium* that is a collagenic sheath that keeps the fibres together (Fig. 2.2).

The muscle fibre is a long cylindrical cell with multiple oval nuclei arranged just beneath its membrane or *sarcolemma*. The *sarcoplasm* of a muscle fibre is similar to the *cytoplasm* of other cells, but it contains an unusually large amount of stored *glycogen* and a unique oxygen-binding protein called *myoglobin*. The myoglobin, along with the rich blood supply, is responsible for the characteristic red colour of skeletal muscle.

The sarcolemma exhibits dark and light bands, which give the cell an overall striated appearance. Consequently, an alternate name for skeletal muscle is *striated* muscle. The dark bands are termed "*A*" (anisotropic) and the light bands "*I*" (isotropic) due to their light polarizing capabilities.

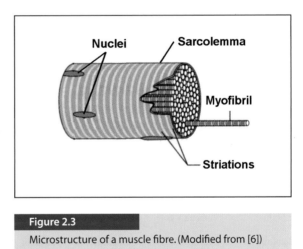

Figure 2.3

Microstructure of a muscle fibre. (Modified from [6])

The structure of a muscle fibre is itself "*spaghetti like*" just as the fibre is to the fascicles. When viewed at high magnification, each muscle fibre is seen to contain a large number of rod-like *myofibrils*. Each fibre has hundreds and even thousands of myofibrils, which contribute to the striated appearance of the muscle fibre. It is these myofibrils that are the base contractile elements of skeletal muscle (Fig. 2.3).

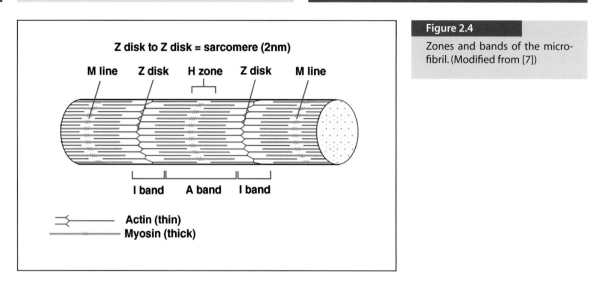

Figure 2.4

Zones and bands of the microfibril. (Modified from [7])

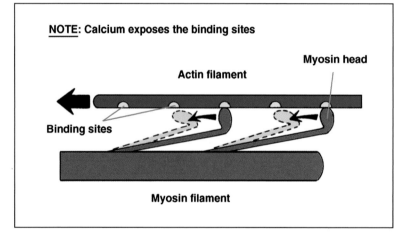

Figure 2.5

Ratchet mechanism of the actin-myosin filaments. (Modified from [7])

2.3 The Contraction Process

The dark A-band of the myofibril is primarily composed of the protein *myosin*, while the I-band is *actin*, another protein. These proteins are arranged in *filaments*, in which the actin overlaps the myosin. The myosin filament is thicker (~ *16 nm*) than that of the actin (~ *8 nm*). Close inspection of the myofibril shows that the dark A-band has a light zone (*H-zone*), which is observable only in relaxed muscle fibres. Similarly, the light I-band has a dark zone termed the *Z-disk*. The Z-disk acts to anchor the actin filaments to one another and other myofibrils.

The region between two successive Z-disks is termed a *sarcomere*, is typically 2 nm in length, and is the smallest contractile unit of a muscle fibre (Fig. 2.4).

The contraction process involves chemical interactions between the actin and myosin filaments. The thin actin filaments slide over the thick myosin filaments, increasing the overlap. The distance between successive Z-disks decrease and the I-bands shorten. "Heads" or *cross-bridges* form between the myosin and actin that successively attach and detach in a ratchet like manner. This pulls the thin filaments towards the centre of the sarcomere. The release mechanism involves the action of adenosine tri-phosphate (*ATP*) binding to the myosin head, which in turn relies on a metabolic pathway (Fig. 2.5).

In the resting state, binding between the filaments is prevented by a protein complex *tropomyosin-troponin* that blocks the active sites on the actin filament. A release of calcium from the *sarcoplasmic reticulum* binds to the troponin that moves the tropomyosin away from the binding site allowing the myosin to cross-link with the actin. The sliding of the actin filament over the myosin results in a shortening of the overall muscle by about 60–70% of its original length. Muscles cannot actively lengthen; only shorten so they tend to work in antagonistic pairs.

Going a Little Further …

In rigor mortis, dying cells are unable to exclude extracellular calcium from infusing into the muscle cells. This triggers the contraction mechanism (rigor); however, as ATP production is halted shortly after breathing ceases, the detachment of myosin from actin is prevented. This leaves the muscles in a state of rigidity for several hours until the proteins themselves break down.

The striated appearance and contraction process of skeletal muscle is well illustrated in the series of photomicrographs shown in Fig. 2.6. In the top picture, (1), the muscle is in a relaxed state and the I and A-bands are clearly visible. The dark Z-band and light H-zone are also visible. With a partial contraction, as in the middle picture, (2), the Z-bands move toward the centre of the sarcomere, as the thin actin filaments are drawn into the A-band by the "ratchet" mechanism. Finally in the bottom picture, (3), the fibre is fully contracted, the light H-zone has disappeared and the I-band is significantly shortened. Note that the dark A-band (myosin) retains most of its original length.

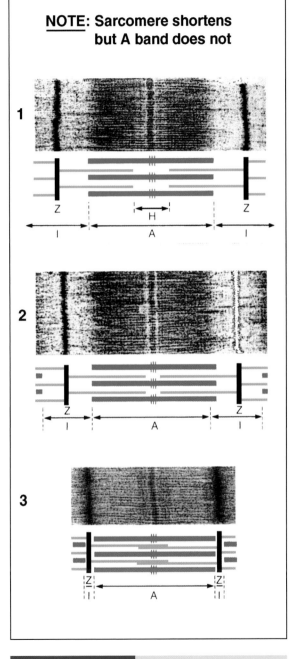

NOTE: Sarcomere shortens but A band does not

Figure 2.6

Photomicrographs of contraction process of striated muscle. (Modified from [7])

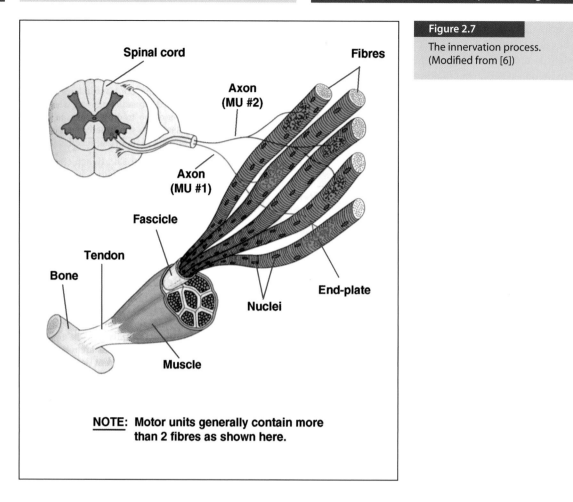

Figure 2.7

The innervation process. (Modified from [6])

Spinal cord

Fibres

Axon (MU #2)

Axon (MU #1)

Fascicle

Tendon

Bone

End-plate

Nuclei

Muscle

NOTE: Motor units generally contain more than 2 fibres as shown here.

2.4 Connections to the CNS

Now that the basic anatomy of the muscle and mechanism of the contraction process has been described, how does the nervous system interact to produce a voluntary contraction?

To answer this question we need to look first at how the nervous system and the muscle fibres are connected. Several muscle fibres are connected or *innervated* from a single *axon* whose cell body lies within the spinal cord of the central nervous system (*CNS*). The junction between the axon and the muscle fibre is termed the neuro-muscular junction (*NMJ*) or *end-plate*. As a rule, each muscle fibre has only one neuromuscular junction located close to the middle.

The collection of a motor neuron cell body, its axon, the NMJs and muscle fibres it innervates is termed a *motor unit*. When an axon is active, all the muscle fibres associated with that motor unit contract. In the muscles for fine control, for example eyelid movement, there are about 1–10 fibres per motor unit. However, for gross movement such as the muscles used for knee extension, this number can be as high as 1000+ per motor unit (Fig. 2.7).

Figure 2.8

Effect of a fixed charged protein on diffusion

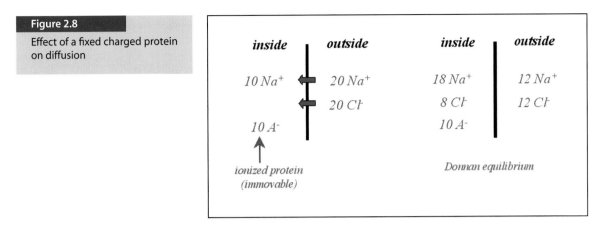

2.5 Fibre Membrane
and the Transmembrane Potential

Both muscle fibres and nerve axons share several similar characteristics. From an electrical standpoint, both can be considered as tubular structures comprising of a *selectively permeable membrane*. This membrane separates the intra-cellular fluid from the extra-cellular fluid. The concentration of ions inside and outside the fibre is different. The three most important ions being:

Potassium: Higher inside than outside   (35:1)
Sodium: Lower inside than outside   (1:10)
Chloride: Lower inside than outside   (1:12)

Diffusion is the term given to the natural tendency of solutions to establish a uniform concentration. For example, a drop of seawater placed in a beaker of fresh water will not remain stationary. It will diffuse throughout the fresh water until the overall concentration of salt is uniform and much lower than that of the original seawater. This diffusion process is more commonly termed *dilution*. The situation with the ionic solutions inside and outside the muscle fibre is no different. There is a general tendency for the potassium inside the fibre to diffuse out, and for sodium and chloride to diffuse into the fibre.

However, there are four mechanisms at play in the biological situation that maintains an ionic concentration gradient across the fibre membrane against the normal diffusion process:

1. Membrane permeability: The free diffusion process is hindered by the selectively permeable membrane. Potassium ions have a smaller hydrated diameter (approximately 50%) than that of sodium; therefore, it diffuses more rapidly across the membrane. Thus, the membrane tends to keep sodium out of the fibre.

2. Membrane polarization: The proteins and fats of the membrane carry ionized groups that give the membrane a negative electrical charge. If charged particles with a "like" charge, e.g. chloride ions, approaches the membrane, they will be repelled.

3. Non-diffusible ions: The existence of a large charged non-diffusible substance on one side of a membrane, such as the ionized proteins making up the sarcoplasm, influences the natural diffusion process. The negatively charged proteins tend to attract the positive sodium ions and repel negative ions. Diffusion will take place until what is termed a *Donnan-Gibbs* equilibrium is established in which the product of diffusible ions is equal on both sides of the membrane. A simple example will demonstrate that this process also sets up an electrical potential across the membrane.

In Fig. 2.8, a situation is shown in which the natural diffusion gradient of sodium (Na^+) and chloride (Cl^-) ions is from right to left across the membrane. If it were not for the presence of the ionized protein, the final distribution of ions would be 15 Na^+ and 10 Cl^- on either side of the membrane. However, the action of the negatively charged fixed protein is to attract positive ions (Na^+) and repel negative ions (Cl^-), thus the ionic distribution is modified. In the Donnan-Gibbs equilibrium situation, the product of the diffusible ions either side of the membrane is equal:

$$Na^+ \times 8\ Cl^- = 144 \ldots inside$$
$$Na^+ \times 12\ Cl^- = 144 \ldots outside$$

However, there is a net imbalance of cations (*positive*) and anions (*negative*) across the membrane, 18/12 and 8/12 respectively. This represents a potential difference across the membrane.

4. Sodium-potassium pump: The final mechanism that can influence the distribution of ions either side of the fibre membrane is an active ion transportation process, termed the *sodium-potassium pump*. This process relies on the metabolic energy derived from ATP breakdown to simultaneously expel sodium that has leaked into the cell and helps to accumulate potassium in the interior. However, the pumping rates are different for potassium and sodium. For every *three* sodium ions expelled only *two* potassium ions are transported into the fibre. Thus, the sodium-potassium pump helps to create a potential difference across the membrane.

The total voltage that appears across the fibre membrane is termed the *transmembrane potential*. Its magnitude is directly related to the nature of the ionic distribution either side of the membrane. This in turn is dependent on the four mechanisms outlined above. In general, sodium ions are discouraged from diffusion due to the selective nature of the membrane. Chloride ions are excluded from diffusion due to the presence of organic anions inside the membrane. This leaves only potassium to consider. The potential developed due to the potassium concentration gradient can be expressed by the Nernst equation:

$$V_m = \frac{RT}{F} \times \log_{10}\left(\frac{K^+_{in}}{K^+_{out}}\right) \approx 90\ \text{mV}$$

This shows that the inside of the muscle fibre is approximately 90 mV negative with respect to outside. Actual measurements show that this value is a little bit lower than this at approximately 80 mV. This is the result of the small amount of sodium leakage, the presence of internal ionized proteins and the effect of the sodium-potassium pump. This potential is termed the *resting membrane potential*.

Going a Little Further ...

It should be noted that the transmembrane potential for axons is somewhat lower from that of muscle fibres. Typical resting potentials are −70 mV, with a threshold point of −55 mV. This is due to slight differences in ionic concentrations.

2.6 Depolarization and the Action Potential

At the NMJ a gap or *synaptic cleft* separates the axon from the muscle fibre membrane. Within the flattened axonal ending are *synaptic vesicles*. These are small membranous sacs containing a neurotransmitter called *acetylcholine* (ACh). The nerve impulse arriving at the axonal ending changes the axon membrane permeability to calcium. Extracellular calcium enters the axon and causes some of the vesicles to fuse with the membrane. The ACh is then released into the cleft by a process of *exocytosis* (Fig. 2.9).

On the sarcolemma of the muscle fibre there is a depression termed the *end-plate* which is highly convoluted. These folds provide a large surface area for millions of *ACh receptors*. The binding of ACh to sites on the end-plate results in changes in the local permeability of the cell membrane, especially to *sodium*. Channels are opened in the cell membrane that allows sodium to flood into the interior. This re-distribution of ions reduces the local transmembrane potential, a process that is termed *depolarization*.

If the nerve stimulus is strong enough, a threshold (∼−70 mV) is exceeded in the cell depolarization that results in *propagation* of an *action potential*. This is the result of ionic currents changing the permeability of the cell membrane near the end-plate. The depo-

Figure 2.9

The neuro-muscular junction (*NMJ*). (Modified from [6])

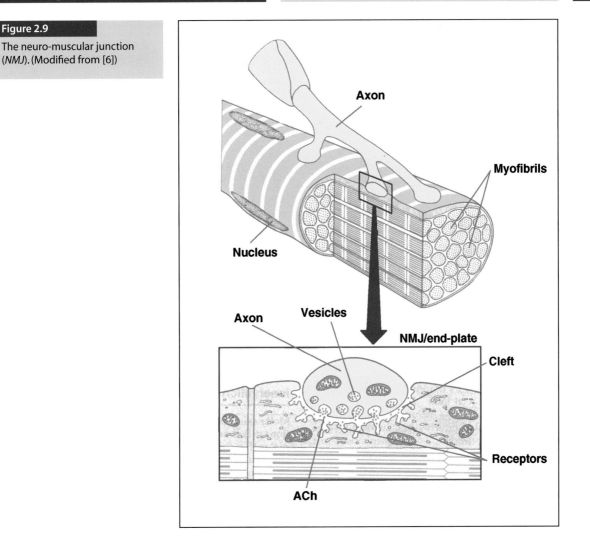

larization region spreads away from the end-plate just as ripples move away from a pebble dropped into a pond. This regenerative effect can be explained by considering a very simple electrical model of the cell membrane. The resting potential can be visualized as an internal negative charge distributed uniformly along the fibre, with a corresponding positive charge outside. Bulk ionic currents are prevented from flowing due to the membrane. When the membrane channels open and allow the local ingression of sodium, the local transmembrane potential is lowered. Ionic currents can then flow internally away

from and externally towards the depolarization region. This ionic current in turn lowers the transmembrane potential in the neighboring region of the initial depolarization zone. In this way, the depolarization region spreads outwards from its initial site (Fig. 2.10).

Once the transmembrane potential has exceeded the threshold point, a full action potential develops. The membrane potential reverses polarity (–90 mV to +30 mV) in about 0.5 ms. This is a positive feedback mechanism whereby the influx of sodium causes a further increase in membrane permeability to

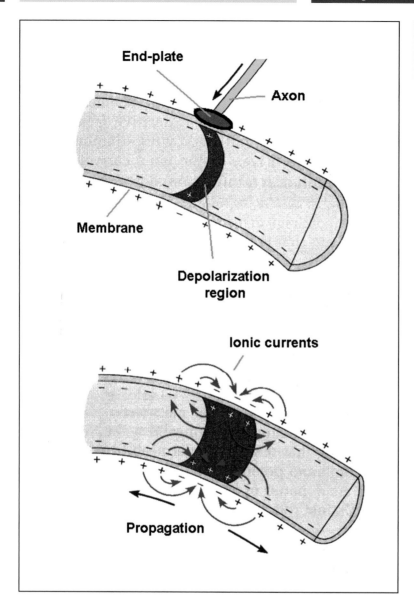

Figure 2.10

The propagation of the depolarization region. (Modified from [6])

sodium. This action is an "*all or nothing response*", in that either no polarity reversal occurs or the full +30 mV potential is developed.

Once the inside of the cell becomes positive with respect to the outside, the electric field gradient opposes further influx of sodium ions. This in turn drops the membrane permeability to sodium – the Na$^+$ gates close. As sodium entry declines, voltage regulated potassium gates open and potassium flows out of the cell. The membrane permeability to potassium increases and the cell membrane potential drops back toward the resting potential. The potassium channels stay open a short while after the sodium channels have closed. This leads to a small *undershoot* in the transmembrane potential (Fig. 2.11).

While cellular depolarization and muscle contraction have both been described from an anatomy and physiological standpoint, how are the two related? The link is the important role that calcium plays in the contraction process. Just as the arrival of nerve impulse at the axonal ending causes an increase in cellular calcium, a similar process takes place in the muscle fibre. On arrival of the muscle fibre action potential, calcium is released from the sarcoplasmic reticulum. This in turn initiates the contraction process.

The calcium is actively transported back to the sarcoplasmic reticulum by an ATP driven pump, with the lowering of calcium responsible for the cessation of the contraction. So, the release of calcium is the final trigger for a muscle contraction.

Going a Little Further ...

Although repolarization restores the resting electrical conditions, it does not restore the original ionic distributions of the resting state. This is done later through the sodium-potassium pump.

2.7 Measurement of the Potentials Associated with Depolarization

The transmembrane potential can be measured by using *microelectrodes*, one of which has to be placed inside the muscle cell. This highly invasive approach is most easily done with isolated cells *in vitro*. *Hodgkin* in the 1950's and 1960's used this approach in his work, whereby he investigated the transmembrane potential of giant squid axons. However, the use of such invasive techniques is not practical in a *in vivo* situation. A far less invasive and delicate method is required.

The effect of the depolarization and subsequent re-polarization can be detected with a pair of electrodes placed outside the muscle cell. The propagation of the action potential can be observed in this manner but its appearance is modified from that shown in Fig. 2.11. If electrodes are placed on the outer surface of the muscle fibre, in line with the long axis of the cell, then a potential difference can be measured as the depolarization region propagates past the electrodes.

Figure 2.11

The action potential and membrane permeability. (Modified from [6])

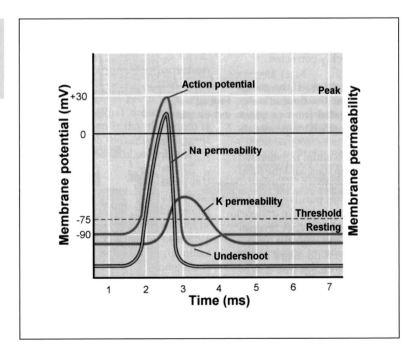

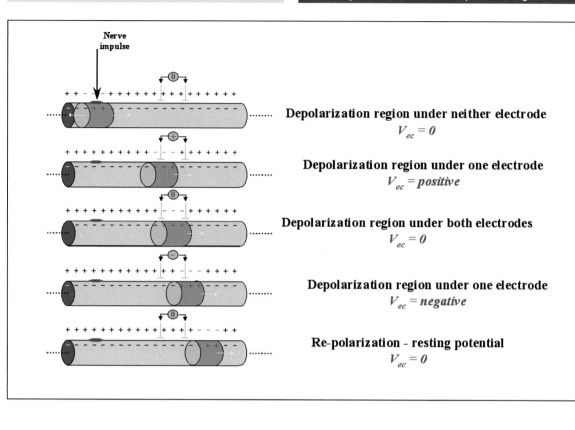

Depolarization region under neither electrode
$$V_{ec} = 0$$

Depolarization region under one electrode
$$V_{ec} = positive$$

Depolarization region under both electrodes
$$V_{ec} = 0$$

Depolarization region under one electrode
$$V_{ec} = negative$$

Re-polarization - resting potential
$$V_{ec} = 0$$

Figure 2.12

A propagating action potential and the associated external potential

This potential differs from the transmembrane potential but it can be detected without breaching the cell membrane. In the resting state, the inside of the cell is approximately 90 mV negative with respect to the outside. However, for two electrodes outside the cell, this potential difference is hidden. Along the outside surface of the cell there is an *isopotential* and so the detected potential is *zero*.

After the cell is stimulated by a nerve impulse, a depolarization region forms around the end plate region. If the electrodes are away from this region, then again the depolarization effect goes undetected. It is only as the depolarization region propagates towards the electrodes that a signal can be detected. As the leading edge of the depolarization region approaches the first electrode, a potential difference develops (Fig. 2.12).

However, when the depolarization region spans both electrodes, this potential returns to zero. As the leading edge of the depolarization region approaches the second electrode, again a potential difference develops but this time with the opposite polarity. Finally, as the depolarization region moves away from the electrode site and the membrane under the electrode re-polarizes, the observed potential returns to zero.

2.8 Spatial Variation in the Arrangement of Motor Units

The muscle fibres of a single motor unit are not clustered together but are spread throughout the muscle. As a result, stimulation of a single motor unit causes a weak contraction of the entire muscle. As all the fi-

Figure 2.13

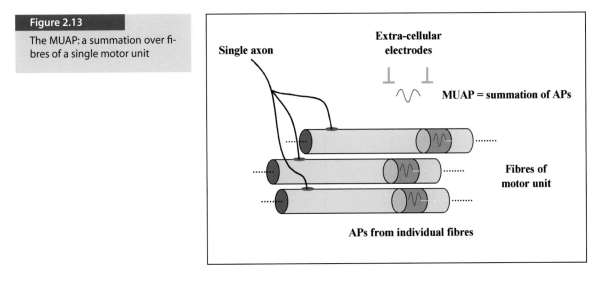

The MUAP: a summation over fibres of a single motor unit

bres of a motor unit are innervated by the same axon, they depolarize or 'fire' *synchronously*. The corresponding externally observed signal, is therefore a summation of the activity from all of the motor unit fibres. This is termed a *motor unit action potential* (MUAP). Although the action potential of each fibre is identical in nature, because of the spatial distribution of the end-plates, the appearance of the resultant MUAP is different from that of the individual action potential. Longitudinal separation of end-plates gives rise to a 'smearing' of the MUAP in time, thus the duration of the MUAP is somewhat longer (4–8 ms) than that of the fibre action potential (1–2 ms). Vertical or depth separation of the end-plates leads to the most.superficial fibres contributing most to the resultant MUAP (Fig. 2.13).

Just as the individual muscle fibres of a motor unit are distributed throughout the muscle, the motor units themselves are distributed throughout the muscle in a random fashion. The observed electrical activity that accompanies a contraction is a spatial summation over all the active motor units. This is what is known as the myoelectric signal: a spatial summation of MUAPs.

2.9 Muscle Force Mediation and the Myoelectric Signal

As all the fibres of a motor unit fire synchronously, the resultant muscular contraction is termed a 'twitch'. This is a sudden jerky shortening of the fibres associated with the unit. To facilitate smooth control of overall muscle tension it is important that not all the motor units fire simultaneously. The CNS therefore controls the firing of the motor units in an *asynchronous* manner.

The overall muscle force can be modulated using two modalities. Firstly, to increase the tension, additional motor units can be selected from the motor pool – *recruitment*. Secondly, the frequency at which the motor neurons are activated can be increased - *firing rate*. In general, the deep motor units are utilized first and as the muscle force increases units that are more superficial are recruited.

The change in muscle electrical activity due to recruitment and firing rate can be observed on the skin surface using surface electrodes aligned along the general direction of the muscle fibres. The identification of individual motor unit activity from this gross myoelectric signal is quite difficult and is an active area of research. The intervening tissue, between the muscle and the skin surface, severely attenuates the

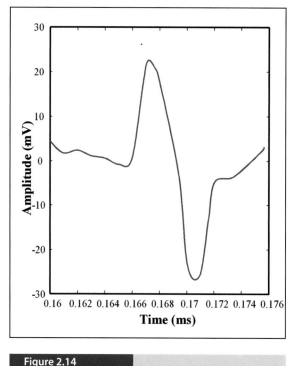

Figure 2.14

Experimentally recorded MUAP

signal and reduces spatial resolution considerably. This results in the signals from individual motor units becoming intermingled and hard to distinguish. This phenomenon, associated with the use of surface electrodes, is generally referred to as the *tissue filtering* effect.

However, it is possible to discern activity from individual motor units using specialized surface electrodes and low levels of contraction. Figure 2.14 shows the appearance of a typical motor unit as recorded from the wrist flexors of the author. It is very similar to the extra-cellular potential, having a biphasic nature. The amplitude however is greatly reduced due to the tissue filtering effect and its time duration is somewhat longer than the typical transmembrane potential, lasting around 6 ms.

In Fig. 2.15, the myoelectric signal from a very low-level contraction is shown. In this figure, three distinct active motor units can be seen and are labeled 1, 2 and 3. Although the electrical activity of every motor unit is identical, the intervening tissue between the active site and the recording electrodes plays an important role. Motor unit #1 is quite superficial. It appears the largest simply because it is closer to the electrode than the other active units. Motor unit #3 is quite deep, as it is more heavily attenuated

Figure 2.15

Experimentally recorded myoelectric signal

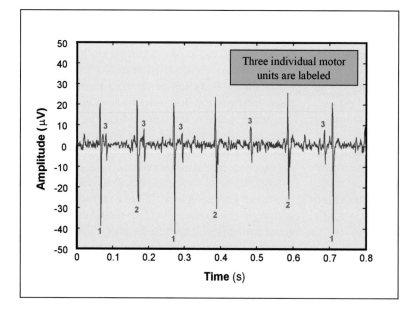

Figure 2.16

Experimentally recorded myo-electric signal (medium contraction)

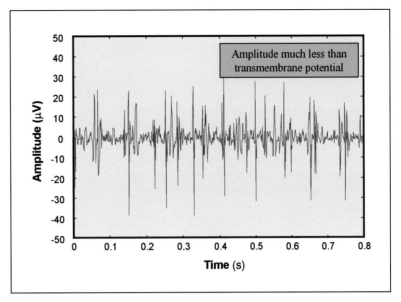

Figure 2.17

Experimentally recorded myo-electric signal (high level contraction)

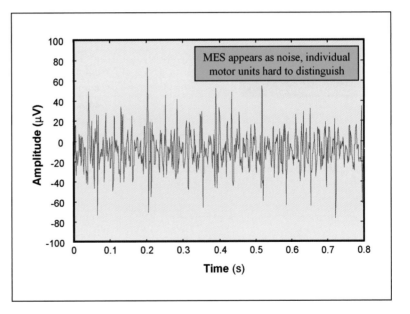

than motor unit #1. The firing rate of motor unit #1 is about 2 Hz (t=0.5 s) while that of motor unit #2 is somewhat faster at about 5 Hz.

As the contraction level increases, it becomes increasingly more difficult to discern the individual motor units. In Fig. 2.16, the contraction level has been increased and more motor units have been activated. It is still possible to determine individual motor units but it is getting more difficult. The firing rate of the motor units is also increasing. The superficial motor units are now firing about every 0.1 s, i.e. 10 Hz. It should be noted that the amplitude range of this signal (~80 µV) is much smaller than the potential developed across the membrane (~130 mV). This is due to the attenuation effect of the overlying tissue and the skin barrier.

Finally, if the contraction level is increased further, as shown in Fig. 2.17, even more motor units are recruited and the firing rate for the deeper fibres increases. It is now impossible to determine the individual motor units and the overall appearance of the signal is that of noise. The large "spikes" are those of very superficial fibres that have been recruited to produce the contraction force demanded by the CNS under voluntary control.

It should be noted that although the vertical scale in Fig. 2.17 has doubled from a 100 µV range to 200 µV, the signal amplitude is still at least an order of magnitude lower than that of the transmembrane potential. In addition, the similarity in the appearance of the MES to that of general noise should not be overlooked. Both of these observations will be re-examined in Chap. 3 where the practical aspects of acquiring the MES with dry surface electrodes in a noisy electrical environment, will be discussed.

Going a Little Further ...

This series of recordings was performed using a specialized concentric ring electrode that is used for research purposes. This type of motor unit discrimination is not generally possible using the electrodes employed in myo-electric control systems.

2.10 Chapter Summary

Skeletal muscle is comprised of fascicles of muscle fibres that are in turn composed of myofibrils. The muscle fibre is a multi-nucleated specialized cell that contains large amounts of stored glycogen in a protein called myoglobin. The major components of a myofibril are the proteins myosin and actin. The sliding of these protein filaments gives the muscle the capability for contraction.

The concentrations of ions inside and outside of a muscle fibre differ considerably. Inside, the concentration of potassium is approximately 35 times larger than outside. Similarly, outside the concentration of sodium is about 10 times larger than inside. This difference in concentration is maintained by the passive action of the cell membrane and the active mechanism of the sodium-potassium pump. A net electrical potential of approximately 80 mV exists across the cell membrane; the cell membrane is polarized with the inside being negative with respect to the outside. This is termed the resting potential.

The start of a contraction is initiated by voluntary CNS action. A nerve impulse travels from a motor neuron located outside the spinal cord, via an axon to a muscle fibre. The termination of the axon is called the end-plate or neuro-muscular junction and it is here that acetylcholine is released that alters the permeability of the muscle fibre membrane. This action causes sodium channels to open and the associated redistribution of ions reduces the local transmembrane potential; this is termed depolarization.

The action of depolarization causes the release of calcium within the cell, which in turn allows the myosin filaments to bind to the actin filaments. This process involves the metabolism of ATP and results in a shortening of the muscle by approximately 65%. In addition, provided a threshold of approximately –70 mV is reached, ionic currents cause the depolarization region to propagate in both directions away from the end-plate. The metabolism of ATP is used to restore the calcium and to return the cellular ionic concentrations to their resting state via the sodium-potassium pump.

In the cycle of resting potential, depolarization and subsequent re-polarization, the transmembrane potential changes from approximately –80 mV to +30 mV and then back to –80 mV in about 2 ms. This is termed an action potential. This electrical activity can be observed either by microelectrodes placed across the membrane or by external electrodes aligned along the muscle fibre. However, the external potential appears as a bi-phasic potential.

Many muscle fibres are innervated from a single motor neuron. The collection of a motor neuron cell body, its axons and associated NMJs and muscle fibres is termed a motor unit. When a motor neuron is activated via the CNS, all the fibres associated with this motor unit fire synchronously. The resultant externally observed electrical activity is termed a motor unit action potential (MUAP). The duration of an MUAP (6 ms) is considerably longer than that of an action potential due to the spatial distribution of the fibres throughout the muscle.

Muscle contraction force is generated through a dual mechanism of firing rate modulation and motor unit recruitment. Just as the MUAP is a summation of the activity of the action potentials from the fibres of a motor unit, the myoelectric signal (MES) is a summation of the MUAP for all active neurons.

The MES can be detected by electrodes placed on the skin surface, however the amplitude of the observed potential is much lower than that of the transmembrane potential. Typical levels are in the range 10 μV to 10 mV. The intervening tissue between the muscle and the skin attenuates and "smears" the signal through the tissue filtering effect.

From an electrical standpoint, the appearance of the MES resembles noise. In fact, researchers dealing with the MES often use band-limited white noise as a model for the MES. However, with the MES the "noisiness" of the signal can be controlled by the contraction level, which is under voluntary control. This aspect of the MES is exploited in deriving a control mechanism for powered prostheses.

2.11 Questions

1. Name three types of muscle found in the human body.
2. What is the smallest contractile element in a muscle?
3. Give one mechanism whereby muscles are attached to bone.
4. Why does a muscle need a plentiful blood supply?
5. What is *myoglobin*?
6. What are the two contractile proteins in a muscle fibre?
7. What is a *sarcomere*?
8. What ion is responsible for the initiation of the contraction process?

9. What powers the sodium-potassium pump?
10. In a resting muscle fibre, is the concentration of sodium greater inside or outside the cell?
11. Approximately how much does a contracting muscle shorten?
12. What mechanism is responsible for the propagation of the action potential?
13. What is a motor unit?
14. What is the name of the axon-muscle fibre interface?
15. Do motor units in a muscle fire synchronously or asynchronously ... and why?
16. By what two mechanisms can muscle force be mediated?
17. What is meant by the term myoelectric signal?

Acknowledgements. During the writing of this chapter, several figures were adapted from previously published material. Two textbooks were used for this purpose, both published by Benjamin-Cummings [6, 7]. The figures were scanned and modified electronically to suit the purpose of this text and are therefore not direct copies. However, it is the view of the author that the origin of these invaluable figures is acknowledged. Figures 2.1–2.3, 2.7, 2.9–2.11 are from [6] and Figs. 2.4–2.6 are from [7].

Suggested Reading

1. Basmajian JV, DeLuca CJ (1981) Muscles alive: their functions revealed by electromyography, 5th edn. William & Wilkins, ISBN 0-683-00414-X
2. Bhullar HK, London GH, Forthergill JC, Jones NB (1990) Selective noninvasive electrode to study myoelectric signals. Med Biol Eng Comp 28:581–586
3. Fox SI (1996) Human physiology, 5th edn. William C Brown, ISBN 0-697-20985-7
4. Green JH (1976) An introduction to human physiology, 4th edn. Oxford University Press, ISBN 0-19-263328-7
5. Katz B (1966) Nerve, muscle, and synapse. McGraw-Hill, ISBN: 07-033383-1
6. Marieb EN (1998) Human anatomy and physiology, 4th edn. Benjamin-Cummings, ISBN 0-8053-4360-1
7. Marieb EN, Mallatt J (1996) Human anatomy, 2nd edn. Benjamin-Cummings, ISBN 0-8053-4068-8

Signals and Signal Processing for Myoelectric Control

D. F. Lovely

Contents

Summary

This chapter explains the way in which the myoelectric signal is used to control powered upper limb prostheses. This first part of the chapter covers the acquisition of the signal and the problems associated with electrodes that can occur in practice. This is followed by a brief description of some signal processing that must be performed to derive a useable control signal. The second part of this chapter describes the various strategies employed to control the terminal device and differentiates between ON-OFF and proportional control. In this part, concepts are explained using examples of some of the currently available technology.

3.1 Introduction

The subject of myoelectric control is a very broad one, ranging from the purely practical objective of providing an amputee with a functional prosthesis to the academic pursuits of modeling and extracting more and more information from the myoelectric signal. It is the intention of this author, to introduce the concepts of myoelectric control building on the foundation of electro-physiology developed in the previous chapter. In addition, from the practical standpoint, examples of currently available hardware will be given, wherever possible, along the way.

In the simplest terms, a myoelectric control system can be thought of conceptually as a switch that controls the power to an electric terminal device. The signal that activates this switch is obtained via surface electrodes from remnant muscles within the residual limb of the user, while the power comes from a rechargeable battery (Fig. 3.1).

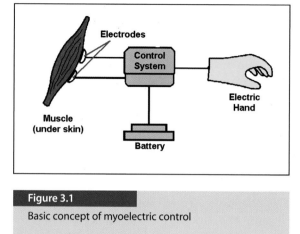

Figure 3.1

Basic concept of myoelectric control

The early myoelectric control systems of the 1970's and 80's were indeed nothing more than "*muscle controlled*" switches. However, today advancement in low-power electronics has led to control systems that can now control more than one function and provide proportional (*speed*) control. Recently, control systems have been introduced which can be programmed at the fitting stage to suit the needs of the client.

Chapter 1 has described this development of myoelectric control systems from a historical standpoint. For the interested reader there are several published reviews of both practical considerations and the research aspects of myoelectric control. Some of these are listed in the bibliography section at the end of this chapter.

3.2 Variation of the Myoelectric Signal with Contraction Level

The concepts of firing rate and recruitment were introduced towards the end of Chap. 2. These are the two main factors that govern the overall tension of a contracting muscle. The force generated depends on the rate at which the muscle fibres are twitching or firing, and secondly how many of them are active. When a muscle contracts all the muscle fibres are not necessarily employed – they only become active when needed. As could be expected, the small motor units responsible for fine control are activated first. Then, if more force is required, the larger motor units begin firing. This is the recruitment process.

As the overall muscle contraction is increased, more motor units begin to become active. At low levels of contraction only the small units deep within the muscle are active. As the contraction level is increased, then more fibres become active and the firing rate increases. Finally, at high levels of contraction, the large superficial fibres begin to fire, giving rise to a large surface signal. Signals such as these are termed motor unit action potential trains (MUAPTs). A summation of these trains is what we know as the myoelectric signal. The most important aspect of the firing rate and recruitment that is exploited in myoelectric prostheses is that they are both under voluntary control.

In Chap. 2 the effect of firing rate and recruitment on the appearance of the surface recorded myoelectric signal was illustrated using small specialized electrodes that are able to resolve individual motor units in low level contractions. If larger electrodes are employed, the summation of the MUAPs is more widespread giving rise to a larger signal. However, this increase in signal amplitude comes at the expense of no longer being able to discern the firing of individual motor units. The overall signal "looks like noise", however, the "*noisiness*" of the signal reflects the contraction level of the muscle.

Figure 3.2 shows a typical MES from the forearm of the author as obtained from a pair of 1 cm diameter stainless steel surface electrodes. The signal shows very little structure as compared to the examples giv-

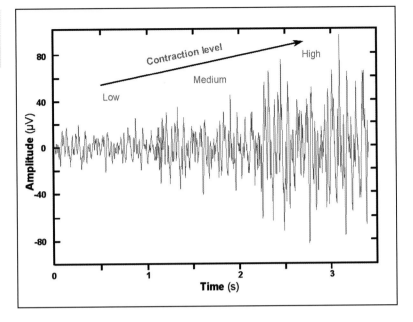

Figure 3.2

Variation of MES with contraction level

en in Chap. 2. No individual motor units can be discerned. This apparent lack of structure or randomness in the MES has led to it being modeled as a white noise source. One such property of a white noise model is a zero mean – ie. the average of the MES is ZERO. On average, the signal is positive for the same amount of time, as it is negative. However, the '*noisiness*' or variance of this signal does change with contraction level (Fig. 3.2).

3.3 Acquiring the Myoelectric Signal

As the signal level obtainable from surface electrodes is so small, the first stage in any myoelectric control system is signal amplification. The design of such an amplifier is a far from trivial exercise due to the environment in which an amplifier must operate.

In any biomedical instrumentation system that involves a subject, there is invariably some unwanted interaction between the subject and the environment. A myoelectric control system is no different. The amputee is always capacitively coupled to the environment – more specifically to the electromagnetic environment. Capacitive coupling exists mainly due

to the proximity of domestic voltage cables and overhead lighting. As capacitive coupling is an electric field phenomenon, current flow in the surrounding environment is not required. All that is required is that the domestic alternating line supply be at a different potential than the body of the subject.

Consider the scenario presented in Fig. 3.3. Here a person is shown coupled to the domestic line supply (*120 V AC in North America*), which in most buildings is concentrated in the ceiling lighting supply. The effective value of this coupling capacitance, C_c, is of the order of a few picofarads[1] (pF). There is also capacitive coupling between the body of the individual and ground. This is termed the body capacitance, C_b. This second capacitance is usually an order of magnitude larger than C_c, due to the widespread nature of the ground as compared with the point source of the domestic line supply.

The two coupling capacitors, C_c and C_b, in series with the body impedance form a simple electrical circuit. A current, I_d, flows from the high potential of the domestic supply, through these capacitors and the

---

[1] 1 picofarad = 10^{-12} of a Farad

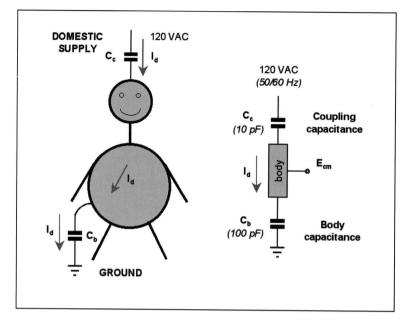

Figure 3.3

Coupling to the environment and common-mode voltage

body, to ground. This current is termed a displacement current and is typically only a few microamperes (μA) in magnitude. This level of current goes undetected by the individual, as it is much lower than what is termed the *threshold of perception*.

However, the effect of this small current is to develop a voltage on the body that is directly proportional to the displacement current and the body capacitance. The value of this voltage is of the order of 5–15 volts – much larger than the amplitude of the surface MES (10μV – 10 mV). This voltage appears all over the body and is present at both surface electrodes and because of this, it is termed the common-mode voltage, E_{CM} – it is common to both electrodes. This common-mode signal is at the line frequency of 50 or 60 Hz (*depending on the country*), which unfortunately is within the frequency bandwidth of the MES, consequently simple filtering of this interference is not possible without distorting the desired signal.

Going a Little Further …

If we assume that the body capacitance is ten times the coupling capacitance, that the internal body impedance is negligible and the line voltage is 120 V AC (60 Hz), then the voltage appearing on the body can be expressed as:

$$E_{CM} = V_{line} \times \frac{X_{cb}}{X_{cc}} = V_{line} \times \frac{|\omega C_c|}{|\omega C_b|} \approx 12\,V$$

The corresponding displacement current can then be estimated as:

$$I_D = \frac{V_{line}}{X_{cb}} = V_{line} \times |\omega C_b| \approx 9\,\mu A$$

This is well below the generally accepted level of perception value of 700 μA.

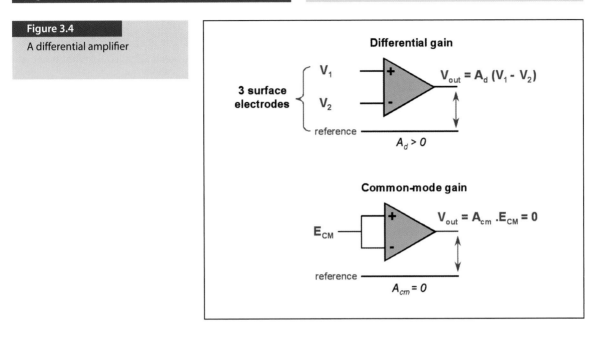

Figure 3.4

A differential amplifier

Because of this frequency overlap, some means of signal acquisition must be employed to reject this large common-mode voltage but at the same time amplify the low level MES signal. This is the role of a *differential amplifier*.

A differential amplifier, as its name suggests, amplifies the difference between two signals as depicted in Fig. 3.4. It has two inputs and rejects any signal that is common to both terminals. In the jargon of electrical engineering, an ideal differential amplifier is said to have zero common-mode gain. In the case of myoelectric control, the two signals are those present at the two electrodes over the site of the controlling muscle group. Provided the external line borne interference affects both electrodes in the same manner, effective cancellation of this common-mode signal can be achieved. For example, let the common-mode signal present on the body be E_{CM} and the small myoelectric signal be expressed as, $\pm V_{MES}/2$, then the voltages appearing on each electrode are:

$$V_1 = E_{CM} + \frac{V_{MES}}{2}$$

$$V_2 = E_{CM} - \frac{V_{MES}}{2}$$

Subtracting these two voltages leaves only the desired MES, which experiences the full differential gain, A_d, of the amplifier. However, as the resultant difference signal is a voltage, then a reference for this potential must be provided. This is the function of the reference electrode. Consequently, all current myoelectric control systems employ three electrodes for signal acquisition. Where this additional electrode is placed is left until Sect. 3.11 where some commercial systems are described.

Some manufacturers do include a notch filter to further suppress the common-mode signal. This very narrow band-reject filter attempts to attenuate only at the line frequency. One obvious disadvantage to this practice is that two versions are required; one centred at 60 Hz the other at 50 Hz to accommodate both the North America and European line frequencies.

Going a Little Further ...

The figure-of-merit for a differential amplifier is termed the common mode rejection ratio (CMRR), which is defined as the ratio of the differential voltage gain, A_D, to the common-mode voltage gain, A_{CM} and is usually expressed as a logarithm:

$$CMRR = 20 \log_{10} \frac{A_D}{A_{CM}} \; dB$$

In an ideal amplifier, the common-mode gain is zero and so the CMRR is infinite. As a rule-of-thumb, for myoelectric control a CMRR of 80 dB (10,000) is usually taken as the minimum accepted standard with most amplifiers encountered having a CMRR of 90 dB or better– measured at the line frequency.

3.4 Motion Artifact

One of the problems associated with surface electrodes is that if they move relative to the skin surface, a 'noise' signal is produced which can be confused with the true MES. This phenomenon is illustrated in Fig. 3.5, in which an electrode placed on the skin surface has been moved sideways. Compare the appearance of this figure to the myoelectric 'spikes' of Fig. 3.2 and note the similarities. In severe cases, this motion artifact completely swamps the MES, but more importantly looks to the control system as a brief large contraction! The major origins of motion artifact are two fold and involve the nature of the interface between the electrode and the surface of the skin along with the variation of electrolyte concentrations in the epidermis.

A surface electrode acts as a transducer in that it converts the ionic activity of the contracting muscle into an electric current. This process sets up a charge double layer at the electrode-skin interface, which can be mechanically disturbed. The situation is analogous to that of a parallel plate capacitor in which the separation of the plates and the area are variable. If this simple model is used, and the charge at the interface is assumed constant, then the artifact developed is dependent on the vertical and horizontal movement of the electrode with respect to the electrolyte/skin. The magnitude of this artifact component is highly dependent on the nature of the electrode material.

The second phenomena that gives rise to motion artifact is termed *skin stretch reflex*. In skin stretch reflex, the various layers of the epidermis set up similar ionic/charge distributions as that present at the electrode-skin interface. Mechanical stretching of the skin displaces these layers and produces surface artifacts that can be up to 5 mV in amplitude. This component of motion artifact is independent of the electrode material.

In the laboratory, skin preparation techniques can be used to minimise the generation of motion artifacts. This usually involves the mechanical abrasion of the *strateum corneum* (*outermost layer of the epidermis*) and the use of electrode gels that are rich in ions. While this approach is valid in the laboratory for short-term studies, it is of limited use in the area of myoelectric control where the prosthesis is used on a long-term basis. In this situation, the only practical approach is to avoid relative movement between the electrode and the skin surface. Hence, a good electrode/skin contact must be maintained at all times, which in turn demands a very good fitting socket. This fit should be such that external loading of the prosthesis does not result in any movement of the residual limb with respect to the electrodes.

If the concept of motion artifact is taken to the extreme, it is possible for an electrode to lose contact with the skin completely. This is termed *electrode lift*, and is largely due to a poor fitting socket or inappropriate mounting of the electrode assembly. With electrode lift, uncontrolled intermittent unwanted operation of the prosthesis often results. This is because the common-mode voltage of the body is present on one electrode and not the other. Consequently, the differential amplifier fails to remove the domestic supply voltage interference and the prosthesis is effectively driven by the 50/60 Hz interference rather than the MES.

Figure 3.5

Motion artifact and electrode lift

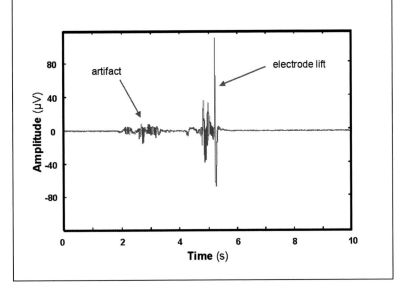

3.5 Processing the MES

To enable the MES to be used as a control means, some feature of the signal must be extracted. This is the purpose of signal processing. As mentioned earlier, the average value of the MES is zero. Consequently, any attempts to low-pass filter the MES, to produce a smoothed signal for prosthesis control; will result in a zero signal. To remedy this situation and to produce a signal that reflects the variance of the MES some form of non-linear processing must be performed. Ideally, what is required is a pulse counter that measures the firing rate of one or many motor units.

Considerable research has been focused on this non-linear element in myoelectric signal processing and several authors have shown independently that a *square law device* is optimum based on error probability. This effectively measures the power contained in the MES. This approach is also particularly adept at extracting pulse-like signals from background noise. As a result, power detectors are the measurement method of choice for highly stochastic signals like neuromuscular pulse trains. Consequently, in the research laboratory power detection is often used to elicit information from the MES with regard to activity level.

The situation in myoelectric control systems is somewhat different. One of the primary design concerns in any myoelectric control system is power consumption. The system must be battery operated and so power consumption must be kept to a minimum. The electronic implementation of a true square law device in analog electronics is not very efficient. Therefore, commercial myoelectric control systems approximate the optimum square law processing by way of a precision *full wave rectifier* (FWR). This is readily achieved with a pair of low power operational amplifiers and signal diodes and so is therefore very meager with power.

Full wave rectification (FWR) can be thought of as taking the negative portion of the MES and folding it along the time axis so that the average value is no longer zero, but some positive value. When this rectified signal is now smoothed or averaged using a low pass filter, the amplitude of the resultant processed myoelectric signal reflects the variance of the raw MES (Fig. 3.6). This new signal, derived from the MES is termed the *processed myoelectric signal*, PMES or more simply the '*myosignal*'. When the individual depolarizations of motor units are closely spaced or su-

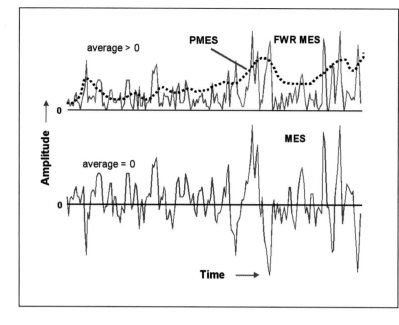

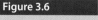

Figure 3.6

FWR and the processed MES

perposed, it is difficult to measure individual firing rates using this FWR measurement technique, however in the majority of cases this approach is more than adequate for providing a control signal for a powered prosthesis.

Therefore, in summary, by amplifying, rectifying and filtering the MES a signal can be obtained which reflects the muscle activity level. All commercial myoelectric prosthetic systems use this PMES to effect control over the terminal device.

3.6 Control of Prosthetic Function

The first myoelectric control systems were targeted towards the replacement of hand function with an electric equivalent. Initially, this was nothing more than an electric hook that provided a basic grasping function with no attention to cosmetic appearance (Fig. 3.7). Today however, there are wide varieties of devices that can be controlled by a myoelectric control system. Electric hands, elbows and wrists are all available in a variety of sizes along with specialized "hooks" for vocational activities. Consequently, the phrase 'terminal device' has entered into the vocabu-

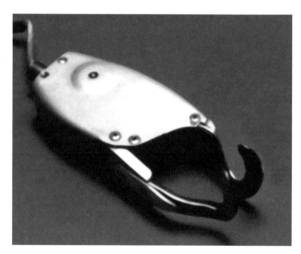

Figure 3.7

Early terminal device – an electric hook

lary of the prosthetic clinic to encompass all the variety of devices that can be controlled from the PMES.

There are many different ways of controlling a terminal device from the PMES. For example, a single

Figure 3.8

Noise threshold in two-site control

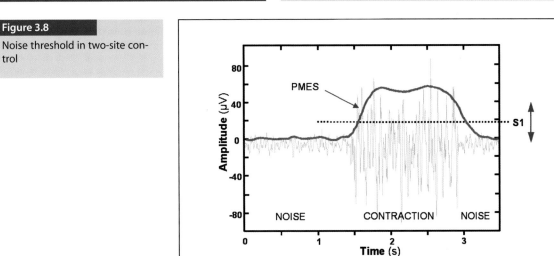

muscle group can be used to control both opening and closing of an electric hand. Alternatively, two different muscle groups can be used; one group for opening the other for closing. In addition, the terminal device can operate at a fixed speed or the speed can be under user control. These variations in how the PMES is employed to control the prosthetic function are termed *control strategies*. Part of the job of the clinical team is to ascertain the best control strategy for the individual client. New strategies are being developed and tried every day to meet the needs of the client and so the area is very dynamic. In this text, only the basic strategies that are available as "*off-the-shelf*" solutions are described.

3.7 Two-Site Systems

As the name suggests, two-site systems use two distinct muscle groups to control the terminal device. Consequently, prostheses employing this type of control are sometimes termed two channel systems as they require two sets of electrodes for their operation and have two PMES. It is usual to use two muscle (remnant) groups that are antagonistic with this type of control system. In this way, the operation of the prosthesis is more natural, especially to the traumatic amputee, as it mimics the natural action of the bi-

ological limb. For example, the PMES from the biceps group can be used to control the flexion of a prosthetic elbow while the triceps PMES activates the extension function.

As it is impossible to design electronic circuitry that is completely free of noise, the MES obtained from any muscle site will be accompanied with a certain degree of noise. As it has been illustrated earlier, this noise looks very similar to a myoelectric signal and so the corresponding PMES will appear as very low-level contraction even with a muscle that is completely relaxed. To prevent inadvertent operation of the prosthesis it is important that any myoelectric control system rejects this 'noise' signal. This is generally accomplished by setting a threshold level, *S1*, for the PMES, as shown in Fig. 3.8, in which the prosthesis remains inactive.

With a two-site system, if the PMES is above the threshold level, the associated prosthetic function is activated. For example, in the case of controlling an electric hand, if the PMES from the extensor site is above the threshold the hand opens. Similarly, if the PMES from the flexor site is above the threshold (*for that channel*) the hand closes. Such a system can be termed a two-site, two-state controller. Each site has its own threshold, which can be individually adjusted for the client. In most cases, this adjustment involves simply increasing the threshold level so that it is

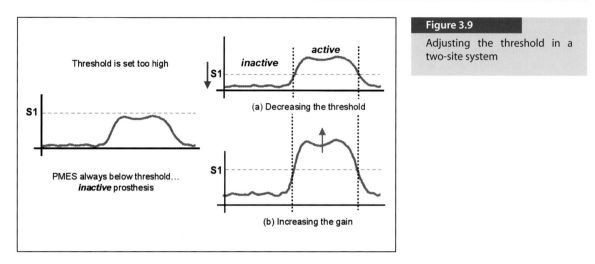

Figure 3.9

Adjusting the threshold in a two-site system

above the noise threshold, ie. no function activation with the control muscle group in a resting state.

Many commercial manufacturers supply systems based on this principle. In practice, the threshold level of each channel is fixed, but the gain of the differential amplifier can be individually adjusted to suit the client. Increasing the gain of the amplifier has the effect of generating a larger PMES for a given contraction level. Consequently, the user does not have to reach the same level of muscle contraction to exceed the fixed threshold level.

As can be seen from Fig. 3.9, increasing the gain of the amplifier (b) has the same effect as reducing the threshold (a). In commercial systems, this adjustment is usually made during the fitting and training phase.

One drawback with two-site systems is that of co-contraction. What happens if both control muscle groups contract simultaneously? The thresholds for both channels are exceeded and the terminal device receives signals to active two functions at the same time. While a problem in early systems, co-contraction issues are now normally taken care of by the drive circuitry of the terminal device (see Sect. 3.9). The terminal device responds to the first signal received and '*locks out*' the co-contraction channel.

3.8 Single-Site Systems

Single-site systems use only one muscle group to control the terminal device. Prostheses employing this type of control are sometimes termed single channel systems, as there is only one set of electrodes to mount in the socket. Consequently, such systems are especially well suited to the young amputee where residual limb area and socket space are limited.

With single-site systems, there is only a single PMES, therefore all the functions of the terminal device must be derived from this single signal. In general, single-site myoelectric control strategies fall into one of two categories; namely, level coded and rate coded systems.

3.8.1 Level or Amplitude Coding

In a level coded system, the function of the terminal device is selected based on the amplitude of the PMES. The available dynamic range (maximum – minimum) of the PMES is divided into three regions. This is achieved by employing TWO threshold levels, S1 and S2, as illustrated in Fig. 3.10. The S1 level is similar to the noise threshold setting of a two-site controller. The S2 level however delimits between two functions or states of the prosthesis.

Figure 3.10

Level coding in a single-site system

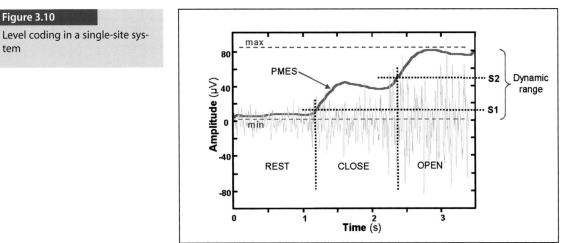

In the case of an electric hand terminal device, the three regions correspond to three functions, namely: REST, CLOSE and OPEN. Consequently, such a system could be termed a three-state controller. A weak contraction of the controlling muscle, below the level of *S1*, causes no operation of the prosthesis; it is in the REST state. With a contraction level between *S1* and *S2* the electric hand closes while a large contraction (*of the same muscle group*) results in opening of the hand.

This technique was pioneered at the Institute of Biomedical Engineering at UNB and was initially targeted towards rehabilitation of the Thalidomide population. This work resulted in the production of a series of UNB myoelectric control systems. In this system, the two switching levels *S1*, *S2* were individually adjustable. Considerable research effort was expended by the same group in the determination of the optimum setting of these switching levels based upon operator error. Although the UNB system has not been available commercially since the mid 1990's, there are many of these systems in the field still functioning as they were designed.

Today, RSL Steeper[2] produces a single-site system based on level coding. However, the method used to divide the dynamic range of the PMES is somewhat different from the original UNB system. The system from RSL Steeper has a fixed separation between the levels and the only adjustment is the amplifier gain. As in the two-site systems, increasing the gain has the same effect as lowering the switching level. However, with this system, both levels are lowered together.

The relative merits of the two systems are that the RSL Steeper single-site controller has only one adjustment for tailoring the device to the client. Consequently, the setup procedure is quick and simple. The UNB system required two adjustments (*one for S1 the other for S2*) and consequently was more time consuming. However, with the UNB system the therapist/prosthetist did have an added degree of flexibility in tailoring the switching levels to the client.

One problem with amplitude coding strategies for myoelectric control concerns the direct activation of the OPEN state (*high contraction level*) from the REST state (*relaxed muscle*) without the inadvertent operation of the CLOSE state (*medium contraction level*). This is achieved by incorporating a small time-delay in the control strategy, such that the user can pass through the CLOSE state without activating the prosthesis. This of course slows the response time of the prosthesis, but does reduce the occurrence of operator error.

[2] RSL Steeper Ltd, Riverside Orthopaedic Center, 51 Riverside, Rochester, Kent, ME2 4DP, England.

3.8.2 "Cookie Crusher" Concept

For very young users, a variation on the level-coding scheme outlined earlier is often employed. Only one threshold level is employed that divides the dynamic range of the PMES into two regions. These regions are generally termed OPEN and CLOSE as this scheme is invariably used with an electric hand terminal device. If the PMES is above the threshold level, the hand OPENS. If the subject then relaxes the contraction, and the PMES falls below the threshold level, the hand CLOSES. Consequently, this scheme can be thought of as an active opening and passive closing control strategy, similar to the conventional split-hook. The automatic closing of the hand gives rise to the popular name for this type of control as the "Cookie crusher".

While the use of only one threshold level makes this system easy to comprehend for a young child, it is imperative that this type of system uses a terminal device that includes some form of battery saving feature (see Sect. 3.9.2). Once the hand has fully closed, the supply to the motor must be shut off automatically, to prevent excessive drain on the battery. Both Otto Bock and RSL Steeper provide systems employing this strategy.

3.8.3 Rate Coding

An alternative to the level coding strategy, which alleviates the necessity of providing a state transition delay, is rate coding. This technique uses a sequential control strategy in which the desired function is first selected and then that function is controlled. The rate coding strategy operates on the principle of how fast the user contracts the control muscle. Function selection is based on the initial slope of the PMES, while an amplitude threshold is used to prevent inadvertent operation of the prosthesis due to noise in the same fashion as a two-site system.

For example, in a below elbow prosthesis, an initial slow contraction rate can be used to select the CLOSE function. Once the function has been selected, then providing the level of the PMES remains above the single threshold, the hand continues to close. Similarly, a fast contraction can be used to activate the OPEN function. This strategy is illustrated in Fig. 3.11. As can be seen in this figure, once the noise threshold, $S1$, is exceeded, a small but finite time is required to ascertain whether the PMES is rising fast or slowly before function selection is activated. Therefore, although a delay is not required for reasons of transiting a state as in a single-site three-state controller, the

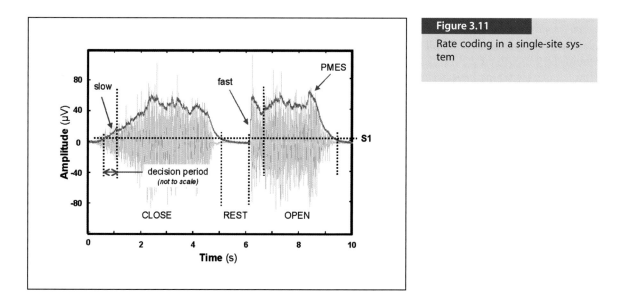

Figure 3.11

Rate coding in a single-site system

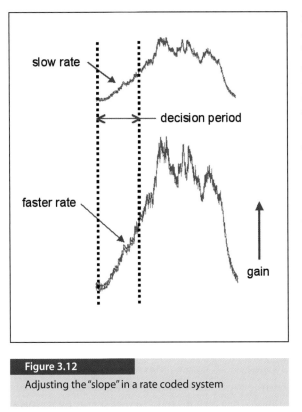

Figure 3.12

Adjusting the "slope" in a rate coded system

multi-function control is given later in this chapter in Sect. 3.11. In addition, rate coding is admirably suited to controlling the speed of the terminal device in a single site system. Once the desired function (*OPEN or CLOSE*) has been selected, the level of the PMES can be used to control the device speed in a proportional manner.

3.9 Terminal Device Electronics

Although the control strategy of a myoelectric control system determines what function is required based on the PMES, it is the terminal device itself, which provides this function. A certain degree of interfacing is required in order for a control system to be able to drive a terminal device.

3.9.1 The Bridge Circuit

All powered prostheses currently on the market employ small rotary direct current (dc) motors to perform the required movement function. To produce the required torque, the output of these miniature motors is fed to a gearbox that reduces the shaft speed. The output from the gearbox is then used to activate the moving parts of the device via further gear arrangements.

The design of small, lightweight gearboxes, which can withstand the substantial wear cycle of the 'start-stop-reverse-start' typical of a powered prosthesis, is far from trivial. It is indeed credit to the mechanical engineering staff of many manufactures' of powered prosthetic components that we have the variety of devices available at our disposal today. Compared to this design challenge, the electronics necessary to control the direction of these motors is very straightforward indeed.

The rotational direction of a dc motor can be controlled by simply changing the direction of current flow. This is most usually accomplished by a set of four electronic switches or relays, as illustrated in Fig. 3.13. This orientation of four switches is often called a '*bridge*' circuit and is controlled from the control logic of a myoelectric control system. These

sequential nature of this control strategy does require a delay to ascertain the initial PMES slope.

This technique is used by Otto Bock[3] in their single-site system. Internally the PMES rate or slope at which the two functions are distinguished is fixed. However, a gain adjustment in this system effectively alters the rate at which the PMES changes for an individual user. The higher the gain, the faster the PMES will rise for a given contraction level, as shown in Fig. 3.12.

One of the advantages of a sequential system is that the number of functions is not limited. This has applications in multi-function control, in which the myoelectric signal can be used to control an elbow, wrist and hand. A more detailed discussion regarding

---

[3] Otto Bock Orthopädische Industrie GmbH, Co, 37115 Duderstadt, Germany

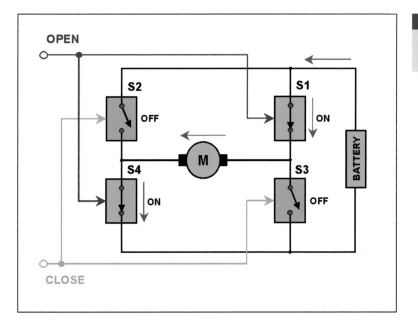

Figure 3.13

Driving the motor: the bridge circuit

switches are arranged so that only TWO can be ON at any instant in time. In Fig. 3.13, when switches S1 and S4 are ON, current flows through the motor from right to left. However, if switches S2 and S3 are ON (with S1 and S4 OFF – remember only TWO switches ON at any given time) then the current flow through the motor is from left to right. By only allowing two switches to be on at any one time, the bridge circuitry takes care of the problem of co-contraction in a two-site system.

All manufacturers of terminal devices locate the bridge circuitry within the device, close to the motor. For example, with the electric hands from RSL Steeper and Otto Bock, removing the soft shell covering of the hand can expose the bridge circuitry. While the bridge circuitry of the Variety Ability[4] hands, the bridge is immediately visible once the hand cosmesis is removed.

3.9.2 Battery-Saving Bridges

For the inexperienced user of a myoelectric control system, inadvertent activation is a common occurrence. Often the situation can exist where the CLOSE signal to an electric hand is active for a prolonged period. However, once the hand is closed, the motor will run in a stalled condition until the control signal is removed. This can lead to rapid battery depletion and a rejection of the prosthesis due to the apparent recurring 'failure' of the battery.

Work at UNB in the 1980's led to a control system which included a '*battery saver*' feature. To be a compatible with as many electric hands as possible, the UNB system used a timing system within the control system which limited the motor running time to that required for full range movement. This approach required no modifications of the motor bridge circuitry and provided extended use for the novice client. It was extremely successful in the rehabilitation of the congenital child amputee and allowed for the very early fitting of a myoelectric prosthesis. Today, manufacturers of powered prosthetic components incorporate similar devices into the bridge circuitry that controls the motor.

---

[4]   Variety Ability Systems Ltd., 2 Kelvin Avenue, Toronto M4C 5C8, Ontario, Canada

The electric hands from RSL Steeper use a different technique than the early UNB battery savers. A current sensing circuit in the motor bridge is used to shut off the motor when running stalled in the closed position. In addition, a small micro switch has been incorporated into the hand to sense the fully open position and interrupt the supply to the motor. A similar arrangement is found on the electric hands from Otto Bock, whereby the motor current is sensed to prevent stalling during the close operation. As an added feature, the level at which this battery saving bridge becomes operable can be adjusted by the prosthetist/therapist. Consequently, a trade off can be made between pinch force and battery life expectancy.

Variety Ability Systems initially took the same approach to battery saving as UNB. Originally, a timing circuit was an option on their electric hands, and was mounted separate from the bridge in the wrist unit. This situation has now been changed in favour of motor current sensing and the battery saver circuitry is now incorporated into the bridge. In this way, more wrist space is made available to accommodate the long residual limb amputee.

3.10 Controlling the Speed of the Terminal Device

In the discussion so far, no mention has been made with regard to controlling the speed of the terminal device. In the early days of myoelectric prostheses, this was not an option, with all systems offering what was termed ON-OFF control. As its name suggests, this is a control mode whereby the electric motor in the terminal device is either ON or OFF. When the motor is ON, its speed is fixed; consequently, the user has no control over the speed of operation of the terminal device.

3.10.1 Proportional Control

Proportional control is the term given to a myoelectric system that supports the speed control of the terminal device. The speed of the device becomes *pro-*

portional to the level of the PMES. In the past, electric hands took up to 2 seconds to go from fully open to fully closed. Thus, a need arose to control the speed at which the fingers moved. However, advances in the electro-mechanical design of hands have reduced this time to around half a second, consequently, today speed control is not a critical issue. However, the situation is somewhat different with regard to powered elbow prostheses.

The range of motion of an elbow is far greater than that of the fingers of a hand. Consequently, it would be more functional if the speed of an electric elbow could be under control so that rapid coarse positioning of the hand could be accomplished. This could then be followed by a slower, finer control of elbow angle to position the hand accurately.

An example of an electric elbow that supports proportional control is the Boston Elbow available from Liberating Technologies Inc.[5] It can be controlled in two ways. Firstly, using a level coded single-site strategy similar to that shown in Fig. 3.10. Two thresholds, *S1* and *S2*, are employed to distinguish between elbow flexion and extension. The amplitude of the PMES above the appropriate threshold then controls the speed of the elbow.

The second control strategy for the Boston Elbow uses two sites. Signals obtained from electrodes located over the biceps and triceps control elbow flexion and extension respectively. This is a more natural arrangement for the traumatic client as it uses the same muscle groups that were used to control the physiological elbow, and may reduce the prosthetic training time. A single threshold level on each muscle site (*S1a and S1b*) is used, just as in the ON-OFF two-site control, to prevent noise from activating the prosthesis. However, now the *difference* in magnitude between the PMES of each site is used to control the speed of the prosthesis. This two-site strategy is illustrated in Fig. 3.14, which shows the activity of the biceps (*Site A*) and triceps (*Site B*) muscles. If the biceps signal is larger than the triceps, then elbow flexion is selected. Conversely, if the triceps activity is higher than the biceps, the elbow is extended.

---

[5] Liberating Technologies Inc., Holliston, Massachusetts, USA

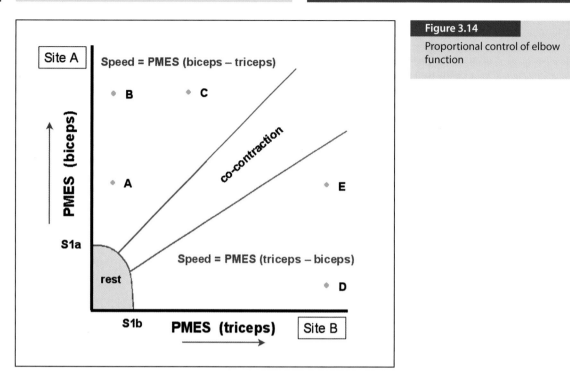

Figure 3.14
Proportional control of elbow function

For example, five specific combinations of biceps and triceps activity levels are shown in Fig. 3.14. These 'operating points' are labeled A to E. While at first thought the elbow flexion speed of points B and C should be the same, as they have similar biceps signals, however as C has a higher level of triceps activity the elbow speed is reduced. To clarify this concept of speed control due to a difference of activity level between two channels, refer to Table 3.1 in which the corresponding prosthesis actions for these operating points are listed.

Another example of a proportionally controlled elbow can be found in the Utah Artificial Arm system from Motion Control[6]. This prosthesis is a two-site system that is compatible with electric hands from Otto Bock. The same two muscle sites that are used to control the elbow can also be used to control the hand. Selection of hand or elbow control is achieved

Table 3.1. Prosthetic function and speed for two-site Boston Elbow

Point	Biceps	Triceps	Function
A	Medium	Low	Slow flexion
B	High	Low	Fast flexion
C	High	Medium	Slow flexion
D	Low	High	Fast extension
E	Medium	High	Slow extension

by using a co-contraction signal. It is up to the user to remember which device is currently active – the elbow or the hand. The original Boston Elbow can achieve the same functional switching via a small body powered switch that is permanently biased to the hand control function. While at first thought, this departure from myoelectric control could be thought of as a retrogressive step, however it does overcome the problem of remembering which device is being

[6] Motion Control, 1290 West 2320 South, Suite A, Salt Lake City, UT, 84119

Figure 3.15

Varying the speed of the motor

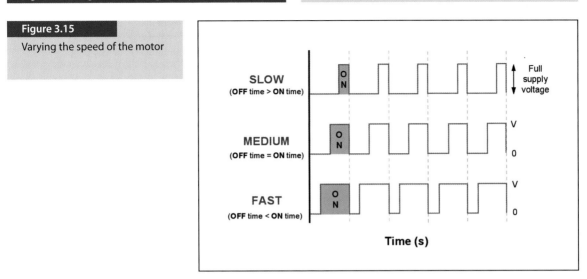

controlled. Recently, the co-contraction mode of switching has been added as an option to the Boston Elbow II.

3.10.2 Terminal Device Speed Control

The maximum speed at which a terminal device will operate is directly related to the speed of the driving motor. The speed of the motor is in turn related to a number of parameters, the principal factors being the load and the supply voltage. For example, an electric hand will operate faster without the cosmetic glove, as the motor does not have to work against the load presented by the stiff outer covering. Likewise, as the battery begins to run down, a noticeable reduction in operating speed becomes apparent with the falling supply voltage.

Although varying the load presented to the motor is somewhat difficult, speed control by altering the supply voltage is a definite possibility. Unfortunately, while reducing the battery voltage will slow down a motor, it also reduces the power (torque) available. This could lead to the situation that we reduce the supply voltage to an electric elbow for precision control, but the corresponding reduction in torque results in the motor stalling under the load of its own weight.

To achieve speed control without sacrificing torque in powered prosthetics, the motor is pulsed on and off with the full battery voltage. The speed of the motor is then related to how long it is pulsed on with respect to how long it is pulsed off. This variation in the pulsing of a motor is termed *pulse width modulation* (PWM) and is illustrated in Fig. 3.15. As the full battery supply is always applied across the motor, no appreciable variation of torque occurs. This method of speed control is often not compatible with conventional ON-OFF bridge circuits. Consequently, manufacturers of proportional systems tend to include specialized PWM circuits within their control systems. These systems (*eg. Boston Elbow*) interface directly to the motor of the terminal device.

3.11 Commercial "Myoelectrodes"

Most manufacturers package the differential amplifier and electrodes together in a single compact package. These are often referred to as 'myoelectrodes'. This is really a misnomer, as the electrode is simply the small conductive disk that makes contact with the skin surface. The role of the true electrode is to convert the ionic activity generated by the contracting muscle into an electrical current suitable for amplification by electronic means. Therefore, it is important

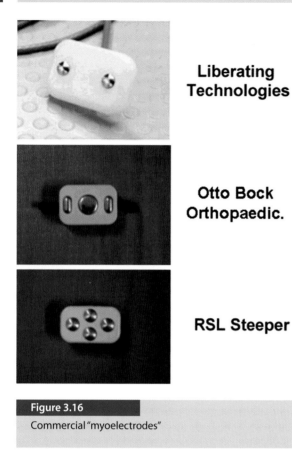

Liberating Technologies

Otto Bock Orthopaedic.

RSL Steeper

Figure 3.16

Commercial "myoelectrodes"

that the reader realizes that when manufacturers of myoelectric components talk about 'electrodes', they are actually talking about the electrode – amplifier combination. In some cases, this even includes the processing circuitry.

As can be seen from the photographs shown in Fig. 3.16, although the package sizes are similar, there is quite a variation in the spacing and size of the actual metal electrodes employed in commercial electrode modules. In the device from Liberating Technologies that is used to control the Boston Elbow, there is no reference electrode, only two small signal electrodes. The reference connection has to be made separately with an additional metal electrode located elsewhere in the socket. This arrangement is admirably suited to two channel systems, as only a single reference is employed. In the Otto Bock electrode assembly, the reference electrode is positioned in be-

tween the two 'signal' electrodes, and has a larger surface area. The large surface area will lower the impedance of the reference electrode and will help to reduce the line-borne interference due to a reduction of the common mode voltage on the body. The electrode module from RSL Steeper takes a similar approach to that of Otto Bock. In this design, a larger reference electrode is achieved by using two electrodes that are connected together internally, but again the reference electrode is placed between the two signal electrodes.

The placing of the reference electrode in between the signal electrodes can have a deleterious effect on the effective common-mode rejection of the differential amplifier. Depending on the surface conductance along the skin surface, the position of the reference electrode can effectively reduce the input impedance of the differential amplifier this in turn has an adverse effect on the ability of the amplifier to reject common-mode signals. However, in most situations this degradation is minimal.

Electrode size affects the acquisition of the myoelectric signal by dictating the volume from which the signal is obtained. In general, a larger electrode will result in a larger signal due to the increase in the pick up volume. In two channel systems, this can lead to problems with cross talk in which the signals from one site become contaminated from activity from the other site. So there is a trade off between size of electrodes and selectivity.

Finally, the spacing between the signal electrodes also affects the appearance of the myoelectric signal. Wide electrode spacing results in a longer time for the depolarization wave to pass between the two active electrodes and, thus, more smearing of the signal will occur. This effectively results in loss of high frequency information in the signal. Conversely, closer spacing will result in a more faithful reproduction of the membrane activity.

In practical myoelectric control systems, the size, spacing and location of the electrodes are dictated more by space considerations rather than by electrical concerns. The smaller the electrode assembly the better the cosmesis and easier it can be accommodated into a prosthesis. So, just as in any implementation of technology compromises must be made to provide a practical solution.

3.12 Multi-function Control Strategies

Controls that can use the same myoelectric system for both elbow and hand control are termed multi-function systems. This is a very active research area presently a hot topic for discussion as there are so many different opinions as to the 'correct' approach. There have been several systems proposed to tackle the problem of controlling several devices from a limited number of myoelectric sites. Attempts have been made to rank their merits by way of error performance. However, most clinics will agree that a fully myoelectric system is often not the best solution for the client. Hybrid systems that combine myoelectric components with switches and conventional harnesses type systems seem to offer the most appropriate rehabilitation solution.

Chapter 9 of this book has been set aside for a discussion on the current research being made in the area of myoelectric control for controlling multi-function prosthetic limbs. This includes some radical ideas to abandon the use of the PMES for control purposes. Sophisticated signal processing techniques have been applied to the MES directly to achieve multifunction control. Although these systems are still in the research stage, they are showing considerable promise especially for the high level amputee. Some systems have been developed that have the ability to adapt or 'learn' specific control patterns from the client; consequently, the control strategy becomes more natural as it is designed by the user. The client trains the prosthesis rather than being trained to use the prosthesis. Other systems provide the terminal device with pressure and slip sensors to provide closed loop autonomous control of grip functions.

3.13 Chapter Summary

In summary, all commercial myoelectric control systems use the contraction level in remnant musculature to control the function of the prosthesis. The MES, which is a summation of muscle action potentials, is detected using surface electrodes and amplified by a differential amplifier. Signal processing is used to derive a signal that reflects the contraction level. This is termed the processed myoelectric signal (PMES) or simply the myosignal. The difference between individual myoelectric control systems is in how this processed signal is used.

All present day, myoelectric control systems can be categorized into either single-site or two-site systems. Single-site systems that use level coding invariably control the terminal device using an ON-OFF function, ie. no control of device speed. To provide proportional (speed) control in a single-site system, selection of prosthetic function is achieved by rate coding. Single-site systems, that employ a single set of electrodes, are admirably suited for the client where space is at a premium, such as the very young user.

In two-site systems, the control options are more varied. Two-site control of an electric elbow generally employs proportional control. ON-OFF control is also available in a two-site system but is usually confined to hand control. Due to the requirement of an additional set of electrodes within the socket, two-site systems are generally more bulky than their single channel counterparts. However, the control strategy tends to be more natural as they tend to employ antagonistic muscle groups, just as in the physiological limb. Thus prosthetic training time may be reduced.

All myoelectric controls need to be adjusted to suit the individual client. In the majority of systems, this is limited to varying the gain, which has the same effect as changing the threshold level/s depending on the type of control strategy being used. Additional information regarding the methods of adjustment for various types of commercial hardware is presented in Chap. 4.

Finally, all modern myoelectric prostheses now employ some form of battery saver to ensure adequate battery lifetime. In the past, this feature was an optional part of some control systems. However, today this feature is usually built into the terminal device where the monitoring of motor current is more easily achieved.

3.14 Questions

1. What is the mean value of the MES?
2. What is a differential amplifier?
3. What is responsible for the common-mode voltage that appears on the body?
4. Explain the difference between a single-site and two-site system.
5. List some terminal devices that may be controlled by a myoelectric system.
6. What is another name for "speed" control in a myoelectric prosthesis?
7. What is the reason for a 'battery saving' device?
8. Lowering a switching threshold is equivalent to decreasing the gain of a myoelectric channel. True or false?
9. What is the purpose of the switching level in a two-channel system?
10. Why is it necessary to pulse the motor on and off to control the speed of an electric elbow, why not simply reduce the supply voltage?

Suggested Reading

1. Daley TL, Scott RN, Parker PA, Lovely DF (1990) A method of comparing operator performance in multifunction myoelectric control systems. J Rehab Res Devel 27 (1):9
2. DeLuca CS (1979) Physiology and mathematics of myoelectric signals, IEEE Trans Biomed Eng, BME 26:313
3. Evans H, Pan Z, Parker PA, Scott RN (1984) Signal processing for proportional myoelectric control. IEEE Trans Biomed Eng, BME 31, PPPP: 207
4. Hogan N, Mann RW (1980) Myoelectric signal processing; optimal estimation applied to electromyography. IEEE Trans Biomed Eng, BME 27:382
5. Hudgins B, Parker PA, Scott RN (1993) A new strategy for multifunction myoelectric control. IEEE Trans Biomed Eng, BME 40:82
6. Lovely DF, Buck CS, Scott RN (1986) An improved battery saving device for use with myoelectric control systems. Med Biol Eng Comput 24:203
7. Parker PA, Stuller JA, Scott RN (1977) Signal processing for the multistate myoelectric channel. Proc IEEE 65:662
8. Parker PA, Scott RN (1986) Myoelectric control of prostheses. CRC Crit Rev Biomed Eng 13 (4):283
9. Perreault EJ, Kearney RE, Hunter IW (1990) A quantitative analysis of EMG amplifiers. 17th Canadian Medical, Biological Engineering Society Conference, 111, Banff, Alberta
10. Scott RN, Paciga JE, Parker PA (1978) Operator error in multistate myoelectric control systems. Med Biol Eng Comput 16 (3):296
11. Scott RN, Lovely DF, Hruczkowski T, Olive MO, Caldwell RR, Hayden J (1986) A new myoelectric control system, J Assoc Child Prosthetic-Orthotic Clin, 21 (2):30
12. Tam HW, Webster JG (1977) Minimising electrode motion artifact by skin abrasion, IEEE Trans Biomed Eng, BME 24:134
13. Williams TW (1990) Practical methods for controlling powered upper-extremity prostheses. Assist Technol 2 (1):3

Commercial Hardware for the Implementation of Myoelectric Control

R. R. Caldwell · D. F. Lovely

Contents

Disclaimer: The information contained in this chapter, especially as it relates to specific vendors and products, is believed to be accurate at the time it was written and is, of course, subject to change with continued advancements in technology and shifts in market forces. Mention of specific products and options is for illustration purposes only and does not constitute an endorsement of any kind by either the authors, editor or the publisher.

Summary

This chapter is a survey of the current components available to the prosthetist and therapist to implement a myoelectric control system. To set the scene, a brief review of the history associated with the development of powered prosthetic components, that has taken place over the last 40 years, is presented. This is followed by an in depth look at current prosthetic components on a manufacturer-by-manufacturer basis. Finally, as sometimes the best solution for the client can only be achieved by mixing components from different manufacturers, the subject of component compatibility is addressed.

4.1 Introduction

In Chap. 3, the various methods of achieving myoelectric control were discussed with regard to the signal characteristics and typical control strategies. In a few instances reference was made to specific hardware. In this chapter, the hardware concepts are expanded further to investigate the prosthetic components currently available commercially to implement a myoelectric control system.

For those readers who have some familiarity with the subject, it is useful to mention some of the earlier manufacturers that are no longer in business. Fidelity Electronics, Leaf Electronics, VA-NYU, Systemteknik and the University of New Brunswick (UNB) are no longer producers of myoelectric control components. It should be noted that UNB is still active in the research and fitting aspect of myoelectric control, which highlights the difficulty in sustaining a manufacturing capability in a market that is extremely small.

Today, the manufacturers of myoelectric control components are limited to seven companies. These are Centri AB, Hosmer, Liberating Technologies, Inc., Motion Control, Otto Bock Healthcare, RSL Steeper and Variety Ability Systems, Inc. In this chapter, each of these manufactures will be profiled in turn, highlighting both established products and those in development. Note that this review is in alphabetical order and in no way implies any ranking based on performance.

To put the achievements of these companies in perspective, this chapter begins with a description of the evolution of myoelectric control from a technological standpoint, rather than the general history as covered in Chap. 1. In this way, the reader will obtain a feel for the progress and advancements made in powered prosthetics over the last 50 years.

The chapter concludes with a discussion of compatibility. As the optimum rehabilitation solution often requires components from different manufacturers, it is useful to have an indication of which products are compatible with each other.

4.2 The Evolution of Myoelectric Control Systems

In Germany, at the end of WWII, a few myoelectric control systems were being used, by amputees in the workplace to accomplish repetitive work. These systems employed vacuum tube technology to process the myoelectric signal, with the prostheses hard wired to a large console housing the electronic circuitry. This type of fixed system had no concern for cosmesis, component weight or power drain but was the beginnings of myoelectric controlled prostheses.

In the late 50's and early 60's, a Russian scientist based in St. Petersburg, A. Y. Kobrinski, developed a self-contained myoelectric control system. This was one of the first stand-alone, battery-powered systems to be used on a number of amputees. In 1965, this system was licensed by the Rehabilitation Institute of Montreal to be used on patients in Canada. Six months later, under a joint effort of the University of New Brunswick (UNB) in Fredericton, New Brun-

swick, and the Ontario Crippled Childrens Centre in Toronto, Ontario, the first all Canadian myoelectric control system was fitted on a patient. This system employed the UNB designed one-muscle 3-state system strategy, as described in Chap. 3.

In the early 70's most fittings were experimental in nature and employed electrodes that had to be regularly injected with paste to provide a good electrical contact with the skin. However, these systems did attempt to address the cosmetic issue by using rechargeable batteries built in to the prosthesis. By the end of the decade, the paste electrodes had been replaced by dry electrodes, which were much more convenient for the wearer. This change was directly attributable to the improvement in solid-state electronics that provided superior noise performance. However, around about the same time, a different approach was taken with the nickel-cadmium (NiCad) battery supply. The internal battery approach was almost universally abandoned for an external battery, mounted on the outside of the forearm section. This not only increased the space available in the prosthesis to accommodate long residual limbs, it also moved the weight of the battery more proximal.

Up until the mid 70's, most fittings were carried out on adults, with electric hands supplied by Otto Bock. The lack of children's fittings was largely due to the lack of a suitable terminal device. This situation was rectified by the introduction of a child-sized hand by Systemteknik in Sweden. Towards the end of the 70's, trials of this hand were conducted both in Sweden, by the University of Gothenburg and in the UK, by RSL Steeper. The results of these trials established the foundation for the regular fitting of children with myoelectric prostheses.

In the early 80's, the results of the Swedish and UK trials led to most clinics fitting children, some as young as 18 months, with myoelectric prostheses. This factor brought clinics from the research state to the routine prescriptions of myoelectric controlled prosthetics. By the middle of this decade many manufacturers were jumping on the bandwagon to develop new lighter weight children's components. These included children's myoelectric control units from UNB and two sizes of child electric hands from Variety Ability Systems Inc. (VASI). At the end of the 80's,

Otto Bock introduced a small "myoelectrode" for applications in both child and adult prostheses.

During the 90's, the myoelectric prosthesis industry began to turn towards computer technology to provide programmable controls systems. These advanced controllers can be adjusted, while on the patient, to give a variety of functions from one or two electrode sites.

Battery technology has also seen substantial advancements in the last 10 years. The ubiquitous nickel-cadmium (NiCad) rechargeable batteries suffer from a drawback due to the chemistry of the cell. If a NiCad battery is re-charged before being completely discharged, then its effective capacity is substantially reduced. This is often referred to as the "memory effect". Consequently, the NiCad battery is beginning to be replaced by both nickel-metal hydride (NiMH) and lithium ion (Li-ion) technology, which do not exhibit a memory effect. In addition, these new technology batteries have a higher capacity-volume ratio that implies a smaller battery for a given capacity. One of the manufacturers, RSL Steeper, has also chosen to include a battery capacity indicator to indicate three levels of charge capacity by the push of a switch.

Terminal device technology has also progressed. Some manufacturers now offer electric hand and hooks that are controlled by two motors. These motors are usually associated with fast and slow movements of finger and/or thumb. However, there are some terminal devices that have one motor for hard control of finger/thumb and the second as a brake for holding pinch forces on an object. Needless to say, the addition of extra motors in the terminal device demands a more sophisticated myoelectric control system.

Finally, the control systems of the 70's and 80's were limited to an ON/OFF method of control. The motor in the terminal device was either ON or OFF; there was no speed control. Today, the patient has the option of proportional control in which the speed of the terminal device is under voluntary control.

4.3 Centri AB

Centri AB is a 2nd-generation family-owned Swedish company that was established in 1948. In the past, Centri AB was known primarily for their passive hands and cosmetic gloves. Today, they currently offer both PVC and silicon gloves for most electric hands on the market. More recently, Centri AB embarked on a program of advanced product development in the area of myoelectric control systems. In the mid 90's, Centri AB introduced a series of Ultra-Lite electric hands, that comprised three sizes ($6\,^3/_4$", $7\,^1/_4$", and $7\,^3/_4$") as measured around the knuckles.

These hands have been recently re-designed to make them more durable. In addition, a $8\,^1/_4$" size has been introduced. Centri AB has also developed custom electronics to control their hands using the active electrodes from Otto Bock for the muscle site signal pickup. Centri have plans to release their own electrode/amplifier module to round off their component line for both teenagers and adults.

The design of the UltraLite hands is unique in several ways. They are made of aluminium and machined nylon to make the units very light (~225 g for the $6\,^3/_4$" size with its wrist unit). Naturally, the larger sizes have slightly more weight. The hands are also

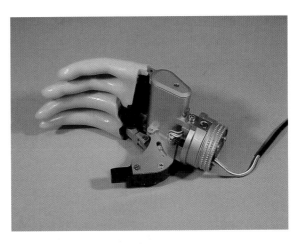

Figure 4.1

UltraLite hand with quick disconncet wrist

Table 4.1. Specifications of UltraLite electric hands from Centri AB

Size (in)	Weight (oz)	Max current at stall (mA)	Pinch force (lb)
6¾	8.4	n/a	12.6
7¼	10.0	n/a	13.6
7¾	10.1	n/a	13.6
8¼	10.4 oz.	n/a	14.0 lbs.

very short from the wrist to thumb tip (~3⅝" for the 6¾") making it an ideal choice for long below elbow (B/E) fittings on those where weight is an important factor (Fig. 4.1).

Finally, the design has a unique movement axis of the fingers and thumb, mimicking the natural hand. This gives the hands a good cosmesis with the geometry of the open hand being much thinner than others on the market. The only disadvantage of the electric hands from Centri AB, may be the small wrist diameter which is approximately 1½" for all hand sizes (Table 4.1).

Contact information:
Centri AB
Datavägen 6
17543 Järfälla
Sweden
Tel: +46-8-58031165
Fax: +46-8-58081128
e-mail: centri@centri.se
Web: http://www.centri.se/main.htm

4.4 Hosmer

Hosmer is the more recent name associated with the Hosmer Dorrance Company which has been making conventional prosthetic components for over 90 years. D.W. Dorrance founded the Hosmer Dorrance Company in 1912 and was the original designer of the split hook terminal device. This product has become so popular in the prosthesis arena that today it still features predominately in their product line.

More recently, from research work conducted at the Rehabilitation Institute of Chicago, Hosmer has moved into the myoelectric control area with their Synergetic Prehensor. This is an electric hook, which employs two motors; one for fast motion, the other for precision. While not a cosmetic solution, the very fast moving jaws, coupled with proportional control gives this device "physiologic speed". However, to achieve this speed requires the use of a 9-volt battery.

Hosmer also supply a line of electric elbows with both exo- and endo-skeletal versions. Their older electric elbow (called the NY electric elbow) also benefits from research at the Rehabilitation Institute of Chicago and can be controlled with myoelectric signals. Finally, their Prehension Actuator (electric forearm rotator) rounds out the components for a prosthetic system for below elbow (B/E) and above elbow (A/E) amputees (Fig. 4.2).

All the above components can be controlled with a proprietary "Myoelectrode" using an external electrode pick-up connected to a small processing unit that can be mounted in any remote space in the prosthesis. This component is available in both single and two-site versions.

Finally, Hosmer has recently introduced a 7.2-volt, 1430 mA.Hr lithium ion battery pack and charger to enhance the performance of their electric elbow. While Hosmer produces a range of powered components for the upper limb amputee, these have been designed with functionality rather than cosmesis in mind. In addition, many of these products operate from different battery voltages (5.0, 6.0, 7.2 & 9.0-volt) and consequently require different charging units (Fig. 4.3).

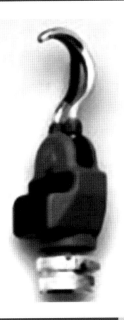

Figure 4.2

Synergetic Prehensor

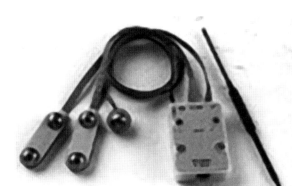

Figure 4.3

"Myoelectric Electrode"

It is interesting to note that Hosmer is owned by Fillauer; a company that specializes in custom fabricated items. This parent company also owns Motion Control and the Centre for Orthotics Design, thus providing a full prosthetics and orthotics service.

Contact information:
Hosmer Dorrance Corporation
561 Division St.
Campbell, California, 95008
USA
Tel: +1-408-3795151
Fax: +1-408-3795263
e-mail: hosmer@hosmer.com
Web: http://www.hosmer.com

4.5 Liberating Technologies Inc. (LTI)

Liberating Technologies Inc. (formerly Liberty Technology) is the originator of the popular Boston Elbow System. However, today LTI are expanding their sphere of interest into new battery designs and programmable control units. In addition, they are currently completing a full revision of the Boston Elbow System using state-of-the-art technology.

The new Boston Elbow System, termed the Boston Digital Arm System, comprises programmable electronics, high capacity batteries, fast chargers and a new forearm lock. As the elbow is programmable at the clinic level, this necessitates the purchase or rent of proprietary software. This feature makes this new product a "change on the go" fitting/training elbow that allows for pre-prosthetic evaluation of the patient.

The Boston Digital Arm system includes five motor controllers for hands, wrists and shoulder joints and several channels of feedback that improves speed and force control. All five motors can operate simultaneously, which was not possible with previous prosthetic arms. It is adaptable to work with all age appropriate hands from all existing manufacturers. In addition, it can be programmed to run in conjunction with traditional 6-volt terminal devices from the internal 12-volt battery pack in both ON/OFF and proportional modes (Fig. 4.4).

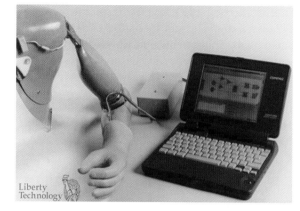

Figure 4.4

Programmable Boston Elbow. (Source: Liberating Technologies Inc.)

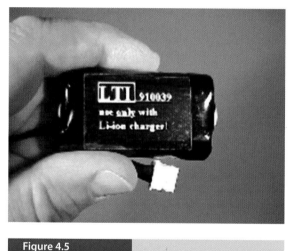

Figure 4.5

Internal Li-ion battery. (Source: Liberating Technologies Inc.)

LTI also designs and manufactures the VariGrip control unit. This is a programmable controller that is compatible with all manufacturers' prosthetic components. This controller can operate up to three powered prosthetic devices such as hands, wrists and elbows. This is especially important if use is to be made of the recently introduced two-motor hands. The VariGrip system is also capable of accepting inputs

from various sources such as force sensitive resistors (FSRs), touch switches, "myoelectrodes" and servo mechanisms, and so provides a very flexible functionality.

LTI also manufactures various types of NiCad batteries suitable for both adult and child powered prostheses. In addition, LTI recently announced a new high-capacity Lithium-ion built-in battery. This device has a 580 mA.Hr capacity (more than twice the capacity of an equivalent NiCad battery) and has an increased terminal voltage (>15%) for more speed and 20% less weight. The battery's small size and low weight results in less bulk and greater comfort for the user (Fig. 4.5).

In keeping with the novel design philosophy of the VariGrip control system, LTI produces or will custom produce every possible combination of adapters to make fitting any component a plug together task.

LTI also distributes products for three of the leading international suppliers of powered prostheses; RSL Steeper of England, VASI of Canada and Centri of Sweden. This enables LTI to provide an excellent array of upper limb components to satisfy each client. The company also supplies powered prosthetic accessories such as: batteries, chargers, hands, wrists, elbows and shoulder joints, electrodes and other input devices as well as silicone and PVC cosmetic gloves and custom high-definition cosmetic covers.

Contact information:
Liberating Technologies Inc.
325 Hopping Brook Road, Suite A
Holliston, Massachusetts, 01746–1456
USA
Tel: +1-508-8936363
Fax: +1-508-8939966
e-mail: info@liberatingtech.com
Web: http://www.liberatingtech.com

4.6 Motion Control Inc.

Motion Control Inc., was established in 1974 by a group of faculty members and researchers at the University of Utah in Salt Lake City, to commercialize the

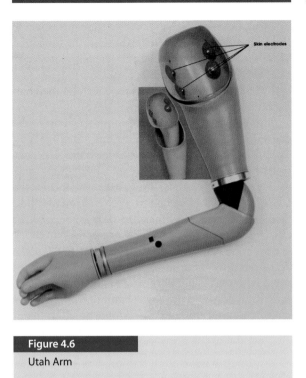

Figure 4.6
Utah Arm

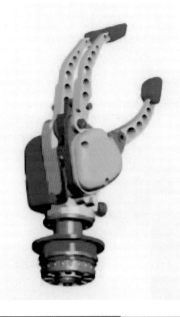

Figure 4.7
Motion Control Hand

medical technology developed at the University's Center for Engineering Design led by Dr. Stephen Jacobsen. As a result of this University-Industry partnership the Utah Artificial Arm was developed.

The first Utah Arm was sold in 1981 and provided a total arm prosthesis that contained its own NiCad battery power supply and myoelectric control system that could operate both the electric elbow and a terminal device. Typically the terminal device was an Otto Bock electric hand or Griefer, while the myoelectric control employed two channels to implement a proportional system. Unfortunately, a drawback of this sophisticated system was the number of adjustments required by the clinic personnel to tailor the prosthesis to the client.

The Utah Arm 2, was introduced in 1997, and was a natural development of the earlier product. This prosthesis retains all the functions of the original Utah Arm, providing full proportional control of both the elbow and terminal device but adds some additional operational features. The terminal device is the default control mode. A quick co-contraction of both myoelectric channels switches control to the elbow, whose position is then controlled by the difference signal between the biceps and triceps channels. On relaxation, the elbow becomes locked in position and control reverts to the terminal device (Fig. 4.6).

Other improvements in the Utah Arm 2 include the use of a nickel-metal hydride (NiMH) battery in place of the standard NiCad and more user-friendly adjustments for setting the various switching levels and operational parameters for the arm. The addition of a quick disconnect wrist module now allows the Utah Arm to be used with both Otto Bock and Hosmer terminal devices, in addition to their own recently announced electric hand.

The Motion Control Hand is similar to an Otto Bock $8\frac{1}{4}$" hand with several modern design improvements. These include the use of light-weight but strong materials, a safety opening release mechanism, extra wide opening fingers, a larger pinch force of 22 lbs. and battery saving electronics. The hand can also be operated from a variety of voltages, up to 18 volts, so that it is compatible with a range of control systems from other manufacturers (Fig. 4.7).

Over the years, Motion Control has also used the original elbow electronics as the basis of a stand alone micro processor control unit with remote electrode pick-up capable of controlling hands and wrist rotators with proportional control from very weak myoelectric signals. This system, called the ProControl is now in its second incarnation and includes an automatic calibration feature that tailors the sensitivity (gain) of the system to the myoelectric signal of the client. The ProControl 2 is supplied with a lithium-ion (Li-ion) battery pack and 2-hour fast charger. The system can also be interfaced to a PC type computer to allow the prosthetist or therapist to visualize the myoelectric signals in real time that is useful for fine-tuning of the system.

Motion Control was acquired by Fillauer Inc., in January 1997 and became part of one of the most comprehensive orthotic and prosthetic research, development and manufacturing companies in the world. Fillauer is headquartered in Chattanooga, Tennessee, while Motion Control continues to operate in Salt Lake City, Utah.

Contact information:
Motion Control Inc.
2401 South 1070 West, Suite B
Salt Lake City, Utah, 84119-1555
USA
Tel: +1-801-9782622
Fax: +1-801-9780848
e-mail: info@utaharm.com
Web: http://www.utaharm.com/index.html

4.7 Otto Bock Healthcare

Otto Bock Healthcare, GmbH was founded in Berlin in 1919 with 20 employees. Today, the company continues to be family-owned and has more than 3,000 employees worldwide. Otto Bock is the world's leading manufacturer/distributor of prosthetic and orthotic components with branches in over 30 countries worldwide.

Otto Bock electric hands are sized with respect to the circumferential dimension around the knuckles. This is the same measurement scheme as used by Centri AB. The adult hands are available in four sizes, $6^3/_4"$, $7^1/_4"$, $7^3/_4"$ and $8^1/_4"$, and are termed the Electrohand series (Fig. 4.8).

Otto Bock has taken the step of moving part of the control electronics into the bridge circuitry (see Chap. 3) that drives the motor of the hand. The control strategy is therefore selected by an appropriate choice of bridge module. Bridges are available for the adult hands that offer rate or level control, using either one or two sites, that can be proportional or ON/OFF in nature. It should be noted that Otto Bock use the term "digital" to describe the ON/OFF method of hand motor control. This should not be confused with a true digital control system that employs a microprocessor in the control unit to allow full flexibility via programming. The proportional mode of operation, in which the speed of the terminal device is controlled, is termed Dynamic Mode Control (DMC) by Otto Bock.

A recent advancement in hand technology by Otto Bock was the introduction of the SensorHand. This terminal device incorporates a slip sensor in the thumb and a strain gauge force sensor to provide a closed loop feedback system. The sensor technology was developed in conjunction with the Schweizerische Unfall Versicherungs Anstalt insurance company and therefore the SensorHand is sometimes referred to as the SUVA hand.

A microprocessor in the hand senses when an object is about to slip, which in turn automatically increases the grip force without client intervention. A brief myoelectric opening signal stops this auto grasp response, while a longer myoelectric signal opens the hand. The SensorHand also incorporates what is termed a Flexi-Grip function. This allows patients to use their sound hand to reposition an object without using electrodes to open and close the hand. In this way the grip appears flexible, like a natural hand. The SensorHand is available in three sizes, $7^1/_4"$, $7^3/_4"$ and $8^1/_4"$ and like the Electrohand series has multiple options with regard to control strategy electronics, which again are located in the bridge unit. However, with the SensorHand, changing a small colour coded

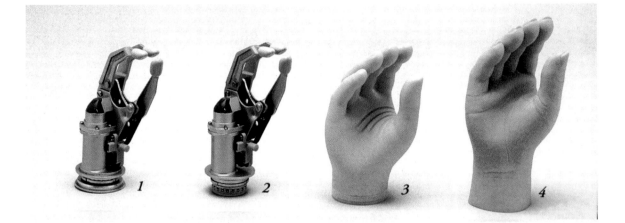

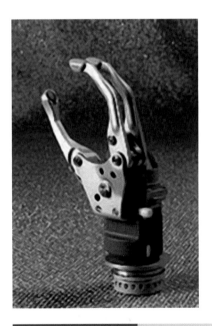

plug in the bridge circuitry changes the control strategy (Fig. 4.9).

Since 1998, Otto Bock has added four sizes of children's hands to their list of components. These devices, termed the Electrohand 2000 system, include 5", 5½", 6" and 6½" models that attain their small size by removing the bridge from the hand and relocating it in the wrist unit. The same colour coded plug concept is used with these hands, allowing the clinic to select the best control strategy for the client. The Electrohand 2000 bridge, termed the 4-in-1 Controller LS, also includes a special high-sensitivity option and a "cookie-crusher" mode. As mentioned briefly in Chap. 3, this strategy uses an active opening and an automatic closing. Otto Bock terms this type of strategy Electronic Voluntary Opening (EVO) and is especially suited for very young users. The bridge uses a laminating ring/wrist connection and operates from a low voltage, 150 mA.hr NiCad (4.8 volt) battery that was specially designed for use with children (Fig. 4.10).

To cope with the long residual below elbow patient, Otto Bock has recently added a transcarpal (TC) electric hand to their product line. The motor is one-third smaller and has been repositioned to take up less room proximally. The result is a hand with the same grip force as a comparable adult hand. The attachment wrist unit has been replaced with a new connection technique that uses cable loops instead of a lamination ring. The Transcarpal Hand is available

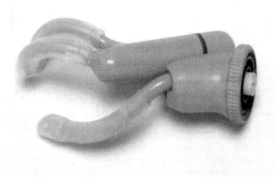

Figure 4.10

System 2000 child hand. (© Otto Bock Health Care)

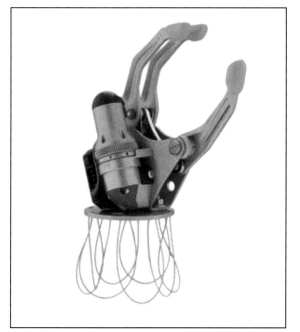

Figure 4.11 ▶

TC hand. (© Otto Bock Health Care)

in the 3 standard sizes (7¼", 7¾" and 8¼") with both ON/OFF and proportional control bridge options (Fig. 4.11).

To round off the terminal device options from Otto Bock, is the Griefer. This is an alternative to an electric hand, which sacrifices cosmetics for robustness and grip strength. The Griefer is an electric hook with jaws that open parallel to about 3½" wide and has a very strong pinch force of up to 29 lbs. The Griefer has proven effective in situations demanding a strong grip and constant reliability. The grip surfaces are adjustable in all planes to allow multiple gripping and holding functions (Table 4.2).

Otto Bock myoelectric "electrodes" are of one size for adults and children and operate on voltage of 4.8 to 6 V. These "electrodes" are used in all Otto Bock control configurations and provide an amplified, processed myoelectric signal in the range of 0–3 volts depending on the muscle activity level. As mentioned earlier, the remaining signal processing and strategy options are defined by circuitry in the bridge electronics. There are two packaging options for these active electrodes; one is a round package that is very robust and suitable for adults, the other is a low profile rectangular package intended for younger individuals.

Otto Bock also manufactures a variety of wrists for regular or long B/E patients. By far the most common with the adult hands are the quick disconnect mechanical passive wrist. This allows a full 360° rotation adjustment by the patient and the quick removal for hand replacement or substitution. In this way, patients can own several terminal devices and select the most appropriate for the task in hand. There is also a less robust passive wrist for the very long B/E patient that does not have the quick disconnect feature. It should be noted that the four sizes of childrens hands (Electrohand 2000 series) only have passive adjustable wrists as the bridge electronics is incorporated as part of the wrist unit.

Table 4.2. Specifications of electric hands from Otto Bock Healthcare

Size (inch)	Age	Weight (oz)	Max current at stall (mA)	Pinch force (lbs)
5	0–2	3.0*	400	3
5 1/2	2–4	4.0*	400	7
6	4–6	4.5*	400	10
6 1/2	6–9	4.6*	400	10
6 3/4	9–12	11.3	500	10
7 1/4	12+	15.0	720	18
7 3/4	Adult	17.0	720	18
8 1/4	Adult	17.0	720	18
Griefer	Adult	18.3	700	29

* These weights do not include the bridge electronics

Contact information:

Otto Bock Healthcare GmbH
Max Nader Str. 15
Duderstadt, 37115
Germany
Tel: +49-55-2784 80
Fax: +49-55-2772330
e-mail: oi@ottobock.de
Web: http://www.ottobock.de

Otto Bock Healthcare
Two Carlson Parkway, Suite 100
Minneapolis, Minnesota, 55441
USA
Tel: +1-800-3284058
Fax: +1800-9622549
e-mail: info@ottobockus.com
Web: http://www.ottobockus.com/index.htm

4.8 RSL Steeper

RSL Steeper was formed by the merger of two companies; Rehabilitation Services Ltd. and Hugh Steeper Ltd. Rehabilitation Services Ltd. was a young company formed by four prosthetists in 1987 with the objective of providing superlative prosthetic services in the UK. Hugh Steeper, a much older company, was established in 1921 and since that time has gained an enviable reputation in the rehabilitation products field.

In the early 80's, Hugh Steeper Ltd. started its own program of designing powered components for children and adults. These included electric hands, battery packs (both Ni-Cad and lithium) battery receptacles (both mounted or external), wrist units, electrodes, cabling and an electric hook called the "Gripper". Over the past 20 years this product line has been refined by the use of lighter weight materials in the hands, new electronics in the hands and electrodes, and new lithium-ion battery technology in the battery packs.

The RSL Steeper electric hands are sized differently to both the Otto Bock and Centri AB products. Instead of measuring the circumference around the knuckles, these hands are specified by the distance

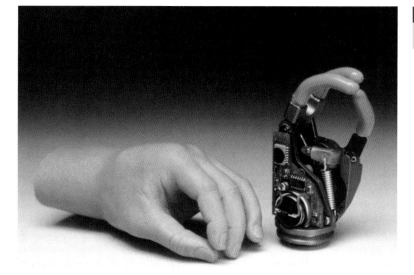

Figure 4.12
Scamp hand for children

across the knuckles. Steeper manufacture seven different sizes of hands ranging from $1^3/4$" through $3^1/4$". The young children's sizes ($1^3/4$" and 2"), called the SCAMP hand, use a single myoelectric signal to activate the open state while using an internal spring for the close function.

While this arrangement is very similar to the "cookie crusher" strategy, the use of a spring rather than a motor drive, allows the child to release a grip on an object by simply pulling away against the spring tension. Another useful feature of these hands is that the fingers and thumb have a compliant sleeve covering the total surface that makes the hands more adaptable to irregular object surfaces without requiring large pinch forces to hold those objects. The disadvantage of these hands is that they are only available in a single function control strategy. Older children generally use a two-function control strategy that provides for voluntary control of both open and close functions (Fig. 4.12).

The older children and adult size of electric hands ($2^1/4$" to $3^1/4$") have an adaptable electronic bridge that can be set via a rotating switch to incorporate single signal activation, dual signal activation at maximum speed of hand, dual signal activation proportional speed to signal strength and a setting for future research strategies. This allows the fitting centre to purchase the correct size hand and decide on the type of control strategy that best suits the patient during the fitting process. The RSL Steeper hands are covered in three types of cosmetic gloves that are available in 11 different colours. The types are regular polyvinyl chloride (PVC), true finish (a more natural look/finish) and silicon. The latter type although a less rigid and tough covering is extremely easy to clean.

The $2^1/4$" to $3^1/4$" hand size ranges are also available with a servo control strategy that is exclusive to RSL Steeper hands. The system uses a transducer mounted as part of a light weight harness that is activated by up to 3/8" extension and up to 1/4 lb. of pull force. This movement matches a similar transducer mounted in the hand that causes the hand to open to the same proportional distance that the harness transducer has been moved. This system is very similar to a conventionally harnessed hook/hand fitting but with much less excursion and pull force requirements while giving the patient the cosmesis and function of an electric hand (Fig. 4.13).

The RSL Steeper hands are connected to the prosthesis through several types of wrist units. The most common is the friction wrist. The other types of wrist units available are for the larger hand sizes and these allow the patient to quickly disconnect the hand and reattach a different device. These are routinely called

Figure 4.13

Adult hand

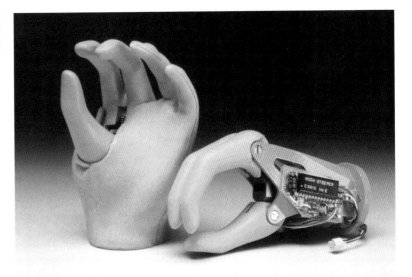

quick disconnect wrists and are similar to those available from Otto Bock Healthcare.

Another optional terminal device from RSL Steeper is the Gripper. This is an electric version of the split hook, which has two powered jaws. One jaw is fast moving with a low pinch force that grips an object lightly. The second jaw can then move up to $^3/_8$" with a very strong grip force when needed. This Gripper can be interchanged with adult hands via a quick disconnect wrist unit. The Gripper comes in two different versions, for use with either 6 or 12-volt systems. This feature is important as most electric elbows run off a 12-volt supply. Consequently, the Gripper can be used both with below elbow (B/E) and above elbow (A/E) prostheses and is compatible with components such as the Boston Elbow (Fig. 4.14).

RSL Steeper also produces a mechanical adult elbow with an electric lock option. This is an excellent option in a hybrid prosthesis in which mechanical (conventional) and powered components are mixed to provide a more functional rehabilitation solution. The electric lock allows the wearer to lock and unlock the elbow using a switch or myoelectric signal (Table 4.3).

To complement the electric hands, RSL Steeper also produces an "electrode" which performs the same functions as the Otto Bock version. The electrode module consists of a small rectangular package that contains the electrodes, differential amplifier and full wave rectifier. This produces an analog signal that is further processed by the electronics in the electric hand bridge circuitry to drive the motor.

RSL Steeper also offers a variety of batteries, cables and connection blocks to interconnect myoelectrodes, touch switches or pull switches with their hands and grippers. In addition, to provide for the ultimate in flexibility, they also make adaptor cables to allow you to mix and match components from other manufacturers with their own products. This includes a new 6 V Li-ion battery with Aon board@ voltage monitor that will fit the Otto Bock battery receptacle which has become a standard over the last two decades.

Contact information:
RSL Steeper
Riverside Orthopaedic Centre
51 Riverside, Medway City Estate
Rochester, Kent, ME2 4DP
England, UK
Tel: +44-01-634297010
Fax: +44-01-634297011
e-mail: paul.steeper@rehab.co.uk
Web: http://www.rslsteeper.com

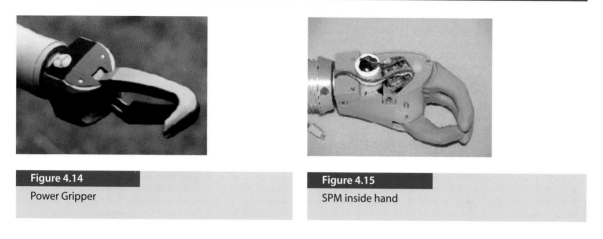

Figure 4.14

Power Gripper

Figure 4.15

SPM inside hand

4.9 Variety Ability Systems Inc. (VASI)

Variety Ability Systems Inc. (VASI) was established in June 1970 through the foresight of Sam Shopsowitz, Frank Strean, and Doug Wells. They, together with other members of the Variety Club – The Children's Charity (Ontario), recognized the growing need for infants and children's prosthetics and so decided to build a production facility to meet those needs. It was recognized that there were many prostheses available for adult usage, due to the vast number of war-related amputations, but manufacturers were slower to address the needs of juvenile amputees. However, in

1971, Northern Electric Company designed and started production and distribution of a mechanical hand. This hand was later replaced by a range of electrically powered hands developed by the Rehabilitation Engineering Department (RED) of The Bloorview Macmillan Children's Centre in Toronto.

Today VASI offer a range of four different sizes of electric hands. Unlike other hands these are labelled according to age group rather than physical size. W0–3, W2–6, W5–9 and W7–11 models cater for ages ranging from infant through 11 years old.

The VASI electric hands have their own interchangeable wrist unit in regular or short versions. All the hands are controlled with a programmable elec-

Table 4.3. Specifications of electric hands from RSL Steeper

Size* (inch)	Age	Weight (oz)	Max Current at Stall (mA)	Pinch force (lbs)
1¾	0–2	5.2	800	12
2	2–4	5.2	800	12
2¼	4–6	8.4	250	15
2½	6–9	8.8	250	15
2¾	9–12	9.8	250	15
3	12+	9.8	250	15
3¼	Adult	10.0	250	15
Gripper	Adult	15.8	n/a	15

* Measurement taken across the knuckles not circumferential

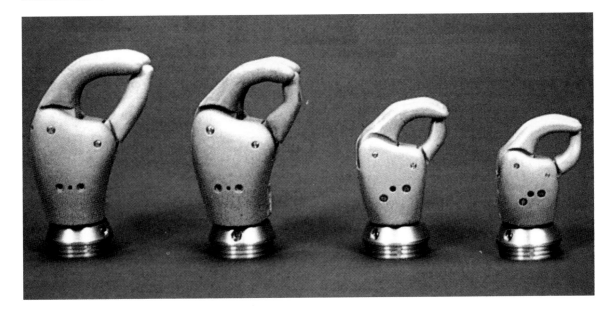

Figure 4.16

VASI range of electric hands

tronic bridge module that fits all four sizes. The SPM (single programmable microcomputer) can be configured during the fitting stage by use of proprietary software and a PC type computer. The SPM can use processed myoelectric signals (from an Otto Bock "myoelectrode" for example) as well as switches and force sensitive resistors (FSR) as the control mechanism. Most control strategies are covered with the SPM. These include both 1 and 2 site, proportional or ON/OFF control in addition to level or rate sensitive options. A "cookie-crusher" mode is also available for very young users. This module also incorporates a parental access switch that allows the opening of the hand by a 3rd party (Fig. 4.15).

The hands have a strong pinch force, but their hard plastic fingers do not enhance hand function, as do compliant fingered hands. On the positive side their hand length is relatively short for fitting long below elbow (B/E) patients and can operate on a wide range of battery voltages from 4.8 to 7.2 volts (Fig. 4.16).

VASI is the only manufacturer that produces two sizes of electric elbows. Just as the electric hands, these devices are targeted towards the child and juve-

Table 4.4. Specifications of electric hands from VASI

Size* (inch)	Age (model)	Weight (oz)	Max Current at Stall (mA)	Pinch force (lbs)
1 3/4	W0–3	3.0	260	4.5
2	W2–6	4.5	340	7.0
2 1/4	W5–9	6.7	1400	9.5
2 3/4	W7–11	7.0	1400	8.0

* Measurement taken across the knuckles for comparison only, selection by age

nile amputee. These elbows incorporate electronic bridges, forearm extensions and the larger size Otto Bock battery receptacle for the power requirements.

VASI also have two different types of wrist modules for use with their electric hands, again tailored to the young amputee. The FLEXIwrist provides for passive flexion/extension when pressure is exerted on the hand and returns to the neutral or in-line position when pressure is removed. This type is best suited to young children. The OMNIwrist provides friction for passive flexion/extension and maintains position while the amputee completes the functional task. Versions of this wrist are available for the Otto Bock Electrohand 2000 system hands, adult hands and RSL Steeper Scamp hands (Table 4.4).

Finally, to assist in the mixing and matching of prosthetic components, VASI produces a wide variety of connectors and adaptors using their own connector technology as the interchangeable standard.

Contact information:
Variety Ability Systems Inc.
2 Kelvin Avenue, Unit 3
Toronto, Ontario, M4C 5C8
Canada
Tel: +1-416-6981415
Fax: +1416-6985860
e-mail: mmifsud@vasi.on.ca
Web: http://www.vasi.on.ca

4.10 Compatibility

Several of the upper limb powered prosthetics companies have tried to make their components workable with other manufacturers. This ultimately is a benefit to the patient as it gives the clinics the ability to mix and match components. In this way the best rehabilitation solution can be implemented for their patients.

However, at least two of these manufacturers have taken the approach that their designs are all that is needed for an optimum fitting. Otto Bock and Hosmer are two such companies. If a clinic wishes to mix and match other vendor products with those from Otto Bock and Hosmer, then it is the responsibility of

someone else to provide the means. Recently, Motion Control has also taken this approach in their newest hand design, which only interfaces with the Utah Arm.

The other manufacturers, namely VASI, RSL Steeper and Centri AB have all designed leads and components to make their system somewhat compatible with others such as Otto Bock. One company, Liberating Technology, has taken the most proactive approach and has dedicated much of their manufacturing efforts to products that will allow mixing and matching of components from all manufacturers. This has extended even to the 2 size NiCad batteries and Li-ion built-in batteries. In addition, the Varigrip control circuits from LTI and the electronics in the Boston Elbow are compatible with all of the electric hands on the market today.

4.11 Questions

1. What two partners were responsible for the first fitting of an all-Canadian myoelectric prosthesis in Canada?
2. The Utah Elbow is the flagship product of what prosthetics company?
3. Which company supplies two different sizes of electric elbows, targeted mainly towards the child and juvenile amputee?
4. How can the myoelectric control strategy be changed in the OttoBock sensor hand?
5. Explain two ways in which electric hand sizes can be specified.
6. What new battery technologies are starting to replace the rechargeable NiCad battery in many powered prostheses?
7. What is a Griefer?
8. Which company was the original designer of the split hook terminal device?
9. Who is the world's leading manufacturer/distributor of prosthetic and orthotic components with branches in over 30 countries?
10. What is the programmable powered prosthetic control system from Liberating Technologies called?

Acknowledgements. The authors would like to acknowledge the assistance given by William Hanson of Liberating Technologies, Robin Cooper of RSL Steeper, Harold Sears of Motion Control and Marty Robinson of Otto Bock Healthcare (CDN) in the preparation of this chapter. Their support through photographs, brochures, permissions and personal contact greatly eased the writing of this chapter for which the authors are extremely grateful.

Meeting the Clients: An Overview

Focus on Prevalence, Psychosocial Issues, Outcomes

S. Hubbard · G. Montgomery · D. Stocker

Contents

Summary

This chapter provides an introduction and framework to the issues and dynamics faced by people with amputations and limb deficiencies at various ages and stages of externally-powered prosthetic fitting. It outlines the prevalence and causes of upper extremity amputation or limb deficiency, introduces some of the psychosocial issues and challenges affecting clients and their families and discusses some of the factors that influence the outcome of the prosthetic fitting process.

5.1 Introduction

Successful rehabilitation for people with amputations or limb deficiencies occurs when each person's individual strengths, challenges and needs are understood and responded to by a supportive and effective team. Further, a prosthesis is not an "off the shelf" product. It is a device that is specifically designed with and for each individual to provide a functional and natural appearing limb replacement. It is essential that the end user, their family and close friends be active participants in this (re)habilitation process. Team members must consider not only physical factors but also the psychosocial, sociocultural and spiritual strengths and needs of the individual during the assessment, design, fitting, training and evaluative process.

5.2 Prevalence/Incidence

5.2.1 Children

Incidence rates are difficult to obtain because most countries do not have a system for mandatory reporting of birth defects and there is little standardization of use of classification systems in clinical practice. A census of 4,105 child amputees in 1980 indicated that congenital limb deficiencies outnumbered acquired losses by a ratio of 2:1 [19].For the congenital population, 49% were unilateral upper limb, 27% lower limb, and 24% were multiple limb-deficient. All together, upper limbs were involved to varying degrees in 62% of cases [20].The congenital, unilateral, upper-limb deficiency was by far the most common single category. Figures for acquired amputations were primarily related to trauma with lower extremity amputations comprising 66% of all cases.

Using survey data from four diverse sources (Canada, United States, Italy, and Scotland), in 1988, McDonnell [20] estimated the incidence of congenital upper-limb deficiencies to be approximately 1:4200 live births. For children likely to be considered for prosthetic fitting, the estimate would be only 1:9400. Anomalies were reported to be more common on the left than the right. In 1998, Brenner [4] reported that approximately 40 children in Canada each year are born with an upper limb deficiency requiring prosthetic treatment. The numbers for Sweden and the United States were projected to be approximately 15 and 402 respectively. Goldberg, in 1989 [13] suggested that 75% of all congenital, unilateral upper-extremity amputees will be missing their left arm below the elbow. The reasons for this are unknown.

In the paediatric age group, the most common causes of acquired amputations are trauma, (varying with the geographic area) and tumors [24].Sources of trauma involving the upper limb are primarily accidents with meat grinders, farm equipment, electrical high-tension wires, explosives, boat propellers, and motor vehicle accidents. Surgery for tumors is most frequently performed for individuals between 11 and 20 years of age.

Recognizing the need for better data concerning the incidence and prevalence of limb deficiency and acquired amputations, the Association of Children's Prosthetic and Orthotic Clinics (ACPOC) [1] has established an international registry of such children. All child amputee clinics in Canada and the United States have been asked to participate.

5.2.2 Adults

The incidence of amputations in the adult population is not well known. One author [34] says it has been estimated that major limb amputations occur in one in 300 people in the United States. Of these, 23% involve the upper extremity and most would be considered candidates for prostheses. Another, [3] estimated that 40,000 persons lose a limb each year in the United States, 30% involving a hand or arm. In both reports the distinction between children and adults, or limb deficiencies and acquired amputations, is not clearly delineated.

Upper limb amputations due to hands being caught in presses, dies and rotating machinery of various types are frequently associated with healthy adult males [9].According to Mooney [22],upper limb amputations among males outnumber those among females by about three to one. There does not appear to be a difference between left or right limb loss. Traumatic amputees tend to be between 21 and 30 years on average. In most of these cases, the surgery takes place immediately after the accident to preserve life and provides little or no time for the individual to mentally prepare for the loss.

Vascular problems requiring amputation are much less common in the upper extremity than in the lower limb. Surgeries for the upper extremity are more frequently performed for management of malignant tumors or severe brachial plexus injuries.

5.3 Psychosocial Impact of Limb Loss

Psychosocial adjustment to limb deficiency or limb loss has received relatively little attention in the literature. The information that does exist tends to be found in anecdotal case studies and clinical experience reports and is not supported by empirical data [21].Clinicians rely on professional judgement and best practices related to individual and family trauma, loss, mourning and grief. These concepts and their accompanying interventions are generalized to limb loss.

Each individual, based on personal psychosocial/sociocultural experience and strengths, adjusts to major crises in their life in their own unique manner. Team members need to be sensitive to these significant major and subtle differences without imposing their own values and time frames. Clients and families appreciate having their stories and the details of their life circumstances witnessed and respected by the treatment team. When heard and valued, clients are more receptive to receiving guidance through the often roller-coaster process of adaptation to limb loss.

5.3.1 Congenital Amputee and Family

Paediatric amputee programs strive to provide the child with a comfortable, cosmetically- appealing prosthesis that is functional and useful. Often overlooked, but equally important, is the goal of providing the child with a positive self-image that will facilitate a productive and satisfying life (Fig. 5.1). This goal is realized by supporting and training the young person to choose when to use the prosthesis and when to adapt and creatively use their residual limb or body [15]. A good program is therefore designed to help a family at birth or time of limb loss to appreciate the whole child and to evaluate the useful role of a prosthesis for cosmesis, comfort and function.

The pre-natal diagnosis and/or birth of a limb-deficient child are known to be points of crisis for families. When a child is born with a congenital absence of one or more limbs, the parent or parents are confronted with the loss of the perfect child they had envisioned. Feelings of guilt, anger, and grief are common. The way in which parents respond to, work through and adapt to their child's limb difference, is a major factor in determining the child's adjustment

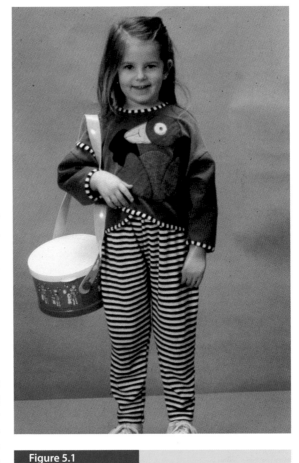

Figure 5.1
Child

and life success including how well the child will accommodate to wearing a prosthesis [4, 5, 10, 11].

The Child Amputee Prosthetics Project (CAPP) team in California was the first to identify the need for professional crisis intervention and to propose a model of care [6]. They suggested that a psychosocial professional should meet with the family in hospital or as soon after birth as possible to provide reassurance, support, information and hope. Grandparents and extended family may also benefit from these interventions and strengthen the whole support network for the child.

The first visit with the amputee team is an opportunity to continue the support initiated soon after birth and to build on family strengths and resiliency. Understanding new technical information and language, dealing with the reality of the appearance and limited function of artificial limbs and the exposure to other clients are challenges that parents face admirably. In fact, many parents report their resolve strengthened by meeting other families. Families have unique and unexpected ways of observing their own situation, no matter how involved or complex, in a positive and affirming way.

Parents need support from all members of the treatment team.

"Professionals must recognize the impact of parents' feelings, perceptions and understanding on the child's outcome. Maintaining consistency and continuity of care helps the professional to realize parents' concerns, address the issues and promote trust and rapport...Addressing parents' needs can increase compliance, enhancing both practitioner success and family satisfaction with treatment". (Swagman and Novotny 1992).

Talbot [27] suggests that the attitude of the clinician is a significant facet of providing psychological support and that an accepting, empathetic, non-judgmental approach is essential. As parents begin to discuss their feelings and concerns, the staff member acknowledges all emotions as understandable and normal. It is important that the clinician provide assurance that the child will develop within the broad range considered normal given no other overt or hidden conditions exist. Providing specific developmental tasks or activities that the child is capable of accomplishing is a good way of promoting competency and reassurance (Fig. 5.2). Supplying parents with information, resources, peer supports and a sense of control – in other words, full partnership in the rehabilitation process is empowering for clients and families. Resources such as "The Child with a Limb Deficiency: A Guide for Parents" [26], the video "Upper-Limb Prosthetic Options for Kids" [25], and the booklet "Children with Limb Loss: A Handbook for Families" [2] were designed specifically to help clinics address the needs of families. The War Amputa-

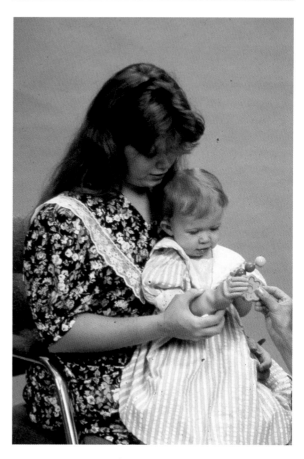

Figure 5.2

Mother and child

tions of Canada CHAMP program [32] also provides a number of services to assist new families.

It is reassuring to note that parents gain comfort and hope from the tender, supportive personal attention received from staff. Family-centered care with an intentional focus on individual and family abilities goes a long way towards demonstrating society's changing attitudes towards disability and differences.

5.3.1.1 Infancy and Pre-school Years

The infancy and pre-school years are particularly challenging for parents. Predictable periods of stress are associated with having to deal with the curiosity of other children in the playground and adults who provide childcare. Each new experience prepares, rewards and encourages parents to continue their societal educational role.

As the young person matures and begins to notice how he or she differs from peers, it is essential that questions are answered with honesty, acceptance and acknowledgement that the youngster, though different is, lovable. Simple, positive explanations will provide the child a model for dealing independently with the world's curiosity.

5.3.1.2 School Age

A child's adjustment to starting school can be variable and may initially pose more stress for the parent than for the child. With acceptance of differences and appropriate accommodations, each child will have the basis for a positive self-image and the resiliency to cope with school enrollment. The family should meet with the child's teacher and principal beforehand to familiarize them with their child's difference, capabilities, needs and any special provisions. An early "show and tell experience" is recommended to satisfy classmate curiosity (Fig. 5.3).

Some teasing is a normal part of interaction for school-age children. The child's sense of self affects and is affected by their ability to deal with the teasing situations [15, 27, 30]. Children should be encouraged to share their school experiences so they may receive support, coaching and role playing tips on how to deal with negative comments. It is recognized that the school culture has much to do with whether bullying is tolerated. Support by school staff and parents must be provided when negativity escalates. The War Amputations of Canada's CHAMP program [32] has some excellent print and video resources to educate and enlighten all young students, whether or not they have a visible limb difference. Schools generally welcome resources such as these to open discussion and celebrate diversity at all levels.

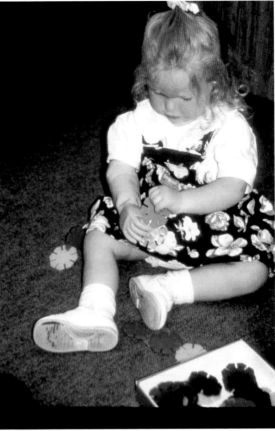

Figure 5.3

Child playing

The most methodologically sound research on children with limb deficiencies thus far has been conducted by Varni and colleagues [30, 31]. Study results suggest that higher levels of classmate, teacher and parent social support are associated with greater self-esteem and that low levels of social support may be significant predictors of depressive symptoms in children with limb deficiencies. It is important to identify those children who are not adapting well to their limb deficiency and ensure that psychological and social interventions are provided.

5.3.1.3 Adolescence

Adolescence is a well-known period of transitional stress for young people. Generally, the predictable problems and behavior patterns associated with this age will be compounded for the teenager with a limb difference. The adolescent is self-conscious about personal appearance and naturally the cosmetic aspects of a prosthesis will assume greater importance. The clinic team must be aware of this and be flexible in prosthetic planning. It is also not uncommon for this age group to discount the functional value of an externally powered limb (temporarily or permanently) in favor of the aesthetics of a more cosmetic, passive device.

During adolescence, communication may be more restricted and inhibited as the teen seeks to do everything on his/her own terms. Also, conflict may arise between the wishes of the parent and adolescent that places the clinic team in the middle of the family dynamics. As it may be harder for adolescents to establish rapport, staff may need to make additional efforts to empathize, understand needs and allow time for decision making.

Adolescents are typically preoccupied with concerns of self-esteem, sexuality and identity. Young people want to know and test out if they are attractive and lovable. The opportunity to speak with a counselor needs to be made available as a usual and positive option for a person of any age. Counseling is indicated if the individual is having difficulty coping and is unusually depressed or angry. Peer contacts and groups for both educational and therapeutic purposes as well as pure fun experiences are vital. Role models play a huge part in fostering hope, direction and advocacy for the future. A short interval of counseling is useful to promote the normality of this period of uncertainty, challenge and transition.

Teens may seek and in some cases require more detailed information about the cause and future implications of their specific limb anomaly or medical condition.

5.3.2 Acquired Amputation

Similar periods of crisis, stress and opportunity occur for the child or adult and their families when an amputation is performed for reasons of illness or trauma. Kohl (1984) states: "there is not only the mourning for the loss of their previous body but a sense of need to reestablish themselves, physically, emotionally and socially". She emphasizes the need for a nurturing rehabilitation environment to provide unconditional positive regard for the client's struggle to deal with all their feelings, fears and unspoken challenges for the future [18].

If possible, a visit by an amputee team member should be made prior to elective surgery or shortly after a traumatic amputation. The individual and family will be concerned with a variety of issues associated with overcoming the loss of a limb or limbs. These include self-consciousness of a changed body image, phantom limb sensation and/or pain, [29] the appearance and function of a prosthesis, the rehabilitation program involved and capabilities for the future. Again, it is essential that they receive simple, honest, accurate information.

The adult is most likely to be worried about the reactions of others, particularly those they love and the effect the limb loss will have on their interpersonal roles and occupational and financial status.

A pro-active stance, involving education and support, perhaps in a group format, alerts clients and families as to common feelings, expectations and solutions. Family or marital therapy sessions focused on the stress and changes ahead can be offered. A priority for clients is often their ability to return to their former employment or career. Providing an opportunity to review job requirements and involve mentors can be reassuring and reduce fears/anxieties about the future.

To facilitate a clearer understanding of the psychosocial adaptations experienced by a person with a traumatic limb loss, Kohl [17] developed a staged analysis of the rehabilitation process through the identification of ten major psychosocial issues. These included: survival struggle, ideations of death, thought disturbances, phantom sensations, mourning, quest for meaning of injury, role relationships, body image, intimacy and vocational options. Professionals should be familiar with this work and that of other authors such as Dise-Lewis [8], Mooney [22], Tyc [29] and Winchell [33] in order to be able to provide an effective rehabilitation program. Much of this information is written specifically for the individual with the amputation and may be useful as a handout or resource material for the client attempting to cope with the normal reactions to limb loss.

Pre-morbid psychological and social characteristics also play a significant role in determining the client's process and success with rehabilitation.

"Occasionally, the amputation event interacts with developmental or character problems such that the patient's coping process and physical rehabilitation are significantly jeopardized. Typically this occurs when the patient has had prior difficulties with issues pertaining to (1) dependence/independence, (2) maintenance of a stable, positive sense of self, or (3) acceptance of one's own and others' limitations" (Dise-Lewis, 1989).

The rehabilitation team needs access to experienced psychosocial staff for an assessment of pre-morbid characteristics and a therapeutic plan to deal with underlying practical and emotional dynamics.

5.4 Acceptance/Rejection Factors

5.4.1 Children

Externally powered prostheses provide an adequate combination of cosmesis and function for many children. However, the acceptance of a prosthesis is based on a combination of individual and multi-dimensional factors. Fisk suggests that there is a difference in acceptance between congenital and acquired amputees.

"In the first instance, the child has no sense of loss and nothing new to get adjusted to. Anything of a prosthetic nature is an aid, and if it is not truly an aid, the child will reject it. Those who lose a limb due to trauma or disease, unless their amputation occurred when they were very young, will have a profound sense of loss and un-

dergo a period of readjustment. How well they manage this change greatly affects their acceptance of replacement prosthetic limbs". (Fisk, 1992)

There are no simple ways to predict individual long-term results or to judge the cost-effectiveness of myoelectric fitting for children. Some children become fully bimanual and feel at a loss when their own prosthesis is not available for use. Other individuals, in preference to a passive prosthetic option, will insist on wearing their myoelectric limb, even though the device is seldom used for active grasp function. A few who have had a long history of skilled prosthetic use will suddenly discard the myoelectric prosthesis and request the fitting of a passive cosmetic prosthesis or specific-need recreational device instead. Some abandon all prosthetic wear.

Although individual outcome cannot be foreseen, it is possible to identify and assess important indicators. These include the level /degree of limb loss, the attitude of the family, age at time of fitting, the personality of the child, the quality of the prosthetic fitting and the location of the prosthetic practice, reliability of components and possibly the predisposition of hand dominance [16].

The degree of limb loss is particularly significant. The most common deficiency occurs at the upper or mid-third forearm level and fortunately, this is the easiest and most successful level to fit prosthetically. Prosthetic designs are relatively straightforward and the trans-radial prosthesis provides balance, body symmetry, and substantial functional gain. Although the child is able to perform most activities of daily living related to school, recreational and household duties with or without a prosthesis, skilled use of a prosthesis is advantageous for bimanual activity. With the prosthesis on, the child can hold the object away from the body and at the midline in order to complete the more complex part of the task with the sound hand.

The child with a longer limb (complete or extensive carpal deficiency) has only limited ability to manipulate objects and a forearm that is usually shorter than the sound side. These children may accept and benefit from the provision of a myoelectric prosthesis, particularly if appearance is an important factor.

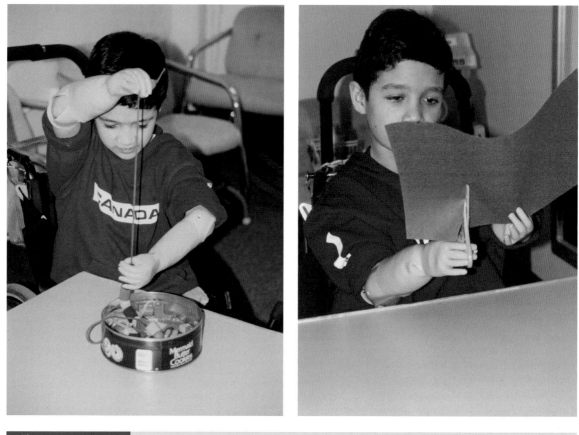

Figure 5.4

Bilateral myoelectric fitting

Results are generally less successful, however, for deficiencies at the partial hand level. Minimal functional gain and questionable cosmetic value (lack of availability of appropriate components), at the expense of loss of sensation, have commonly resulted in less wear and high rejection figures [16]. Promising advances in technology (partial-hand designs, smaller electronic boards and battery packages) may change the outcome for this group of clients in the future.

Trans-humeral fittings are relatively well accepted by clients and can provide both functional and cosmetic benefit. The mid to two-thirds humeral deficiency is the ideal length to accommodate the need for adequate muscle sites, shoulder motion and sufficient leverage to bear the weight of the prosthetic components.

The needs of the high level amputee are more complex and less well served by prosthetic devices since restorative function becomes increasingly difficult to achieve for higher levels of limb or bilateral limb loss. External power is generally easier to operate and therefore more successful than body-powered for these clients. However, the complexity, control and weight of components required as substitutes for the loss of multiple degrees of freedom, generally results in lower acceptance rates [16, 28]. In the case of the juvenile amputee, it is essential that devices be kept as simple and lightweight as possible and functional expectations kept realistic.

The child with multiple limb deficiencies presents a tremendous challenge to a prosthetic clinic team.

"Ironically, although the functional need increases with more anatomic absence or loss the tolerance for wear of prostheses decreases. Loss of sensation, heat-dissipation problems and energy consumption required for wear alone not even counting energy required for functional operation, are significant. Personality differences affect gadget tolerance, ability to concentrate and ability to persevere". (Clark et al, 1998)

Should one prescribe prostheses that are as high-tech as possible or is it more cost-effective to direct resources toward environmental control and aids for living? The debate is longstanding and unresolved. Experienced clinicians generally agree that children should be allowed to try prostheses at a time when the prostheses will help them experience developmental milestones and perform age-appropriate tasks [7]. These children may require the opportunity to experience the prosthetic fitting process in order to evaluate the advantages and disadvantages afforded by prostheses before they and their parents will be able to accept their disabilities and limitations. The need for cosmesis, particularly at periods of crisis such as school entry and adolescence should not be underestimated (Fig. 5.4).

Assuming comfort, fit and function of the prosthesis are optimal, the influence of family attitudes and commitment in a child's acceptance of a disability and assistive devices is crucial. Parental responsibility for encouraging use of the prosthesis, monitoring growth changes and attending to repair needs demands heavy involvement. Parents that perceive tangible benefits of powered prosthetic wear – comfort, ease of use and function and who also like the appearance, find it much easier to reinforce and reward their child's prosthetic learning and to carry through with training goals [16] (Fig. 5.5).

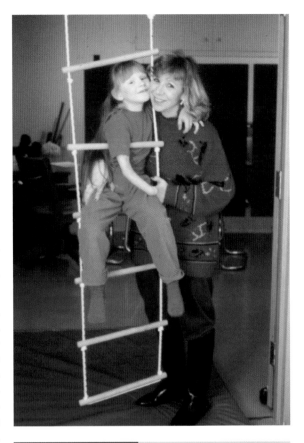

Figure 5.5

Parent and child

5.4.2 Adults

The decision to use and wear a prosthesis is determined more by individual choice and less by family and external factors as a person ages. Winchell [33] suggests that there are several factors that influence whether a person will choose to wear a prosthesis and under what conditions, for how long etc.

As with children, the level and severity of amputation may influence the choice to use a prosthesis. The higher the level of amputation and the number of artificial joints required, the more weight and less degree of freedom of motion are afforded. This, however, does not preclude a person from becoming an efficient user of a prosthesis if they are strongly motivated to do so.

The fit of the prosthetic socket and the appropriate choice of components (chosen with input from the individual) can make a significant difference to the outcome. The individual must feel comfortable while wearing the prosthesis. Arm amputees are much less tolerant of discomfort than leg amputees, since their function is better with one hand than it would be with one leg [12]. They must also be able to be confident that the device will perform in a reliable and predictive fashion. The use of both a hook and a hand may be required for some individuals depending on their job and lifestyle.

People perceive pain and discomfort in various ways. A person with an extremely low tolerance to pain and discomfort may not be able to tolerate the wearing of a prosthesis, no matter how well the prosthesis fits.

Unrealistic individual expectations derived from emotional factors and/or misunderstanding of what function a prosthesis provides, may cause a person to reject a prosthesis. The media sometimes provides the basis for unrealistic expectations for powered prosthetics. Most powered prostheses function best as a non-dominant holder as opposed to a dominant manipulator. Careful education as to the benefits and limitations of the prosthesis and training in functional use can help to reduce the frustrations and disappointments that contribute to rejection of a prosthesis.

A person may develop vascular or neurological complications that are unrelated to the amputation but can restrict or prevent the use of prosthetic devices. Similarly a person who has developed a neuroma, may for a time choose not to use a prosthesis until the pain from the neuroma has subsided or the neuroma has been surgically excised.

Some people may choose to wear a prosthesis in certain situations and not in others. Many people wear the prosthesis to work or school but choose to remove it when they return home in the evening. This selective wear pattern is not dissimilar to the choice of clothing or footwear. A decision to cease wearing a myoelectric prosthesis must be respected and not

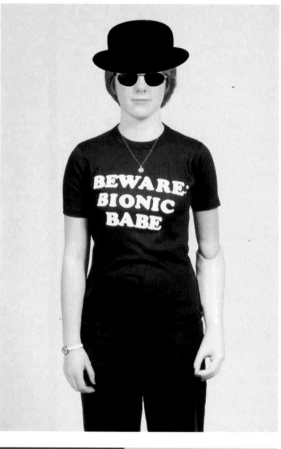

Figure 5.6

Bionic babe

considered a failure either for the individual and family or for the clinic itself. Needs change over time and it is not at all uncommon and perhaps may be the norm, for an individual to opt in and out of prosthetic wear over the years.

Cost and reliability of components may become a factor for prosthetic rejection as well. Individuals who received funding, initially, for provision of a prosthesis may not have the ability to pay for cosmetic glove replacements and ongoing maintenance/repair costs. Clients who regularly participate in activities that place constant and significant torques and pressures on the powered prosthetic hands may become disillusioned when they discover that the electric hands are not designed for or capable of being used for their needs or particular lifestyle.

Individual personality factors, motivation, and ability to persevere determine the outcome of prosthetic fitting to a great extent (Fig. 5.6). The best technology, training and prosthetic skill in the world will not provide a positive result without strong client motivation and the will to succeed.

5.5 Chapter Summary

In this chapter we have outlined many of the needs of the individual with limb loss and the myriad of factors that determine successful prosthetic wear/use patterns. Professionals working with the child, adult and family need to be cognizant of the influence they have on the outcome of a prosthetic fitting. Not only can the time of rehabilitation be shortened through a coordinated approach but also the nature of the team support will influence each individual's success.

The fitting of a prosthesis is best conceptualized as a nonlinear process where individual team members work in partnership with each other and with the client/family throughout the whole process of fitting, training and follow-up evaluation. In order to have a prosthesis that fits and is functional, it is important there be frequent consultation and discussions amongst members of the team. Colleagues, working in close proximity, are able to problem solve and effectively achieve client goals.

5.6 Questions

1. How is the development of a child's positive self-image best facilitated by the clinic team?
2. Identify the major challenges faced by families i) at the time of diagnosis of limb deficiencies, ii) during school age and iii) during adolescence. What is the best way for clinicians to support clients and families at these crucial times?
3. List several psychosocial factors related to clients and families that the prosthetic team must take in-

to account when assessing a client's suitability for a prosthetic device.
4. What are the major issues and emotional reactions for those who have an acquired amputation as opposed to a congenital limb deficiency? Describe the types of interventions and supports that would benefit this population.
5. Identify the major factors related to acceptance/rejection of a prosthesis. In your opinion which are the most crucial?
6. What factors make the fitting of high-level amputees complex and challenging?

References

1. Association of Children's Prosthetic and Orthotic Clinics (ACPOC). 6300 N. River Road, Suite 727, Rosemont, IL 60018-4226
2. Area Child Amputee Center. Mary Free Bed Hospital and Rehabilitation Center, 235 Wealthy SE, Grand Rapids, Michigan 49503.
3. Atkins D, Meier R (1989) Preface. In: Atkins DJ, Meier RH (eds): Comprehensive management of the upper limb amputee. Springer, Berlin Heidelberg New York
4. Brenner CD (1993) Population estimates for new congenital upper limb deficiencies. Notes from paper presentation, Myo-Electric Control Symposium, Fredericton, New Brunswick.
5. Brooks B, Beal L, Ogg L, Blakeslee B (1962) The child with deformed or missing limbs: his problems and prosthesis. Am J Nursing 62(1): 89
6. Brooks M, Setoguchi Y, Thue J, Beal L, Tom D (1965) Crisis intervention. Inter-Clin Info Bull 4(11):7–15
7. Clark M, Atkins D, Hubbard S, Patton J, Shaperman J (1998) Prosthetic devices for children with bilateral upper limb deficiencies: when, and if, pros and cons. In: Herring J, Birch J (eds) AAOS/Shrine Symposium: the limb deficient child. American Academy of Orthopaedic Surgeons, Rosemont, IL, pp 397–404
8. Dise-Lewis JE (1989) Psychological adaptation to limb loss. In: Atkins DJ, Meier RH (eds) Comprehensive management of the upper limb amputee. Springer, Berlin Heidelberg New York, pp 165–172
9. Fernie G (1981) The epidemiology of amputation. In: Kostuik J, Gillespie R (eds) Amputation surgery and rehabilitation: the Toronto experience. Churchill Livingstone, New York, pp 13–15
10. Fisk J (1992) Introduction to the child amputee. In: Bowker JH, Michael JW (eds) Atlas of limb prosthetics: surgical, prosthetic and rehabilitation principles, 2nd ed. Mosby-Year Book, St Louis, pp 731–734

11. Friedman LW (1978) The limb-deficient child. In: The psychological rehabilitation of the amputee. Charles C Thomas, Springfield, IL, pp 77–83
12. Friedman LW (1978) Prosthesis limitations and rejection. In: The psychological rehabilitation of the amputee. Charles C Thomas, Springfield, IL, pp 67–73
13. Goldberg MJ (1987) The dysmorphic child: an orthopedic perspective. Raven Press, New York
14. Hubbard JL (1996) The self-concept of children with congenital upper-limb deficiencies. MA Thesis, York University, Toronto
15. Hubbard S (1981) Social and psychological problems of the child amputee. In: Kostuik J, Gillespie R (eds) Amputation surgery and rehabilitation: the Toronto experience. Churchill Livingstone, New York, pp 395–401
16. Hubbard S, Kurtz I, Heim W, Montgomery, G (1998) Powered prosthetic intervention in upper extremity deficiency. In: Herring J, Birch J (eds) AAOS/Shrine Symposium: the limb deficient child. American Academy of Orthopaedic Surgeons, Rosemont, IL, pp 417–431
17. Kohl S (1983) The process of psychosocial adaptation to traumatic limb loss. In: Krueger D (ed) Emotional rehabilitation of physical trauma and disability. Spectrum (S.P. Medical and Scientific Books), New York, pp 113–145
18. Kohl S (1984) Emotional coping with amputation. In: Krueger D (ed) Rehabilitation psychology: a comprehensive textbook. Aspen Systems, pp 273–282
19. Krebs D, Fishman S (1984) Characteristics of the child amputee population. J Pediatr Orthop 4:89–95
20. McDonnell PM, Scott RN, McKay LA (1988) Incidence of congenital upper-limb deficiencies. J Assoc Child Prosthet Orthot Clin 23(1):8–13
21. Minnis P, Stack, D (1990) Research and practice with congenital amputees: making the whole greater than the sum of its parts. Int J Rehab Res13:151–160
22. Mooney RL (1995) The handbook: information for new upper extremity amputees, their families and friends. Mutual Amputee Aid Foundation, Lomita, CA
23. Novotny M, Swagman A (1992) Caring for children with orthotic/prosthetic needs. J Prosthet Orthot 4(4) July: 191–195
24. Setoguchi Y (1989) Evaluation of the paediatric amputee. In: Atkins DJ, Meier RH (eds): Comprehensive management of the upper limb amputee. Springer, Berlin Heidelberg New York, pp 227–239
25. Swagman A, Novotny M (1992) Upper limb prosthetic options for kids. Video and accompanying guide. The Area Child Amputee Center at Mary Free Bed Hospital & Rehabilitation Center of Grand Rapids and the Variety Children's Amputee Program at the Rehabilitation Institute of Chicago
26. Talbot D (1979) The child with a limb deficiency: A guide for parents. Child Amputee Prosthetics Project, Shriners Hospital for Crippled Children, Los Angeles, CA
27. Talbot D (1990) Helping the limb-deficient child deal with social reactions to physical difference. J Assoc Child Prosthet Orthot Clin 25(3) Winter:76–80
28. Trost F, Rowe D (1992) Externally powered prostheses. In: Bowker JH, Michael JW (eds) Atlas of limb prosthetics: surgical, prosthetic and rehabilitation principles, 2nd edn. Mosby-Year Book, St Louis, pp 767–778
29. Tyc V (1992) Psychosocial adaptation of children and adolescents with limb deficiencies: a review. Clin Psych Rev 12:275–291
30. Varni JW, Setoguchi Y (1991) Psychosocial factors in the management of children with limb deficiencies. Phys Med Rehabil Clin North Am 2:395–404
31. Varni JW, Pruitt SD, Seid M. (1998) Health-related quality of life in paediatric limb deficiency. In Herring J, Birch J (eds) AAOS/Shrine Symposium: the limb deficient child. American Academy of Orthopaedic Surgeons, Rosemont, IL, pp 457–473
32. War Amputations of Canada, CHAMP Program. National Headquarters. 2827 Riverside Drive, Ottawa, Canada, K1V0C4.
33. Winchell, Ellen (1995). Coping with limb loss. Avery Publishing Group, Garden City Park, New York
34. Wright TW, Hagen AD, Wood MB (1995) Prosthetic usage in major upper extremity amputations. J Hand Surg 20A (4): 619–621

Powered Upper Limb Prosthetic Practice in Paediatrics

S. Hubbard · W. Heim · S. Naumann
S. Glasford · G. Montgomery · S. Ramdial

Contents

Summary

Powered upper-limb prosthetic practice in paediatrics is based on the principle of family-centered care. Children have unique prosthetic needs that are best addressed by a multidisciplinary team approach. This chapter outlines: the procedures used in myoelectric fitting; the availability and nature of child-sized components; the basic concepts and applications of myoelectric control systems for children and adolescents; socket designs and paediatric considerations; and the need for supplementary devices for sports, recreation and special activities.

6.1 Introduction

The physical, emotional and prosthetic needs of a child are very different from those of the adult and must be understood and addressed. Successful powered prosthetic fitting requires the coordinated approach of an experienced multidisciplinary team.

Limb anomalies in children are classified as congenital limb deficiencies or acquired amputations resulting from trauma or disease. Although the needs of the two groups may vary, family involvement is an integral part of any treatment program.

When a child is born with a limb deficiency parents may initially be overwhelmed by shock, grief, feelings of guilt (need to identify a cause, assign blame, etc.) and concern for the possibility of other anomalies or intelligence being affected. In addition, there may be worries about financial implications and future independence of the child. Parents may at first be unwilling to accept the reality of or need for a prosthetic solution to the problem. Parents frequently ask about transplantation or reconstruction of the abnormal limb. The ultimate hope of any parent is to be able to provide a "normal" arm or leg for their child [23].

The impact of parental feelings and perceptions on the child's long term adjustment, self-acceptance and outcome related to prosthetic wear must be recognized by both parents and professionals [13]. Professionals willing to address families' needs for repeated reassurance, support and information, undoubtedly will contribute to better outcomes and overall adjustment/acceptance. The resolution of guilt and acceptance of the situation are ongoing challenges for families as they continue to provide the support and nurture needed to promote healthy development for their children. Professional counseling should also be made available. Introduction of parents to other families with children of similar diagnoses and parent support groups can be very helpful adjuncts at this and other important stages of development.

Early goals of prosthetic care, therefore, are first to assist with the acceptance and bonding processes between parent, child and siblings, emphasizing strengths and abilities rather than focusing on deficiencies, and second, to assist the child with accepting and assimilating a prosthetic device into a developing body image (Fig. 6.1).

In time, attention shifts from the families to the physical and emotional needs of the children themselves. It is important to always include the children in any discussions about their care. Even very young children need to be involved in answering questions, evaluating fit and function and asked for their suggestions and input. Clinicians need to be knowledgeable of normal child development and sensitive to issues associated with specific stages. Treatment approaches are adjusted according to age and individual needs.

Upper limb amputations acquired in childhood usually occur as a result of disease or trauma and are

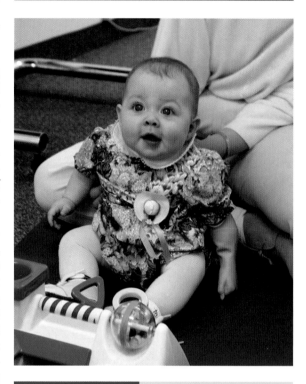

Figure 6.1

Fig. 6.1. Paediatric prosthetic practice

highly stressful for children and families. Unlike children with congenital limb deficiencies, children who have acquired an amputation mourn the loss of the missing limb, have a myriad of conflicting feelings and may have difficulty accepting an artificial replacement. Complications associated with oncology treatment, including nausea, fatigue, weight loss and tissue healing present additional challenges for individuals with childhood cancer. Knowledge, support and compassion are required to assist the children and families through this process.

6.2 Procedures

Prosthetic fitting and training programs can usually be provided on an outpatient and home/community basis. Prosthetic prescriptions are kept simple at first and gradually increased in complexity over time. Devices have to fit well and enhance function if they are to be accepted by children. Cosmetic appearance must also be acceptable to both the child and family. Components used for children need to be size appropriate, made of lightweight materials and designed for rugged durability. Component modules enable re-use of parts when growth changes are required.

6.2.1 Age of Fitting

Prosthetic prescriptions are based on developmental needs, including the social, emotional and recreational requirements of the child. Studies of normal development [5] indicate that patterns of hand use begin very early and it is reasonable to assume that the younger the age of fitting, the more likely the child is to integrate the use of the prosthesis into body image and functional activity [9, 15, 24]. It is common practice to have a child with a congenital, unilateral upper-limb deficiency fitted with a passive prosthesis between three to six months of age as the child begins to develop trunk and sitting balance. The passive prosthesis conditions the child to wearing a device, assists balance and gross motor development and satisfies the parental need for some restoration of normal appearance.

The optimal age to begin myoelectric fitting is still somewhat contentious. However, if one subscribes to the theory that early fitting promotes better acceptance and functional skill, then a myoelectric limb can be provided as early as the child's physical size allows. The smallest electric hands are considered suitable in size for infants sometime between 9 to 15 months of age. A single-site, voluntary opening control system is most effective for use with this age group. The electrode is usually placed proximally on the forearm extensors for a trans-radial deficiency; and over the triceps muscle in the case of a trans-humeral deficiency [8].

6.2.2 Check Socket

Prosthetic practices do vary from one facility to another. Following casting, for example, some prosthetists proceed directly to the production of a laminated socket and finished device. Others prefer an interim step and fabricate a clear check socket to assess the fit, comfort and suspension. In this case, a control system and hand can be attached and hand activation can be observed to ensure that the electrode placement is effective in detecting EMG activity and that the child is able to tolerate the weight of the components. Once the team is satisfied that the socket fitting, loading factors and control site are satisfactory, the final prosthesis can then be fabricated.

6.2.3 Operating the Control System

With the voluntary opening control system, the young child easily learns how to operate the prosthetic hand in a self-discovery manner. At first, only inadvertent action is observed, but very quickly, the infant acquires the ability to intentionally open the hand. A safety/parental access switch discretely mounted on the prosthetic forearm can be used by the clinician or parent to open the hand and place objects in it. The child is encouraged to try to open the hand and release the grasped object. As the child becomes accustomed to wearing the prosthesis and more conscious of the control strategy, the electrode sensitivity can

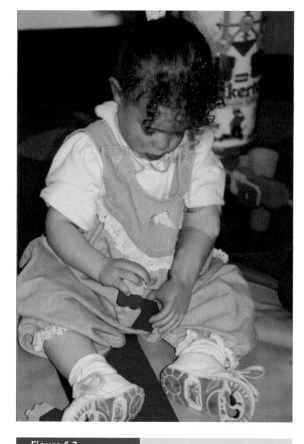

Figure 6.2

Infant fitting

opening system to a two-site, two-function system without much difficulty. Occasionally, it is not possible to identify a second site, and a one-site, two-function control strategy is required. Procedures used are similar to those employed for older children or adults. These include muscle site identification, control system selection and calibration, muscle control training and functional use training. (See Chap. 8, "Training of Children", for further details.)

Once the prosthesis has been completed, the family is instructed on the donning/doffing procedures, skin care, battery charging and ongoing service needs. Regular follow-up appointments are scheduled to monitor need for growth adjustments, component maintenance, training or other services.

6.2.4 Multi-limb Deficiencies

Management of the child with multiple limb-deficiencies or amputations requires special consideration. Although the rejection rate for upper-extremity prostheses is known to be high, it is generally agreed that any child who is motivated to use a prosthesis or prostheses should be given the opportunity to do so. Psychosocial benefits are not trivial [4]. Needs must be addressed on an individual basis and considerable experimentation and innovation is required. These children have a low tolerance for mechanical gadgetry and often, understandably, cannot tolerate the weight, heat, loss of sensation and restrictive nature of prosthetic devices.

be reduced and use of the hand encouraged in play activity. The development of bimanual skills is a gradual process and best achieved with the guidance of an occupational therapist, who works with the family to provide ideas, such as suitable play activities, to stimulate the child's awareness and use of the prosthesis (Fig. 6.2).

Children generally become more cooperative, with improved communication and attention skills, between three to four years of age. This makes it easier to apply effective evaluation strategies for optimal myoelectric fitting and training of a more complex control strategy. In most cases, children are able to make the adjustment from a one-site, voluntary

6.3 Components

Manufacturers such as RSLSteeper, [18] Otto Bock Health Care GmbH, [14] and Variety Ability Systems Inc. [27] offer a comprehensive line of components to accommodate the needs of children of various ages for externally powered prostheses. The following section outlines the features and benefits of these products.

6.3.1 Hands and Wrists

Currently all electric hands on the market are designed with opposition of the thumb to the index and middle fingers. Each manufacturer offers a range of product sizes to accommodate age-specific requirements from infancy to adulthood. All electric hands need a cosmetic glove to provide a protective covering and an aesthetic appearance. Each manufacturer of electric hands offers a selection of glove sizes and colors to customize their products to the needs of the individual child.

6.3.1.1 RSL Steeper Ltd. Products

The Scamp hand, designed for younger children, is available in two sizes: the $4\frac{1}{2}$ – suitable for 6–36 months of age and the $5\frac{1}{2}$ – suitable for 2–5 years of age. The hand is constructed of aluminum, making it durable and lightweight. The finger group and thumb have covers to provide finger compliance and, therefore, a more secure grip and extended glove life. Both hand sizes can be opened manually to release the grip, providing an added safety feature for the user (Fig. 6.3, Table 6.1).

RSLSteeper also offers three larger electric hand sizes to accommodate older children. These include the size 6 for 5–8 years, $6\frac{3}{4}$ for 8–12 years, and $7\frac{1}{4}$ for youth to adult.

The larger hands have a different drive system that allows the hand to maintain finger opening in any given position. This mechanism ensures accurate finger positioning and eliminates the possibility of the fingers closing on their own with the applied resistance of the cosmetic glove. A soft foam shell protects the hand mechanism and the electronic module. The shell provides a softness of texture for both the Scamp and the other RSL Steeper hand series.

Three types of wrist unit are available for the RSLSteeper electric hands. These wrist units include a friction wrist, a wrist connector and an electrical disconnect unit. The friction wrist is available for use

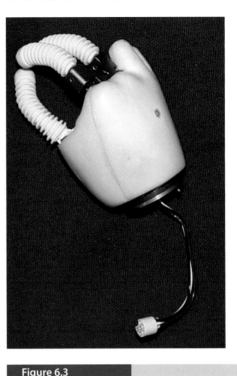

Figure 6.3

SCAMP hand

Table 6.1. Scamp hands (printed with permission of manufacturer)

Hand specification		
Hand Sizes	Scamp $4\frac{1}{2}$	Scamp $5\frac{1}{2}$
Operating Voltage	6	6
Running Current – Less than	150 mA	150 mA
Weight with harness – including cosmesis	143 g–148 g	143 g–148 g

Table 6.2. VASI hands (printed with permission of manufacturer)

Hand specification				
Hand Sizes	VV 0–3	VV 2–6	VV 5–9	VV 7–11
Operating Voltage	4.8 V/6 V	4.8 V/6 V	4.8 V/6 V	4.8 V/6 V
Current consumption	260 mA	340 mA	1.4 A	1.4 A
Opening width	53 mm	51 mm	70 mm	69 mm
Grip force	3.5 lbs / 4.5 lbs	5.0 lbs / 7.0 lbs	6.0 lbs / 9.5 lbs	6.5 lbs / 8.0 lbs
Weight with electrical harness, no wrist unit or cosmetic glove	86 g	126 g	190 g	198 g

with all RSLSteeper hands. It provides 320 degrees of rotation and adjustable friction-tension. The wrist connector is used for individuals with a long trans-radial or wrist-disarticulation residuum. The wrist connector fixes the hand in place, and the child uses forearm supination/pronation motion to change the position of the hand. The third unit, an electrical disconnect wrist, is available for size-6 hands and larger. This wrist allows the user to interchange the hand with other Steeper devices. The Scamp and other Steeper hands can be operated by any of the Steeper input devices. It is also possible to use the Otto Bock electrode as an alternative input device.

6.3.1.2 Variety Ability Systems Inc. (VASI) Products

VASI offers four child-sized hands, the VV0–3, VV2–6, VV5–9 and VV7–11 (see Table 6.2).

The product codes correspond to the nominal age range of the child for whom they are intended. The entire hand series is based upon the same design principles, with each element proportionally enlarged. The hand body and finger groups are made of a durable injection molded plastic. Since the VASI electronics are housed in the hand body, the self-contained, compact design of the hands makes it possible to provide a cosmetic appearance even when space is limited. The VASI hands are compatible with most electronic switch, FSR and myoelectric control systems (Fig. 6.4).

VASI carries a wide array of wrist units that can be used with their hands to accommodate varying residual limb sizes. Of particular note is the Omni wrist, a multi-positional component that allows the hand to be passively rotated in addition to placement in flexion, extension and radial or ulnar deviation. The Omni wrist comprises a ball and socket system with friction adjustment that allows the user to manually position the terminal device at a functionally advantageous angle.

VASI also offers an electric wrist rotator that is particularly useful for children with high level and/or bilateral upper-limb deficiencies. The electric wrist rotator can be used with the VV2–6, VV5–9 and VV7–11 hands and can also be combined with an Omni wrist to provide maximum functionality (Fig. 6.5).

Liberating Technologies Inc. [12] carries the Flexi Wrist, a self-adapting product for young children. This wrist can accommodate an infant's crawling activities, allowing the hand to adapt to the surface of contact. When the arm is lifted, the hand moves back to a neutral position.

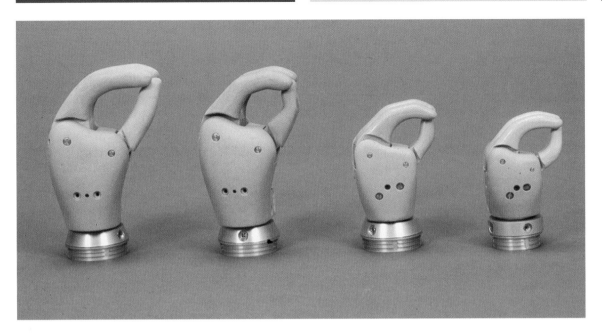

Figure 6.4

VASI hand series

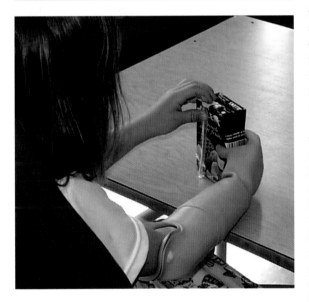

Figure 6.5

OMNI wrist

6.3.1.3 Otto Bock Health Care GmbH (Otto Bock) Products

Otto Bock has taken a different mechanical design approach towards the development of its child-sized electric hands. The 2000 series comprises four sizes, the size 5 hand – ages 18 months to 3 years, the size $5^{1}/_{2}$ hand – ages 3 to 6 years, the size 6 hand – ages 5 to 10 years, and the size $6^{1}/_{2}$ hand – ages 8 to 13 years (see Table 6.3, Fig. 6.6).

The Otto Bock 2000 series hands are made of lightweight aluminum and have a grasp concept that differs from those seen in all other production electric hands. The finger group rotates with the thumb on an angled axis, making a sweeping motion when the hand is opened or closed. This results in a more natural looking grasping motion. The product assumes a hand shape and soft texture once the cosmetic glove is applied. Despite their fragile appearance, the 2000 series hands are durable and resistant to moderate sand and moisture exposure. The length of the hand body should be taken into consideration when fitting a young child with a long residual limb as it may cause the prosthesis to be too long compared to the sound side. In addition to Otto Bock's own EMG con-

Table 6.3. Otto Bock 2000 series hands (printed with permission of manufacturer)

Hand specification				
Hand sizes	OB 5	OB 5 1/2	OB 6	OB 6 1/2
Operating voltage	4.8 V	4.8 V	4.8 V	4.8 V
Current consumption	200 mA	200 mA	200 mA	200 mA
Opening width	33 mm	35 mm	54 mm	56 mm
Grip force	15 N	35 N	55 N	55 N
Weight – no cosmetic glove or power bridge	86 g	115 g	125 g	130 g

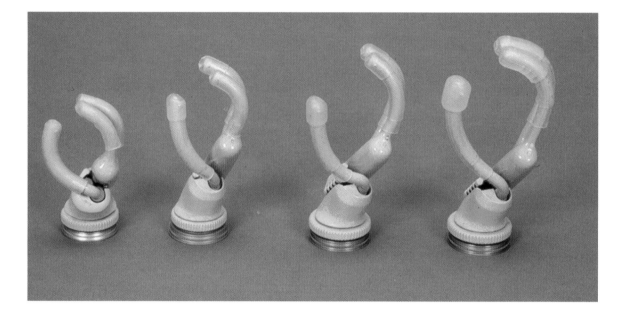

trol devices, Liberating Technology's VariGrip III system (see Sect. 6.4) can be used with this hand series when switch or FSR control is desired.

The wrist is a passive friction type. The friction is adjustable for individual preference by adding rubber o-rings within the wrist. A threaded collar at the end of the hand is used to assemble the hand to the wrist unit. As there are no wires connecting the hand to the wrist, the hands can be removed or installed easily, making it convenient to service the device. VASI offers a modified version of the Omni wrist for use with the 2000 series hands.

Figure 6.6

OB 2000 hand series

6.3.2 Elbows

Mechanical and electrical options are available for children. The choice of component is dependent on the child's age, physical size, control ability and residual limb length.

6.3.2.1 Side Joints

Side joints are commonly used for the longer residual limb lengths associated with amputations or deficiencies close to the elbow. These hinges, mounted on the outside of the socket, keep the elbow level close to that of the contralateral side. The side joints are available in various sizes, and can be free swing with locking option or friction operated. The disadvantages are that they add bulk to the prosthesis, they are not cosmetic in appearance and they do not provide humeral rotation. VASI has recently introduced friction controlled side joints that are slimmer in shape, improving the look of the finished prosthesis (Fig. 6.7).

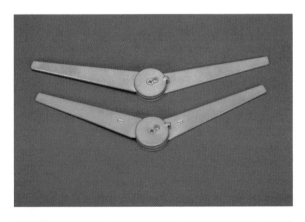

Figure 6.7

VASI friction side joints

6.3.2.2 Elbow Components

Elbow components are available in many sizes and shapes and incorporate a turntable, providing passive humeral rotation. Elbow components can be categorized as passive, locking or electric.

Passive

For younger children, passive friction elbows are commonly used in combination with electric hands. RSLSteeper [18] offers child-sized passive friction elbow components in 2 sizes, both allowing humeral rotation and flexion-extension. Hosmer [7] provides a friction elbow for older children.

Locking

Various manufacturers such as Hosmer, [7] RSLSteeper [18] and Otto Bock [14] provide mechanically operated elbows for children of approximately 7 years of age and older. These elbows can be locked and unlocked using a cable and harness system. Children may experience some initial difficulty learning how to lock and unlock these joints due to the need to counteract the distal loading effect of the heavier electric hands.

Electric

An electric elbow may also be considered a viable option for the child amputee. The decision to use an electric elbow depends on the child's ability to tolerate the additional weight and the degree of operating complexity the child can manage. VASI offers two sizes of electric elbows for children; the VV3–8 and the VV8–12, with the numbers representing the approximate ages for use. Most electronic control systems and terminal devices are compatible with these two elbows. The elbows have a passive-friction humeral rotation component. The VV8–12 elbow has the added feature of free-swing motion when the elbow drive disengages in full elbow extension (Fig. 6.8).

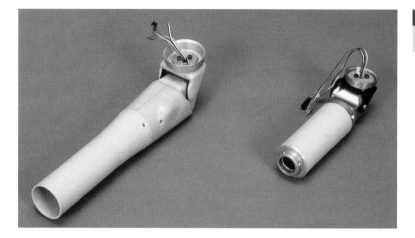

Figure 6.8
VASI electric elbows

6.3.3 Shoulder Joints

Components for shoulder joints are available from several sources: RSLSteeper, VASI, Hosmer, and Liberating-Collier. The RSLSteeper [18] elbow components for children work very well in providing a cosmetically acceptable shoulder joint for small children (see Fig. 6.9). As an alternative, it is possible to use the VASI Omni wrist as a shoulder joint, with some modification of the joint required to fit a humeral section.

The Hosmer FAJ 100 [7] is a lightweight shoulder joint mainly used for adults. However, due to its low profile physical shape, it can also be used on school-aged children. The FAJ 100 provides friction-controlled flexion and extension as well as abduction and adduction control.

For very active children the Liberating-Collier shoulder joint [12] is another option to consider. This product provides free swing, allowing positioning of the arm under gravity, and can be locked into the desired position using a notch switch or electric powered control switch. Abduction and adduction are friction controlled. The Liberating-Collier shoulder joint is appropriately sized for teenagers and adults. There are no electrically powered shoulder joints currently available.

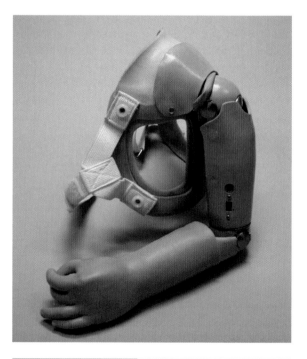

Figure 6.9
Steeper elbow used as shoulder joint

6.3.4 Batteries

The operation of any externally powered prosthesis depends on batteries as the power source. Over the years, battery cells have decreased in size and weight and gained more capacity, allowing a longer use of the prosthesis before recharging is required. The smaller battery size also enables a more cosmetic manufacturing of prosthetic forearms. The batteries used are rechargeable and are specially packaged for safe and easy prosthetic use. The manufacturer's charger must be used to recharge the batteries. Choosing the right size and capacity of battery depends on the requirements of the electrical components used in the individual child's prosthesis.

All major upper limb prosthetic suppliers offer different varieties of batteries including nickel cadmium or lithium ion, with 6 volt or 4.8 volt outputs. Batteries can be classified as external or internal, depending on how they are located in the prosthesis.

6.3.4.1 Internal Batteries

Internal batteries, housed inside the prosthesis, may improve the cosmetic appearance of the prosthesis. Internal placement also eliminates the possibility of the child removing and losing or misplacing the battery. A charge plug is integrated into the outside of the prosthesis together with an on/off switch. Using an external charger, recharging of the battery is performed overnight when the prosthesis is not worn and switched off. The disadvantage to using an internal battery is that if the prosthesis runs out of battery power during the day, the battery cannot be simply interchanged.

6.3.4.2 External Batteries

External batteries can be physically removed from the prosthesis and interchanged with a freshly charged battery for continued use of the device. A battery case is integrated into the outer shell of the prosthesis and holds the battery securely in place. If the battery does not sit flush with the surface, its visibility may make the prosthesis less attractive.

If there is insufficient space to locate the battery within the prosthesis, a remote battery holder can be used to clip onto the child's clothing. With this system the weight of the battery is removed from the prosthesis, but the need to have a cable connecting the battery to the prosthesis can be cumbersome and prone to breakdown problems.

6.3.5 Input Devices

The input device controls an electromechanical prosthesis. Selection of the appropriate input device depends upon the physical ability and level of amputation of the individual. The main approaches considered are electromyogram (EMG) control and switch control.

6.3.5.1 Electrodes

EMG control uses surface electrodes to pick up a myoelectric signal from an underlying, contracting muscle. There are different types of electrodes available and of these, two child-sized versions are available from Otto Bock [14] and RSLSteeper [18]. Both the Otto Bock 13E125 electrode and the RSLSteeper D12839 electrode are small in size and feature an integrated amplifier. The 13E125 electrode is thinner than the D12839 enabling improved cosmetic finishing of a prosthesis for small children.

6.3.5.2 Switches

Switch input devices are mainly used for higher level amputations where more control options are required. Different types of switches such as pull, push and rocker switches are available. Switches can have different control configurations: namely, single action, dual action and momentary action (Fig. 6.10).

Pull switches are used in conjunction with a harness for activation. A shrug motion of the shoulder or flexion and abduction of the residual limb activates

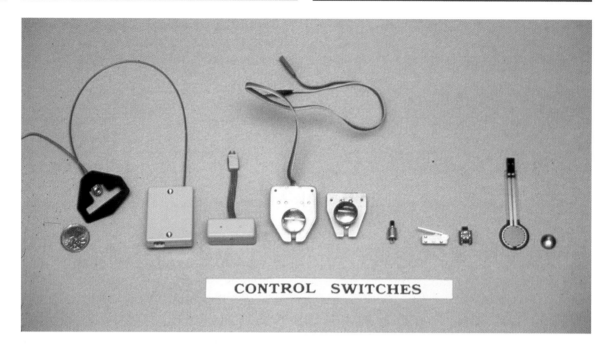

CONTROL SWITCHES

Figure 6.10

Electric switches

ments. The FSR is used in the same locations as the conventional push switches, and because of its physical shape, less mounting space is needed, enabling more cosmetically appealing prosthetic designs.

the pull switch and operates the electric component (i. e. elbow). Push switches are used in shoulder disarticulation prostheses and are activated by shoulder girdle elevation, depression, protraction and retraction motions. Phocomelic digits can also be used to operate switches if they have sufficient strength and mobility (Fig. 6.10).

6.3.5.3 Force Sensing Resistors (FSRs)

The Force Sensing Resistor (FSR) is another type of push switch that differs from the conventional mechanical switches in both appearance and function. The FSR is a touch pad that is spoon-shaped and wafer thin. The output produced is proportional to the pressure exerted on the pressure pad. The FSR is sensitive to moisture and may not function properly when exposed without protection to humid environ-

6.4 Control of Electrically Powered Prosthetic Systems

6.4.1 Introduction

This section begins with a brief review of some of the basic concepts related to control of electrically powered, upper-limb prosthetic components and then describes the currently available control systems, the options they provide and the ways in which they can be applied.

6.4.2 Control System Components

There are three components needed for control of an electrically powered prosthesis: system input, controller and output (Fig. 6.11).

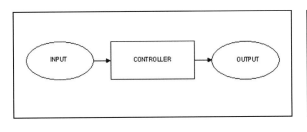

Figure 6.11

Control system components

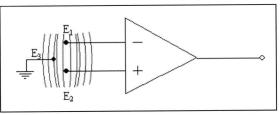

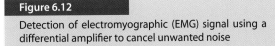

Figure 6.12

Detection of electromyographic (EMG) signal using a differential amplifier to cancel unwanted noise

6.4.2.1 System Input

The first component is the control signal, or input to the system, which allows the user to voluntarily control the prosthesis. The input signal can be derived from a number of different sources using different types of transducers. For example, trans-radial prosthetic devices use the electromyographic (EMG) signal recorded from underlying muscles via electrodes as the input to the control system. There are three electrodes in each EMG transducer. As depolarization potentials travel along individual muscle fibres during a muscle contraction, they will first pass beneath one electrode (i.e. the positive electrode), as shown in Fig. 6.12, and then a second electrode (i.e. the negative electrode). These two electrodes are referenced to a third electrode, called the ground electrode, so that the signal recorded from the first electrode is automatically subtracted from the signal recorded from the second electrode. This 'differential' arrangement will ensure that signals common to both electrodes, such as that from heart muscle, are cancelled out, leaving just the EMG signal.

6.4.2.2 Controller

The second component is the electronics controller, which will condition the input signal. Figure 6.13 illustrates how the 'raw' EMG signal is processed so that it can be used to control the motor of a prosthesis. The EMG signal shown in Fig. 6.13a is first rectified, i.e. the negative components of the EMG signal are flipped up by making them positive (Fig. 6.13b). The high frequency components of the signal are then filtered out (Fig. 6.13c), so that an 'envelope' of the EMG activity is left. This envelope represents the strength of contraction of the muscle, in other words, how hard the muscle was contracted. There can still be a small signal present when the muscle is inactive. There might also be inadvertent muscle activity as the arm is moved around during activities other than grasping or holding an object, such as reaching towards an object.

The amplitude of an EMG signal is in the order of a few millionths of a volt, and can be amplified by adjusting the gain of the EMG amplifier. The distance of the electrodes from the muscle's motor point (perhaps due to varying thickness of a fat layer) will also affect the amplitude of the EMG signal. Therefore, the adjustable gain of the amplifier needs to be set so that the resultant signal allows the user to operate the prosthesis without undue effort. A threshold EMG value is set to prevent unintentional activation of the prosthesis. If the EMG signal is below the threshold, then the controller will ignore the input signal and will not activate the prosthesis. If the EMG signal exceeds the threshold, then the prosthesis will be activated. Setting the gains and thresholds to suit a particular user is called calibrating the control system.

Other inputs to the control system might come from a force-sensing resistor (FSR), for example, that transduces the force as one presses against the FSR into an electrical control signal that would resemble the waveform shown in Fig. 6.13(c).

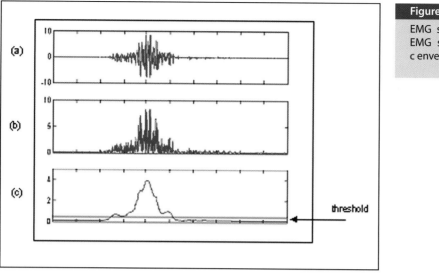

Figure 6.13 a–c
EMG signal processing. a 'raw' EMG signal; b rectified signal; c envelope of EMG activity

The controller will also execute the strategy that the amputee will use to control the prosthesis. For example the strategy may be a 'single-site voluntary opening' one. In this strategy, a control signal that exceeds the threshold would cause the hand to open. When the signal drops below the threshold or is absent, the hand will close. The various control strategies are detailed below. The controller should also incorporate an 'energy-save' circuit, which is responsible for turning the motor in the prosthesis off if the mechanical movement has reached a limit, such as the hand being fully open. This ensures that the battery in the prosthesis is not unduly drained when the prosthesis is not operating.

Some prostheses feature multiple modalities that a controller should be able to accommodate. For example, the Otto Bock 2000 series of hands has one motor to provide increased speed during opening or closing of the hand and another motor to provide increased pinch force once an object has been grasped. For such systems the controller needs to sense what mode the hand is operating in, so that the appropriate motor can be activated.

6.4.2.3 Output

The third component is the output. The output signal from the controller will go to the motor in the terminal device, resulting in, for example, the hand opening. A power bridge within the controller ensures that an appropriate level of power is delivered to the motor.

6.4.3 Control Strategies

The control strategy determines how the inputs from the person are used to create the desired motions with the prosthesis. The type of control strategy that is chosen for a particular user will depend upon a number of factors. These include the number of prosthetic components the amputee wishes to control, the number of muscle sites or switches the amputee can control independently, the characteristics of signal generated by the muscle(s), FSRs, or other input devices and the cognitive ability of the user.

The control system can control the prosthesis in one of two ways, digitally or proportionally. In digital control, the speed of the motor will be constant at its maximum, once the input signal exceeds the threshold. In a proportional system the speed of the motor

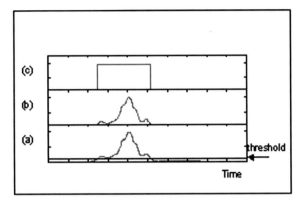

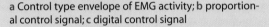

Figure 6.14 a–c

a Control type envelope of EMG activity; b proportional control signal; c digital control signal

will change in proportion to the change in magnitude of the input signal. This is illustrated in Fig. 6.14.

Since the amputee can control the speed of a prosthetic component in a proportional system, it is used for those individuals who want more precise control of movement e.g., finger-thumb positioning on a delicate object. Proportional control is more helpful for larger hands where travel distance between fingers and thumb is greater. It is also beneficial in controlling the flexion and extension speed of an electric elbow.

The child's abilities must also be considered when deciding between proportional and digital control, since proportional control requires the additional ability to sustain the input signal (e.g., an EMG sig-

nal) steadily after crossing the threshold. Digital control, although less refined, is easier to master and may be a more appropriate choice for a younger child. The child may start with digital control and later switch to proportional control after gaining skill and experience.

The most commonly used control strategies are described below:

6.4.3.1 Single-Site One-Level Voluntary Opening

The single-site voluntary opening strategy, also known as the 'cookie crusher', has a single input source, such as an EMG electrode, FSR or switch. The presence of an EMG or FSR signal that exceeds the threshold, or closing of the switch, results in a hand opening; whereas, any signal below the threshold or absence of a signal results in the hand closing, as shown in Fig. 6.15. Alternatively, the controller can be set so that instead of the action being voluntary opening, it is voluntary closing.

This 'cookie-crusher' strategy is most suitable when fitting a child under 3 years of age. At this age the child does not have the communication skills or cognitive ability to learn to use a system that can independently control opening and closing of the hand. Rather, the child will intuitively connect arm muscle activity with opening of the hand. If not, a parental switch can be provided that will allow the clinician or parent to open the hand independently of the child and to place toys and objects in it. The child can then be encouraged to open the hand to release the

Figure 6.15

Single-site 1-level voluntary opening control strategy

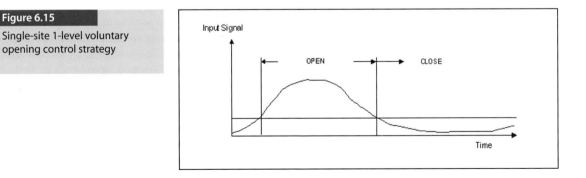

grasped object. The gain is initially set high and then decreased gradually as the child becomes more skilled at operating the hand.

6.4.3.2 Single-Site Two-Level-Sensitive

Similar to the single-site, voluntary opening control strategy, a level sensitive strategy has only one input source. However, this strategy allows the user to control either the opening and closing of a hand or the rotation in two directions of a wrist or the flexion and extension of an elbow. A prosthetic hand will be used to illustrate the concept. In the 2-level-sensitive strategy, two thresholds are set (Fig. 6.16). If the input signal has an amplitude that is less than that of the lower threshold, the prosthesis will not operate. If the input signal is between the two thresholds, then the hand will close. If the input signal exceeds the higher threshold, then the hand will open. A slight delay between the input and output signals is introduced when the input signal is in the middle region to avoid inadvertent hand closing during transition from the lower threshold to above the higher threshold.

6.4.3.3 Single-Site Rate-Sensitive

The rate-sensitive control strategy is an alternative to the level-sensitive control strategy. Instead of using the amplitude of the signal to control which function (e.g., opening or closing of a hand) occurs, the rate at which the user contracts a muscle or presses against an FSR will determine the direction of the motor. As shown in Fig. 6.17, when the input signal crosses the lower threshold, the system waits for a preset period of time (tens of milliseconds) and then compares the signal to the upper threshold. If the signal is still below the upper threshold after the preset time delay, it is considered to be a slowly rising signal (low rate) and the hand closes. If the signal exceeds the upper threshold before the end of the delay, it is considered to be a quickly rising signal (fast rate) and the hand opens. Rate-sensitive control can also be proportional, allowing for variable control of the speed of movement, while level-sensitive control is strictly a digital

control strategy, moving the prosthesis at a fixed speed in one direction or the other.

6.4.3.4 Single-Site Alternating

The alternating strategy will automatically allow the user to switch between opening and closing of a hand, using successive muscle contractions or FSR activations from a single site. Using a hand as an example, the first input exceeding the threshold will cause the hand to open, the second input exceeding the threshold will cause it to close, the next suprathreshold input will cause it to open again, and so on. The user should be able to select the option that control will always default to the same function, (e.g., hand opening) after a predetermined time lapse since the last activation. This ensures that the user will always know what action the hand will perform when next activating the input (see Fig. 6.18).

6.4.3.5 Two-Site Level-Sensitive (Two-Site, Two-Function)

This is the most commonly used control strategy. With a hand prosthesis, for example, the input from one site is used to open the hand and the input from a second site is used to close the hand (Fig. 6.19). The two-site control strategy can be used in the following two ways depending upon the abilities and preferences of the user.

First-Come-First-Served

In this strategy, if the flexor muscles contract first, the hand will close and if the extensors contract first, the hand will open. In this scheme, the second muscle group to contract is ignored. See Fig. 6.19.

Difference Control

Similar to the first-come-first-served strategy, if the flexor muscle contracts, the hand will close and if the

Figure 6.16

Single-site 2-level sensitive control strategy

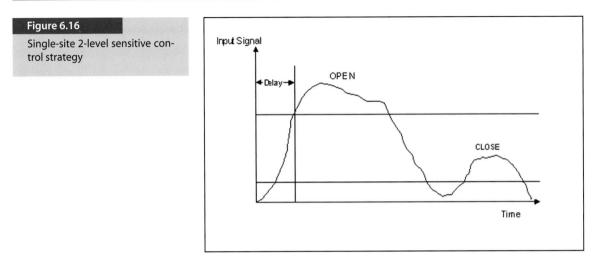

Figure 6.17

Single-site rate-sensitive control strategy

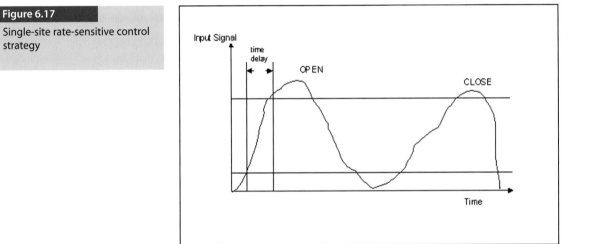

Figure 6.18

Single-site alternating control strategy

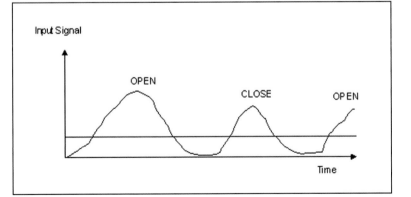

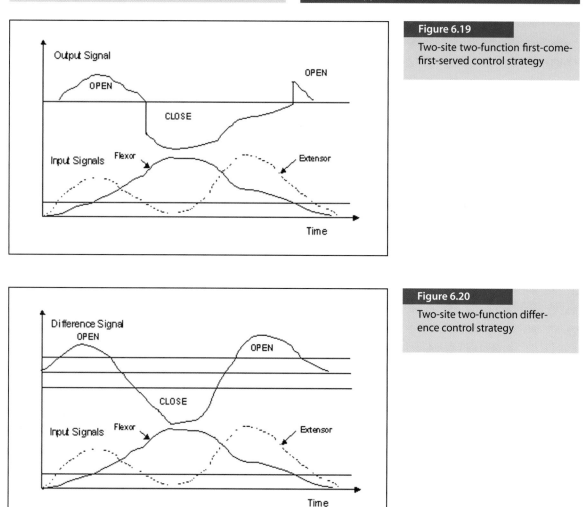

Figure 6.19

Two-site two-function first-come-first-served control strategy

Figure 6.20

Two-site two-function difference control strategy

extensor muscle contracts, the hand will open. However, if both muscle groups contract (co-contraction), then the speed and direction of the motor will be governed by the difference in amplitude between the flexor and extensor muscle input signals (see Fig. 6.20).

The two-site level-sensitive strategy can be implemented either in digital or proportional form.

6.4.3.6 Mode Switching

In mode switching, two input signals are used to control more than one device, e.g., a hand and a powered wrist. For example, when using EMG control, the flexors would close the hand and the extensors would open it. The user can then switch control from the hand to the wrist by co-contracting the two muscle groups. Now a flexor signal will supinate the wrist and an extensor signal will pronate the wrist. To switch control back to the hand, the user can co-contract again. If no signal is received for a preset period of time, control will automatically revert to the hand. If the user produces inadvertent contractions, the scheme can be altered so it only responds to rapidly initiated contractions. Similarly, FSRs can be used to generate the input signals in place of EMG electrodes. This control scheme can be extended to also include an elbow, so that two muscle co-contractions or simultaneous activation of the two FSRs would sequentially switch control from hand to wrist to elbow, and then back to hand.

Several variations of this mode switching strategy are possible. If the user can access an auxiliary switch input in addition to the standard electrode or FSR inputs, the auxiliary input can be used to sequentially switch control between hand, wrist and elbow in conjunction with any of the control strategies described above.

6.4.3.7 Hybrid Systems

For users with trans-humeral, shoulder disarticulation or forequarter amputations, a variety of input methods can be used to provide control of a hand, wrist or elbow. For example, biceps and triceps can be used for hand operation and a pull switch could be used to control elbow flexion and extension. Commercial systems should be flexible enough to allow for a mixture of different input types in combination with different control strategies to allow the clinician to configure the prosthetic system to the needs and abilities of each client.

6.4.4 Commercial Control Systems

There are currently three types of commercially available control systems. Each type is discussed below. With the advent of microprocessors and the miniaturization of electronic components, newer systems provide the client and clinician with flexible, multifunctional control options.

6.4.4.1 Fixed Single Strategy

In the past, circuit boards were designed to implement a particular control strategy. An example of this that is still available is the controller for the RSLSteeper Scamp hand, [18] which is a single-site voluntary opening strategy. Some programmable controllers can be ordered with a single strategy, in a non-programmable configuration at a lower cost than programmable modules. This option would be chosen if the control strategy for a particular client is already known and unlikely to change in the future. An example of such a system is the Variety Ability Systems Inc. (VASI) SPM (Single-motor Programmable Module), [27] which can be factory set with a particular strategy. The clinician can still modify the gain and threshold parameters by linking the controller to a Personal Computer via a cable (see Fig. 6.21). Preprogrammed strategies available from VASI at the time of writing include single-site voluntary opening, single-site level sensitive, single-site rate sensitive, single-site alternating and two-site level sensitive either proportional or digital. The system can be used in conjunction with EMG, FSR or switch inputs. If a change in strategy were required later, the controller would have to be returned to the supplier for reprogramming.

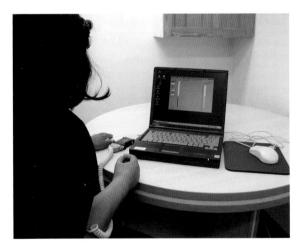

Figure 6.21

Client with prosthesis connected to computer

6.4.4.2 Selectable Strategies

Most manufacturers of powered upper-extremity prosthetic products produce controllers that allow the clinician to select one of several pre-programmed control strategies. This option would be desirable if the clinician was not sure which strategy would best meet the needs of a particular client or if it is known, that given time, the child will proceed from one strategy to another (e.g., from a single-site voluntary opening strategy, to a more advanced strategy such as a two-site, two-function system).

RSLSteeper provides the Multi Control [18] for their child-sized hands (children ages 6 months to 12 years). This controller can be configured for digital or proportional single-site voluntary opening, single-site level sensitive and two-input control using a switch selector. Input sources are EMG, switch, and slide potentiometer.

Otto Bock HealthCare GmbH [14] has a 4-in-1 controller in which one of four control strategies and left or right side can be selected by means of colour coded plugs. The four available strategies are single-site 1-level voluntary opening, two-site level sensitive digital, two-site level sensitive proportional and two-site level sensitive proportional with low EMG input signal (~20 μV). Eight plugs are available – one for each of the control strategies in combination with left or right arm selection. In order to change the strategy or side, a different plug corresponding to the choice of side and strategy would be inserted into the controller. This system does not allow the clinician to modify any of the control parameters such as gains (except using the gain control on the electrode) and thresholds and is meant to be used with EMG as the input signal source(s).

6.4.4.3 Selectable and Adjustable

Variety Ability Systems Inc.[27] and Liberating Technologies [12] have been instrumental in developing controllers and computer software that enable the clinician to select the strategy from a pre-programmed list of control strategies and then to adjust the control parameters (e.g., gain and threshold) to customize the system for the individual user. These systems are also user friendly and allow the clinician to select different input control signals, including EMG, FSR and switch. VASI's SPM system allows for control of a single motor device. This type of controller would be selected when, for example, a young child begins with a single-site voluntary opening strategy and later graduates to a two-site level-sensitive system after learning agonist-antagonist muscle control.

Liberating's VariGrip III [12] allows for control of 1 to 4 motors. For instance, it could be used to control a VASI hand, wrist rotator and elbow (3 motors) or an Otto Bock 2000 series hand (2-motor system) in combination with a wrist and elbow (4 motors). Depending on the input control source, gains and thresholds for either amplitude or rate control can be set independently. These systems also have an optional autocalibration routine in which the system will monitor the user's input signals and set gains and thresholds to take advantage of the full operating range of the user's input signals while minimizing the effects of cross-talk between agonist and antagonist muscle signals. These systems also incorporate visual feedback to the clinician and user about the relationship between the input signals and the motor outputs. As an example of this, Fig. 6.22 shows software which displays the input signals from biceps and triceps and a third channel permitting one to switch between hand, wrist and elbow using an external switch and also shows the hand, wrist and elbow motor responses. An example of how this system could be used clinically is the fitting of a young child with a trans-humeral amputation. The child may begin with an electrically powered hand together with a passive wrist and elbow. As the child's competency increases, the board could be reprogrammed to accommodate an active elbow and eventually an active wrist, as well, if desired.

The available SPM control strategies are listed in Sect. 6.4.4.1. VariGrip III strategies, in addition to the SPM strategies, include mode switching and hybrid control.

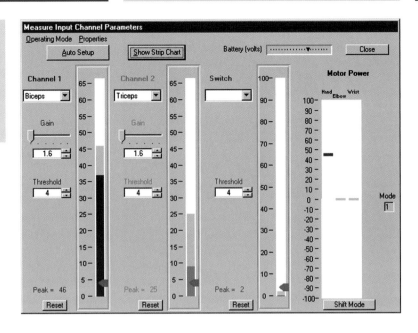

Figure 6.22

MyoAssistant computer program showing biceps and triceps input channels, indicator for switching between hand, wrist and elbow, and; hand, wrist and elbow motor outputs

6.4.5 Conclusions

The availability of microprocessor-based controllers that can fit within prostheses has revolutionized powered upper limb prosthetic systems by providing a range of easily configured control strategies for prostheses. This allows the clinician to tailor the system to the user's needs, resulting in a fitting that is more likely to be accepted and used. Such a system can be more cost effective in the long run, as it is simpler for the clinician to adapt the original system to changing physiological or cognitive conditions.

6.5 Sockets

6.5.1 Paediatric Considerations

Congenital amputees, particularly those with longitudinal deficiencies, often present with unique physical characteristics that require imagination and ingenuity to fit with a prosthetic system. Socket designs need to be customized to meet the needs of the individual child.

Myoelectric prostheses are designed to be as self-suspending as possible, allowing maximum range of motion while maintaining adequate suspension for the electrical components. In the case of children, sockets need to suspend securely enough to withstand the forces exerted by children engaged in active play.

Growth consideration is an important factor. Growth tends to occur in spurts, especially in the first two years and again in pre-adolescence. Growth changes are not predictable or uniform. It is not at all uncommon for a child to first experience an increase in stump volume, resulting in an uncomfortable tight socket and then, shortly after, to experience a gain in axial length resulting in the socket becoming loose and poorly suspended. The fit of the socket must be monitored and adjusted frequently, with the socket being replaced as often as needed to maintain comfort. In many cases it is possible to re-use the more costly electrical components such as electrodes, hands and elbows at the time of a socket replacement.

Children have low tolerance for lengthy socket donning/doffing procedures. Compromises may need to be made to ensure that the socket can be applied and removed with ease but can still provide

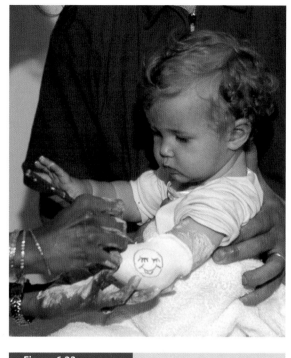

Figure 6.23

Casting an infant

adequate suspension and consistent electrode contact.

Sockets must be lightweight but durable. Hard acrylic resin laminated sockets are preferred in paediatric practice. The material is considered non-toxic, it is easy to fabricate and it can be modified as needed for growth. As the acrylic laminate is heat formable, pressure points can be remolded to provide relief and comfort. In the case of small children, the sockets can be fabricated with fewer layers of reinforcing material to allow easier adjustment. The sockets can also be split open longitudinally and/or extended proximally to adjust for minor circumferential and axial growth.

Casting the very young child can present some challenges (Fig. 6.23). Parent and child need to be assured that the casting procedure will not cause discomfort. A child usually has a short attention span and, therefore, needs to be distracted to keep the af-

fected limb still during the casting procedure. It may be helpful to have the mother nurse or bottle-feed an infant during the casting procedure. For toddlers and older children, singing songs, talking about friends or things they like to do, and playing with toys can help to keep them occupied.

6.5.2 Trans-radial

6.5.2.1 Assessment

Children born with transverse trans-radial limb deficiencies constitute the majority of clients in a paediatric caseload. Fortunately they are also the easiest to fit with an upper limb prosthesis. Prosthetic designs are relatively straightforward and appropriate-sized components are available. Generally the rate of acceptance is high as the children are able to derive benefit from the combined cosmesis and function that a myoelectric prosthesis affords.

Residual limbs of the children in this group usually have healthy skin and ample soft tissue covering. In fact, as younger children tend to have an excess of fatty tissue and bony landmarks may not be well defined, achieving supracondylar suspension can often be a challenge. Children with transverse deficiencies frequently have some form of vestigeal tissue or "nubbins" that need to be accommodated by providing additional space within the socket. In some cases, this tissue is loosely attached and susceptible to trauma, especially in donning the prosthesis, while in other cases it may be quite rigid and contain bony segments.

Other anomalies may be evident as well. For example, elbow hyper-extension of 20–30 degrees and radial head subluxation are also quite common and should be addressed when designing the socket. In some cases the distal radius and ulna may be fused with a resultant curvature of the forearm segment. In this case, the limb may be very wide at the elbow (prominent radial head) and taper significantly to a bony tip or mass of undeveloped tissue (see Fig. 6.24).

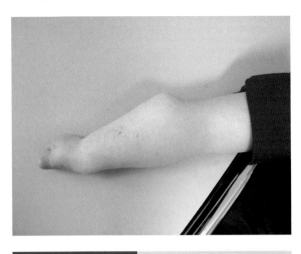

Figure 6.24

Residual limb anomalies

6.5.2.2 Design

Sockets are generally designed to be self-suspending using some modification of the Muenster approach. Some prosthetists prefer the snug, lower rim A-P fit (Muenster style) [10], while others prefer the M-L (Northwestern University supracondylar) design [2]. In many cases a combined approach is the most effective with suspension forces distributed between the two dimensions (M-L and A-P) according to individ-

ual preference and length of the residual limb. For example, the forces may be almost equally divided between medial-lateral and anterior-posterior for the shorter limb but more focused on medial-lateral suspension for the mid-forearm or longer limb.

Likewise, the anterior brim is extended proximally to the distal cubital crease area for the shorter limb but lowered and elongated for ease of application for a longer limb. The opening in the volar area should be just sufficient to allow easy application and removal but secure enough to discourage the younger child from removing and discarding the prosthesis at will. For the very short stump, the posterior proximal brim of the socket may be brought up more than 1/2 inch above the olecranon fossa to increase the suspension surface. The medial and lateral brims extend above the epicondyles and are well defined for young children since the epicondyles are not fully developed. There is a need for generous flares and rolled edges to avoid pinching tissues.

It is important to maintain as much elbow flexion as possible. Lowering the anterior brim will help to increase elbow range for the longer length limb. If it is not possible to obtain 100 degrees or more in cases of very short residual limbs, the prosthetic forearm can be pre-flexed during fabrication to help compensate for the limited elbow range.

The posterior/superior quadrant may be cut out (see Fig. 6.25) to facilitate and improve ventilation [20]. This modification reduces perspiration, associ-

Figure 6.25

3/4 Trans-radial socket

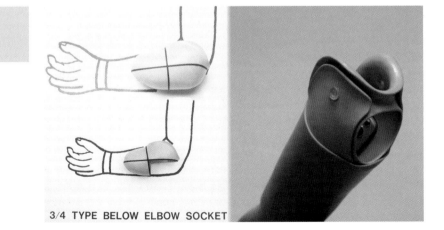

3/4 TYPE BELOW ELBOW SOCKET

ated skin and control problems and improves comfort/wearing tolerance. It is also advisable to reinforce the narrow posterior brim for the active child.

Additional space is provided distally for prosthetic growth allowance and to avoid distal end discomfort when weight-bearing on the prosthesis. It is also important to ensure that there is sufficient circumferential room to accommodate distal stump tissue motion required for control purposes. Various types of removeable socket liners have been used with mixed success in an attempt to prolong the life of a socket for a growing child [3, 21]. However, due to the bulkiness, this approach may not work well with the very young children for whom it would be most beneficial.

In the case of a longer amputation or limb deficiency at or just below the wrist, the socket must still enclose most of the forearm to ensure that electrodes are located over adequate muscle sites. Supracondylar suspension can be used but it effectively eliminates forearm pronation and supination. Another option may be to try to eliminate the supracondylar brim and have the proximal trimlines cut down distal to the humeral epicondyles to preserve some of the forearm's natural pronation and supination motion. This type of socket provides stability at the distal portion and transmits rotation. Suprastyloid suspension options include the use of an expandable inner liner or an obturator door to allow entry of the residual limb into the socket. One of the major challenges for fitting at this level is to keeping the overall length of the prosthesis equal to that of the contralateral arm. It is important therefore to select components that minimize the total length of the prosthesis.

6.5.2.3 Check Sockets

Since the prosthesis is intended to be self-suspended and worn without a stump sock, the fit of the socket is critical. Clear polycarbonate check sockets (Fig. 6.26) can be used as a diagnostic tool. The transparent socket material allows the prosthetist to observe the pressure distribution and modify the socket accordingly. The clear socket also makes it easier to transfer the identified electrode site markings accurately. Depending on the method of application

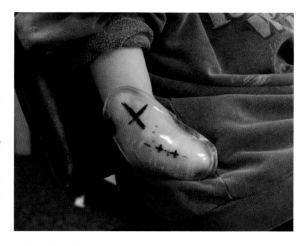

Figure 6.26

Clear check socket

(push-in or pull-in techniques), the tissues may shift and cause the electrode site markings to appear in different positions than that which was intended. The check socket provides an opportunity to assess the implications of this tissue distortion and allows for a more accurate determination of the electrode sites. Holes can be cut out and electrodes placed in the socket for control training and to assure proper placement and calibration.

The preferred way of donning an externally powered prosthesis is the *pull-in* method. With the help of a piece of nylon stocking, the residual limb can be gently pulled into the socket. This is done so that the limb tissues can be properly positioned into the socket and also so that the electrodes are in ideal locations for optimum control. For infants and very small children, the caregiver is responsible for this activity. It is essential that they receive adequate instruction and practice. Older children become quite adept in applying the sockets themselves.

Once the socket appears to be fitting comfortably, a weight check can be carried out to assess the loading effects on suspension and control. The skin is checked again, and once any required modifications have been completed and evaluated, the definitive prosthesis can be manufactured.

If the team has any doubts as to the outcome of the fitting, it is possible at this stage to temporarily attach components to the check socket to create a preparatory prosthesis, which can be sent home on a trial basis before continuing on to finish the device.

6.5.3 Trans-humeral

6.5.3.1 Design

Conventional socket designs have not proven to be very satisfactory for myoelectric fittings of children with trans-humeral level amputations or limb deficiencies. The increased weight of the externally powered components and their mass distribution in the prosthesis alters the biomechanics to a point where it is not possible to obtain sufficient axial stability and rotational control with standard approaches. Operating control problems due to loss of electrode contact and rotation of the residual limb within the socket generally result in frustration and lack of use.

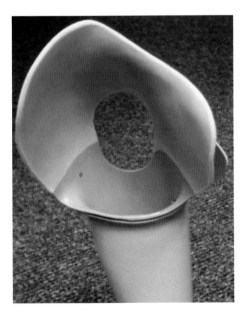

Figure 6.27

1/2 and 1/2 THDSS socket

A more effective socket design, often referred to as the 1/2 and 1/2 socket [22], was developed in an effort to improve the wearing comfort, suspension and functionality of the conventionally made trans-humeral socket. Later known as the THDSS, the trans-humeral dynamic suspension socket is a unique interface that resolves many of the former fitting/control problems. The design consists of a hard acrylic total contact socket distal to the axilla (medial side flattened to prevent pressure on the side of the chest) combined with an integrated, laminated silicone extension that encompasses the shoulder complex (see Fig. 6.27). A lateral obturator is cut out over the deltoid area for better ventilation and increased flexibility of the silicone portion.

Rotational stability is obtained from the semi-flexible anterior and posterior extensions extending from the socket anterior to the deltopectoral groove and posterior to the lateral portion of the infraspinatus. A simple chest suspension strap is used to keep the socket from sliding off the shoulder. This socket has enhanced rotational stability, reduced harnessing and, most importantly, the weight of the components is distributed over a greater area thereby enhancing comfort and wearing tolerance.

Congenital residual limb shapes vary considerably. In some cases, the distal part of the limb may be quite bulbous compared to the proximal aspect and the child may have difficulty donning the prosthesis. Special care will be required in the cast modification to ensure that soft tissue choking does not occur. Bony overgrowth of the humerus is also not uncommon. In this case additional space has to be allowed, first at the distal end of the socket to protect the bone tip in the event of a fall, and second at the distal lateral area of the socket to minimize distal end stump pressure when the child abducts the shoulder. Whenever possible, growth allowance at the end should be added. Growth change may also occur circumferentially rather than axially. In this case it may be possible to heat and stretch the socket once or twice before a complete socket refit is required.

At the elbow disarticulation level, it is preferable to use a socket designed to encapsulate the epicondyles of the humerus in order to preserve humeral rotation. The bulbous end is used for suspension, and an expandable liner or an obturator allows the residuum to fit into the socket. Cosmetic finishing of the prosthesis at this level is more difficult because of the larger circumference at the distal end. In many cases the limb deficiency will include some degree of hypoplasia which in time will result in the residual limb becoming somewhat shorter in length and easier to fit cosmetically.

6.5.3.2　Check Socket

Similar to the process described for trans-radial fitting, a clear check socket is used to assess the ease of socket application, fit, comfort, pressure points and electrode sites. Due to the complexity of a trans-humeral fitting, it is also helpful to proceed further and assemble a mock-up prosthesis to adequately evaluate the loading factors of the child's own components on the fit and comfort of the socket as well as establishing proper alignment of components. Weight distribution is very different when the elbow and forearm are in place and positioned at different elbow angles. The loading effect on electrode contact and control operation can be assessed as well.

6.5.4　Shoulder Disarticulation/Forequarter

Difficulty in upper limb fitting increases proportionately with the degree of limb loss. Designing an appropriate interface for the young child with a shoulder disarticulation or forequarter deficiency is a major challenge due to the small body mass, the weight of the prosthetic limb, the lack of a child's tolerance for any restriction of body movement and problems with heat dissipation.

For the infant or toddler's first passive prosthesis, a flexible thermoplastic basket style interface is recommended because it is light, comfortable, easy to apply and allows the child to become accustomed to wearing a device without too much restriction. However, once the child is ready for an active prosthesis it then becomes necessary to stabilize the socket on the chest wall so that the child can use the clavicle or acromion to operate the control switches and a more rigid interface material is required.

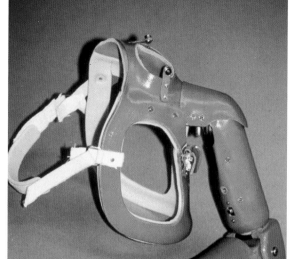

Figure 6.28

Sauter frame

The basket interface is particularly well suited for the very young child because the integrity of the material aids in stability. The laminated socket completely encapsulates the shoulder and some aspects of the thoracic area and has the advantage of distributing the weight of the prosthesis over a broad surface area. This interface does, however, limit air circulation and can be very hot to wear.

Thermoplastic materials have been tried in an attempt to reduce the weight and manufacturing time, but they have done little to address the problem of heat build-up. Venting holes can be drilled into the basket and fenestrations can be created to try to improve the air circulation problem. Care must be taken though not to cut out too large an area or the structure will lose its strength.

A frame style socket design, often called the Sauter frame, [19] is a more effective interface for the older child or adolescent who does not require the same degree of socket conformity to the body for active play as does the younger child. The frame (see Fig. 6.28) contours the rib cage and rests on the shoulder area. Due to the nature of the design, there is much less socket material encompassing the body, thereby allowing more air circulation.

Laminated frames with carbon reinforcement can strengthen the structure but add the disadvantage of greater weight and bulkiness. Also, only limited changes can be made after the device has been finished.

An aluminum frame interface is lighter in weight and, therefore, more comfortable to wear. It is made from aircraft grade aluminum that is hammered and bent to form a sturdy but lightweight frame. It also has the advantage that it can be changed or modified. Extra growth allowance can be built into the frame interface by adding a thicker cushioned liner on the inside of the frame initially and then changing to a thinner liner when extra room is required.

Flexible leather straps or laminated silicone patches can be incorporated in the shoulder suspension area for increased comfort, flexibility and loading surface. A chest strap is used to keep the shoulder frame secured. In some instances, a lateral support pad may be added to prevent the chest strap from cutting into the axilla and aid in distributing the opposition forces over a larger area.

6.6 Recreational Devices

Any discussion of paediatric prosthetics practice must address the need for recreational devices. Children require social contact with their peers and the opportunity to engage in the same activities. Through sports and recreation, children with limb deficiencies can develop psychological, social and physical skills that will be valuable assets throughout their lives [1]. Children of all ages learn through play. They can learn sportsmanship, teamwork and leadership in athletic competition. They can express a passion for music or the arts or they can engage in a diversity of leisure activities such as golf, fishing, swimming, skating, bodybuilding, woodworking and auto mechanics. Each child has the right to participate to the best of their ability. This may mean that throughout the child's life he or she may wish to do certain activities that will require the use of a variety of prostheses or assistive devices.

While the myoelectric prosthesis provides significant functional benefit for most activities of daily living, it does have some limitations. Water, sand, impact and vibration easily damage powered prostheses. Hand size, grip strength and reaction time may be insufficient for sporting activities. Alternative approaches will likely be needed to enable the child to be a full participant in sports and recreational activities.

Prosthetic options include the use of traditional body powered prostheses, manufactured specialty products or custom-made solutions. Body-powered prostheses, particularly the voluntary-closing systems, can be very useful. They offer a number of positive benefits including durability, speed of activation and variable grip strength. Unfortunately, children accustomed to wearing self-suspended myoelectric prostheses are often unwilling to accept the need to wear harness and cable systems even though they may provide functional advantages for certain activities that they wish to engage in. In some cases neither the body-powered nor the myoelectric prostheses are of benefit for a chosen activity and a specialized terminal device is required.

There are a number of commercially available terminal devices for clients with upper-extremity amputations or limb deficiencies. Although the majority of these devices have been designed for the adult population there are a few options that can be of benefit to children. One of the best examples is the TRS Super Sport/ Freeflex device [25] (made of soft, flexible, tough elastic polymer and shaped like a cupped hand). It is particularly useful for gymnastics and ball sports (see Fig. 6.29).

In many cases, a commercial product is not available that fulfills the child's needs and it becomes necessary to make a custom device. The activity itself

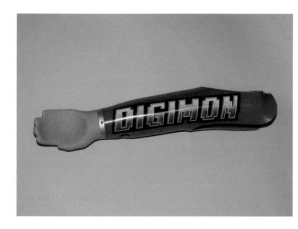

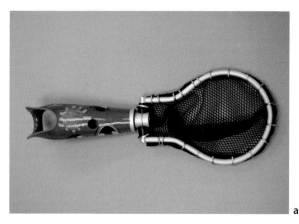

a

Figure 6.29
TRS Free Flex TD

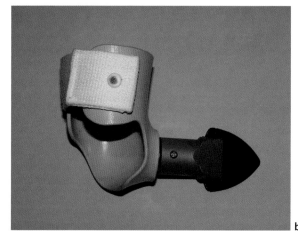

b

must be studied and the needs of the device considered [16]. For example, a hockey device is required to be strong and resilient, whereas a violin attachment needs to be lightweight and more delicate. Innovative problem-solving and engineering support can make it possible to fabricate a variety of special devices (Figs. 6.30 a–c). For example, equipment has been designed and fitted for sports and recreational activities such as hockey, ball catching, weight lifting, golf, fishing and skiing. Musical instrument adaptations include devices for piano, trumpet, guitar, drums and violin. Many of these devices are now commercially available by special order [17].

As children grow into adulthood, their needs become more focussed. They may not require as many different devices but demands and expectations for performance will be higher (Figs. 6.31 a–c). Teenagers can be very competitive and small changes can make a significant difference. Articles by Anderson [1] and Radocy [16] are recommended for further reading on this topic.

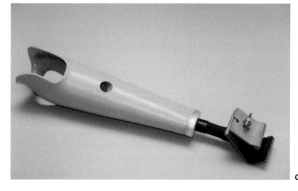

c

Figure 6.30 a–c
a Ball catching net. b Guitar pick. c Weight-lifting device

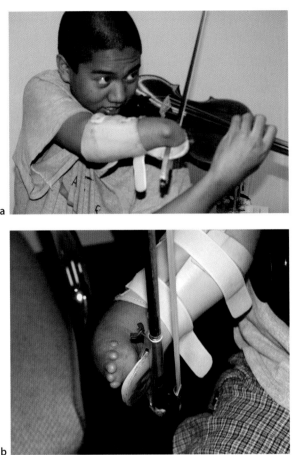

a

b

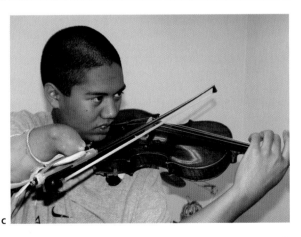

c

Figure 6.31 a–c

Individual using spatula to play a violin

6.7 Chapter Summary

The fitting of a myoelectric prosthesis is a complex partnership between client, family and team. A successful outcome is dependent on a host of dynamic interdependent factors that must continually be reviewed and acknowledged as the process develops. The client's own life circumstance (congenital/acquired, age, developmental stage, residual limb function, family dynamics, psychosocial and socio-cultural factors) as well as the treatment team's experience and expertise, must interact successfully to produce a dynamic, challenging and ultimately satisfying outcome.

The major appeal of a myoelectric prosthesis for a child is its natural appearance. Other advantages include the superior grip strength of the electric hands, ease of control, reduced energy expenditure, the lack of harness and control cables and the ability to operate the limb in any position [3]. Disadvantages include the cost, inability to use the prosthesis in sand/water situations, durability (gloves in particular) and the limited hand opening size of the smaller hands. Further research and development is needed to improve the electric hand's prehensile capability to produce a glove that is both durable and stain-resistant, to miniaturize components further, to decrease overall weight and to seal systems in order to allow children to engage in water/sand play activities.

Options for children with high level or bilateral limb loss are still insufficient to meet their needs. Multifunctional control of lightweight components that have multiple degrees of freedom are required to improve the functionality of electromechanical devices for this population.

Also, the rising cost of health care is becoming an important concern in all countries. Because there is no documented evidence of benefit of myoelectric fittings, controversy exists as to the appropriateness of providing such expensive technology, especially to young growing children. Although it is believed that early fitting is conducive to prosthetic acceptance and skill and that a cosmetic prosthesis contributes to enhanced self-image and improved self-esteem, these hypotheses have not been demonstrated empirically

[3, 6, 9, 11, 28]. Clinicians must provide scientific evidence that myoprosthetic practice is effective and essential. Empirically-based outcome assessments/measurements are needed to assess and compare practices, to determine the predictors for acceptance and use and to measure the functional and psychosocial benefits of prosthetic use.

6.8 Questions

1. Why is paediatric practice considered a specialty?
2. Name the three types of upper-extremity prosthetic components that can be activated electrically?
3. What are the advantages of external versus internal batteries in a powered, upper-extremity prosthesis?
4. What are the different components of a powered upper-extremity prosthetic control system?
5. Under what circumstances would you select a single-site control system for a client?
6. Why might you select a digital control system over a proportional control system for your client?
7. What are the advantages of a THDSS socket?
8. Give three reasons for using a non-powered upper-extremity prosthesis?

Acknowledgements. This chapter is dedicated to the memory of William Sauter, pioneer, advocate and innovator in myoprosthetic practice, mentor, colleague and friend.

References

1. Anderson T (1998) The limb deficient child. In: Herring J, Birch J (eds) AAOS/Shrine Symposium: the limb deficient child. American Academy of Orthopaedic Surgeons, Rosemont, IL, pp 345–352
2. Billock JN (1972) The Northwestern University supracondylar suspension technique for below elbow amputations. Orthot Prosthet 26(4):16–23
3. Brenner CD (1992) Electronic limbs for infants and preschool children. J Prosthet Orthot 4:24–30
4. Clark M, Atkins D, Hubbard S, Patton J, Shaperman J (1998) Prosthetic devices for children with bilateral upper limb deficiencies: when, and if, pros and cons. In: Herring J, Birch J (eds) AAOS/Shrine Symposium: the limb deficient child. American Academy of Orthopaedic Surgeons, Rosemont, IL, pp 397–404
5. Exner CE (1989) Development of hand functions. In: Occupational therapy for children, 2nd edn. CV Mosby, Toronto, pp 235–244
6. Fisk J (1992) Introduction to the child amputee. In: Bowker JH, Michael JW (eds) Atlas of limb prosthetics: surgical, prosthetic and rehabilitation principles 2nd edn. Mosby-Year Book, St. Louis, MO, pp 731–734
7. Hosmer Dorrance Corporation, 561 Division Street, Cambell California, USA 95008–6905
8. Hubbard S (1991) Prosthetic considerations: pre and school-age children. In: VASI manual. Variety Abilities Systems Inc., Toronto, Ontario, Sect. 2.1–2.2
9. Hubbard S, Kurtz I, Heim W, Montgomery G (1998) Powered prosthetic intervention in upper extremity deficiency. In: Herring J, Birch J (eds) AAOS/Shrine Symposium: the limb deficient child. American Academy of Orthopaedic Surgeons, Rosemont, IL, pp 417–431
10. Kay H, Hartmann G, Cody K, Casella D (1965) A Fabrication manual for the muenster type below elbow prosthesis. Prosthetics and Orthotics Research Division, School of Engineering and Science, New York University, New York
11. Krebs D, Edelstein J, Thornby M (1991) Prosthetic management of children with limb deficiencies. Phys Ther 71:920–34
12. Liberating Technologies Inc. 325 Hopping Brook Road, Suite A, Holliston, Massachusetts, USA 01746–1456
13. Novotny M, Swagman A (1992) Caring for children with orthotic/prosthetic needs. J Prosthet Orthot 4 (4):191–195
14. Otto Bock Health Care GmbH Business Units Orthopedic Industry Max-Nader-Str. 15 37114 Duderstadt Germany
15. Patton J (1989) Developmental approach to pediatric prosthetic evaluation and training. In: Atkins DJ, Meier RH (eds) Comprehensive management of the upper limb amputee. Springer, Berlin Heidelberg New York, pp 99–120
16. Radocy B (1987) Upper-extremity prosthetics:considerations and designs for sports and recreation. Clin Prosthet Orthot 11(3):131–153

17. Rehabilitation Engineering Department: Mechanical Services, Bloorview MacMillan Children's Centre, 350 Rumsey Rd., Toronto, Ontario

18. RSL Steeper Riverside Orthopaedic Centre, 51 Riverside, Medway City Estate, Rochester, Kent ME24C, UK

19. Sauter W (1981) Myoelectric and Microswitch upper extremity prostheses. In: Kostuik J, Gillespie R (eds) Amputation surgery and rehabilitation: the Toronto experience. Churchill Livingstone, New York, pp 367–383

20. Sauter W (1986) A 3/4 type below-elbow socket for myoelectric prostheses. Prosthet Orthot Int 10:79–82

21. Sauter W, Dakpa R, Galway R, Hubbard S, Hamilton E (1987) The development of layered "onionized" silicone sockets for juvenile below-elbow amputees. J Prosthet Orthot 22(3):57–59

22. Sauter W (1991) Powered upper extremity prosthetics programme: Current clinical practice. In: Rehabilitation Engineering Annual Report, Hugh MacMillan Rehabilitation Centre, Toronto, pp 36–43

23. Setoguchi Y (1991) The management of the limb deficient child and its family. Prosthet Orthot Int 15:78–81

24. Sorbye R (1989) Upper extremity amputees: Swedish experience concerning children. In: Atkins DJ, Meier RH (eds) Comprehensive management of the upper limb amputee. Springer, Berlin Heidelberg New York, pp 227–239

25. Therapeutic Recreation Systems Inc (TRS) 3090 Sterling Circle, Studio A, Boulder, CO 80301, USA

26. USMC 180 N. San Gabriel Blvd. Pasadena, CA 91107 USA

27. Variety Ability Systems Inc.(VASI) 2 Kelvin Avenue, Unit 3, Toronto, Ontario, Canada M4C 5C8

28. Varni J, Pruitt S, Seid M (1998) Health-related quality of life in pediatric limb deficiency. In: Herring J, Birch J (eds) AAOS/Shrine Symposium: the limb deficient child. American Academy of Orthopaedic Surgeons, Rosemont, IL, pp 457–470

Powered Upper Limb Prosthetics in Adults

R. D. Alley · H. H. Sears

Contents

Summary

This chapter will discuss pre- and post-delivery assessment methodologies, rehabilitation strategies, prosthetic componentry, interface design and system application for adults requiring powered upper limb prosthetic intervention. The aim of this chapter is to familiarize the reader with the many facets of upper limb prosthetic care, allowing the clinician to expand his or her cache of available strategies with which to ensure the success of the individual in need of prosthetic intervention.

7.1 Introduction

Truly a specialized blend of art and science, the field of upper extremity prosthetics demands a great depth and breadth of knowledge in order to maximize a patient's rehabilitation potential. Yet this specialized field offers limited opportunities in which interested clinicians can obtain such experience. This is a direct result of not only the relatively small number of individuals requiring upper limb prosthetic intervention but also of the limited number of these individuals who *pursue* such intervention. It is estimated that the typical practitioner cares for an average of one to two individuals with upper limb loss or amelia per year and many clinicians see even less. Indeed, in the author's view, the difficulty in the utilization of electrically powered upper extremity prostheses stems not from inadequate technology but rather from a lack of familiarity with the proper and selective use of such technology. The misconception, held by some, that functional outcome comparisons between cable-operated systems and electrically pow-

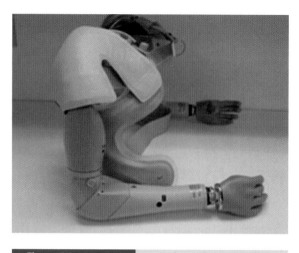

Figure 7.1

Bilateral myoelectric shoulder disarticulation system

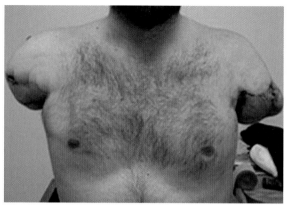

Figure 7.2

Individual with bilateral high level amputations

ered systems, for example, can be ascertained without proper consideration of applied assessment methodologies, practitioner experience, the degree and character of family support and the richness and range of rehabilitation strategies among other critical factors, is inappropriate. In the author's opinion, for this and a variety of other reasons, there were many inherent flaws in earlier comparison studies on usage and success rates of electrically powered upper limb prostheses (Fig. 7.1).

Another critical aspect concerning upper extremity prosthetics is the degree to which its approach and application differ from that of lower extremity prosthetic care.

The prevalence of adverse psychological and psychosocial issues inherent in the individual with upper limb loss and even amelia is typically far greater than in those who have lower limb involvement. The majority of upper limb amputations are secondary to trauma, whereas the majority of lower limb losses are related to issues of inadequate circulation. The abrupt loss of an upper limb results in either a complete absence or at best a severe degradation of the preoperative stage, impeding the psychological preparation usually present with a prolonged illness and

subsequent elective surgery for the amputation of a lower limb. For this reason alone, the psychological impact is usually much more severe in the traumatic and sudden loss of an upper limb. Add to this the fact that upper limb loss is visually more apparent and the appearance of the limb is often aesthetically unpleasant due to the effect of trauma (Fig. 7.2).

It is imperative then, that the rehabilitation team members consider the impact of all of the relevant issues in developing their strategy and that during the evaluation, which typically marks the initial contact with the patient, significant attention is given to psychological and psychosocial support.

7.2 Pre-prosthetic Assessment

Perhaps the most critical aspect of the evaluative process is the knowledge that even individuals with similar levels of amputation or amelia have different interests, needs and desires and hence each requires a unique methodology in precipitating prosthetic success. It is indeed not enough for the clinician to be armed with this knowledge but rather to implement it within a framework based on careful and comprehensive assessment of those specific factors that will lend themselves to the individual's adoption of an optimal rehabilitation strategy. Many successful outcomes hinge more significantly on the initial assessment and the subsequent care plan than they do on the level of limb loss or the type of prosthetic control used.

There are differing thoughts surrounding the use of electrically powered prostheses experienced by some of the prosthetists in clinical practice today. When evaluating an individual requiring upper limb prosthetic intervention, it is imperative that the clinician is familiar with not only the physical characteristics and properties of upper limb prosthetic systems and componentry but the operational parameters as well as the inherent advantages and limitations of each. This knowledge and its dissemination to the patient during the assessment will help lay the foundation for a rehabilitation strategy tailored to the individual's needs and desires and allows the patient's active participation in its development. Although each individual assessment must be personalized, it is crucial that some standardization of the assessment methodology exist in order to create a correlation between the evaluation and prosthetic outcomes. This is especially significant when considering electrically powered applications, as the data concerning successful utilization of these control systems for adults is generally limited. As mentioned previously, psychological issues are extremely prevalent in upper limb cases, most significantly with adult traumatic amputations. It is therefore essential that a bond is first established between the prosthetist and patient.

After the establishment of a positive relationship, the next phase of the assessment should center around the clinician becoming acquainted with the individual's specific needs and desires. These should be based on factors including, but not limited to, medical history, previous prosthetic history (if applicable), past, present and future vocational requirements and avocational desires, prior, current and anticipated activity level with and without prosthetic utilization as well as any and all extenuating psychological and psychosocial considerations (Fig. 7.3). Enough time should be taken here in order to allow

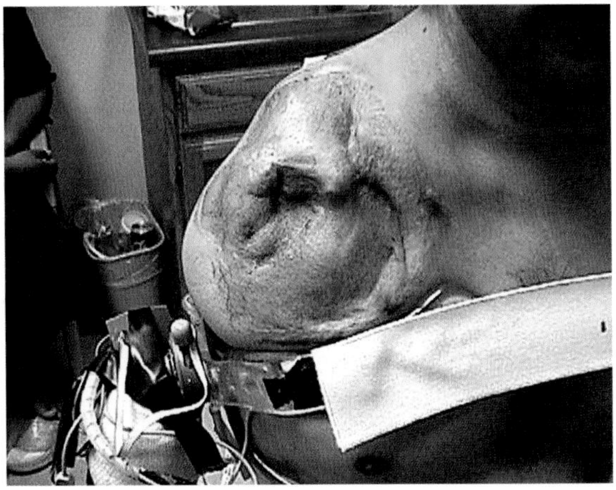

Figure 7.3
Severe shoulder trauma

an in-depth understanding of where the patient has been physically and mentally, where he or she is currently, and where the individual would like to be and in what time frame. This phase of pre-prosthetic assessment revolves around the clinician becoming educated about the patient. The next phase, education of the patient, is an important aspect of the assessment. It is also perhaps the most significant in its relationship to successful outcomes, for without it the patient relies solely on the evaluating prosthetist to decide the methodology and system(s) to be utilized. Without an adequate understanding of available technology and the processes intrinsic in prosthetic provision, the patient is restricted in the ability to contribute to his or her overall rehabilitation strategy. This patient involvement increases the odds of identifying optimum prosthetic pathways that could achieve success.

It is vital then, that the evaluation consist of a detailed discussion of the inherent advantages and limitations of each available prosthetic option. The patient's rehabilitation level, lifestyle requirements and personal issues can be extremely dynamic and it is important to discuss options applicable to this particular evaluation, which is a snapshot in the individual's life at a critical point. Although a detailed de-

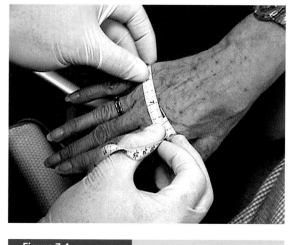

Figure 7.4

Critical measurement during evaluation

7.3 Prosthetic Options

For the patient to gain an understanding about whether or not an electrically powered prosthesis is appropriate, it is essential that the evaluating prosthetist discuss not only the physical attributes of such a system but what its functional parameters are and how they compare to and contrast with other types of prostheses. In order to do this most effectively, the clinician should feel confident with his or her ability to discuss, in detail, the entire range of options available. What follows will be a brief analysis of non-electric options relegated to specific references on how they differ from externally powered systems (Figs. 7.6).

It must first be realized that not wearing a prosthesis is an option. For many years the prosthetic community regarded a successful fitting as one in which the patient wore the prosthesis on a regular basis and for extended periods of time throughout each day. It should be understood that some individuals simply utilize their prosthesis only when they absolutely require it in order to assist with an activity. If the prosthesis effectively fulfills this role when tasked, even if called upon rarely, then it should be considered a successful strategy. In this regard, a practitioner should understand the reasons one might have for not wearing a prosthesis frequently. Issues which are not unique to externally powered prostheses are the individual having an unsatisfactory first experience, a lack of knowledge about available options, and no or minimal gain in functional advantage with utilization of a prosthesis.

Discomfort is certainly a significant reason for an individual to not wear a prosthesis. More specific to externally powered systems, the added weight of electric components can cause discomfort in those areas responsible for bearing it. In addition, this weight combined with the torque produced during operation of an electric elbow, for example, requires a stable frame and the inherent intimacy that is typically required for stability. This increased intimacy usually results in an interface with greater contact pressures in those areas responsible for preventing rotational instability. Furthermore, a larger "footprint" in

scription of specific evaluation techniques unique to each level of limb loss or amelia is outside the scope of this chapter, it is important to note that differences in the approach one should take to each level of limb absence do exist. For simplicity's sake, however, we will discuss certain universal aspects of pre-prosthetic assessment that apply to most, if not all, individuals requiring powered upper extremity prostheses (Fig. 7.4).

Although we will first look at the physical characteristics of both the individual and the prosthetic systems themselves that lead to establishing the efficacy of the utilization of electric power, it is important to note that when evaluating an individual it is best to have a clear understanding of the indications and contraindications inherent in the psychological and psychosocial environment as well. Put more simply, it is not enough to confer the suitability of an electrically powered prosthesis based on simple limb length or the availability of sufficient EMG signals. This is because the goal of prosthetic intervention is not merely adequate operation, but rather successful, sustained *utilization* of the prosthesis, and this demands a much more careful analysis of all the factors which may be relevant in determining such an outcome (Fig. 7.5).

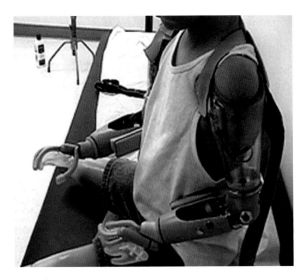

Figure 7.5

Common humeral hybrid configuration

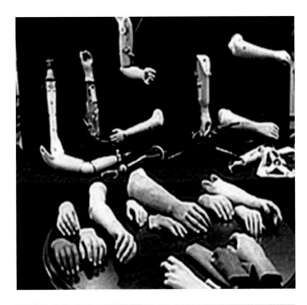

Figure 7.6

Miscellaneous UE componentry

contact with the skin is usually required and hence heat dissipation becomes a major concern, particularly in those individuals with higher levels of involvement where the ability to dissipate heat is more greatly affected.

Another strong reason for an individual to choose not to wear a prosthesis involves the loss of tactile sensation experienced with wearing a prosthesis, particularly with those individuals who have retained the ability to use their residual limb adequately for assistance and rely on their sense of touch to successfully perform certain functions. This is especially true when working with the blind or with an individual whose sight is limited and must rely much more heavily on their other senses in order to cope with their environment.

Finally, although an electrically controlled prosthesis can assist in increasing an individual's functional envelope, there may be many cases in which the interface actually restricts their physical range of motion and this restriction is severe enough or causes enough discomfort to warrant not wearing it.

The idea of discussing the advantages of not wearing a prosthesis with a patient during the initial evaluation may be thought of as controversial but if an accurate description of expectations is to be given, then it is imperative to include this discussion in the assessment.

A passive (inactive prehension or semi-prehensile) prosthesis often compares favorably to an electrically powered system in the areas of weight, cosmesis and cost, (although silicone cosmetic coverings can add a significant amount of weight and cost to a passive prosthesis), both in terms of initial outlay as well as maintenance. The most significant functional limitations of passive prostheses are their lack of active prehension and pinch force, although some designs enable limited pinch with manipulation of passive digits for example (Fig. 7.7).

As stated previously, the most common comparisons are made between cable-operated prostheses and electrically powered systems. Cable-operated prostheses typically cost less initially and require fewer funds to be set aside for maintenance and repair. The nature of most cable-operated hook prehensors allows greater visibility during the reaching,

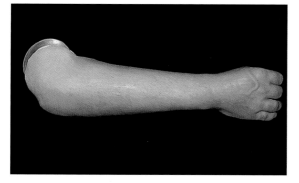

Figure 7.7

Passive (semi-prehensile) prosthesis

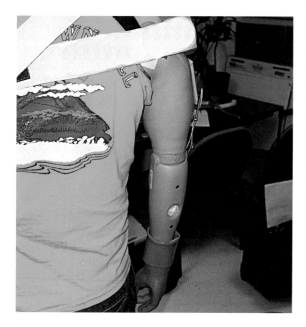

Figure 7.8

Cable-driven humeral prosthesis

acquiring and manipulative phases of small objects. It is important to note, however, that the cost of this greater visibility is a reduction in prehensile contact area, which can be a great disadvantage when manipulating certain shapes or materials.

A significant advantage of cable operation is its ability to provide feedback to the user. The advantage to the user of being able to sense the position of the terminal device in space or the degree to which it is open or closed can be tremendous. It should, however, be noted that feedback, particularly with experienced users, is a property of electrically powered systems as well. This feedback is delivered to the user through vibrations created by the running motor in the hand, wrist or elbow and by sound when the motor stalls at the end of its component's range of motion (in addition to any inherent feedback mechanisms supplied by the manufacturer(s) of system components to signal a mode switch such as that between hand and wrist operation, for example) A time component can also be measured by the experienced user, as he or she knows the opening or closing speed of their prehensor, for example, in digital systems (and in proportional systems, provided the prehensor is moving at maximum velocity or the user is familiar with gauging muscle effort to prehensor speed). Feedback of this nature is limited to active operation of the electrical components and apart from kinesthetic proprioception in the human limb available to users of all options; it is the feedback from the cable that, in many cases uniquely provides positioning information while components are static (Fig. 7.8).

These mechanical devices are more environmentally resistant, provide kinesthetic and proprioceptive feedback and in almost every case, weigh significantly less than their electrical counterparts. The one exception to this occurs in pediatric myoelectric prostheses utilizing the Otto Bock System 2000 hand, often weighing about the same as a comparable cable-driven design.

When comparing a cable-operated elbow to an electrically powered one, it is almost always found that an individual is capable of generating greater flexion velocities by utilizing cable control. This characteristic can range from being mildly advantageous to absolutely critical depending on either the individual or situation.

Cable-operated systems are devoid of the need for battery maintenance, installation and removal as well as any requirement for activation or deactivation (powering up or down), all of which can demand increased dexterity and cognitive function.

There are also significant disadvantages to be found when comparing a cable-operated system to electrical systems. In general in the cable-operated system, pinch force is drastically reduced. Functional range of motion, particularly when compared to myoelectric systems, is typically reduced, primarily due to the nature of gross body movement and its relation to harness design. The harness required to operate a cable-controlled prosthesis is generally more restrictive and uncomfortable. This is because it is usually required to not only suspend and control the prosthesis but is often required to stabilize it as well. As the axilla is often used as an anchor point for the harness, nerve entrapment syndrome is frequently prevalent in varying degrees, resulting in tingling and numbness in the contralateral hand (if present) and in severe cases, may even require surgical intervention. An excellent way around this problem is demonstrated with the "vertically arrayed dual ring" harness. Developed as an improvement over both the Northwestern Ring harness and the horizontally arrayed dual ring harness, Fig. 7.10 shows how the control strap is maintained in an inferior alignment for increased efficiency. In unilateral applications, the axilla anchor angle is opened up considerably to reduce axillary compression. The author further suggests that tabs are placed on each ring to deter rotation, further increasing efficiency. Cable-operated prostheses, even those with hand prehensors, have poor static and dynamic cosmesis. In addition, the gross body movement required to operate not only cable-operated systems but all commercially available non-myoelectric prostheses results in atrophy of muscle and other soft tissue within and around the encapsulated limb. Myoelectric control almost always requires the activation of intrinsic muscle (muscle within the prosthesis), hence maintaining and even improving mus-

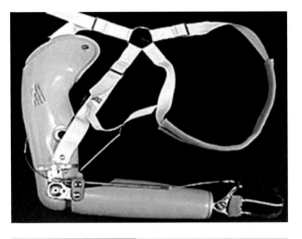

Figure 7.9
Cable-driven humeral prosthesis

cle condition within the limb as well as improving circulation and the health of associated soft tissue (Fig. 7.9).

Gross body movement utilized in cable-operated prostheses often requires more energy expenditure than activation of intrinsic musculature via myoelectric control or in cases where less of it is required for control of other externally powered systems. This is extremely important to the elderly, to individuals whose energy capacity has been reduced by medications or disease and for those individuals who simply dislike expending energy to a significant degree.

A related yet often overlooked aspect of gross body movement regarding acquired limb loss is its almost complete disassociation from any correlation between the muscular system and neural network utilized for prosthetic action and those initially involved prior to amputation. This is of great importance, not only for growing girls and boys, whose neural networks are undergoing significant development but also to adults, where it has been shown that these networks are dynamic and respond in a similar fashion to muscles, which follow the S.A.I.D. (specific adaptations to imposed demands) principle. Myoelectric control typically ensures at least some stimulation occurs via pathways established prior to amputation, even if the trauma or subsequent surgery has altered it significantly.

A hybrid prosthesis, the most common configuration being the utilization of a cable-operated elbow and an electric prehensor, fits neatly between a conventional prosthesis and a fully electric system and incorporates the advantages and disadvantages of both types of control (Fig. 7.11).

Similar to a more conventional design, the hybrid system almost always requires a control harness, an exception occurring when ballistic movement is used to flex the elbow, as can be achieved in some cases with the Otto Bock "Ergo" elbow. All of the disadvantages that typically accompany the use of a control harness as described above apply to the hybrid system; however, because the prehensor is commonly electric, the control strap can be less restrictive as it is incorporated for elbow flexion alone. Nevertheless, it is important to note that because of the additional weight of an electric prehensor, it does place an additional load on the harness, although this is usually not enough to offset the advantage gained by not having to control a mechanical hook.

The weight of a hybrid system is greater than a conventional prosthesis in nearly every case, again the exception being the use of an ultralight terminal device, such as the System 2000.

The hybrid system, as it incorporates electric components, is more susceptible than a conventional prosthesis to environmental hazards as well as the shock incurred by impact with the ground or other objects.

The cost of a hybrid is invariably greater than a cable-operated system, both in terms of initial cost and maintenance.

Because of its similarities to a fully electrical system, the hybrid enjoys many of the advantages inherent with electric control, namely increased pinch force and functional envelope as well as a reduced harness involvement. Its utilization of a cable-driven elbow (the most common configuration) results in the wearer being able to experience and utilize feedback, increased elbow flexion velocity, reduced initial and maintenance costs of a fully powered system and reduced weight, again with respect to a fully powered system.

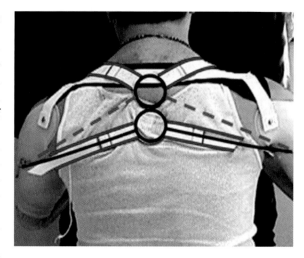

Figure 7.10

Vertically arrayed dual ring harness

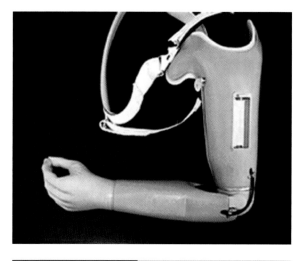

Figure 7.11

Humeral hybrid prosthesis with ballistic elbow

A unique characteristic of the hybrid not commonly realized with either cable-operated or fully electric control is its ability to provide synergistic operation of both elbow and hand.* This allows the user to adjust the opening width of the hand, for example, while simultaneously positioning the hand in space, more closely imitating the human grasping process.

Because comparisons have been made previously between cable-operation and electric power, only a brief summary of the advantages and disadvantages will be made here. The fully electrically powered prosthesis possesses increased pinch force, increased functional envelope, improved static and dynamic cosmesis over that of both a cable-operated hook and hand and enlarged contact area for prehension. Two unique advantages with respect to all other options are that the prosthetic action typically requires the least amount of energy expenditure and in myoelectric systems, a control strap or cable for prehensor or elbow operation is not required. This allows the prosthetist to utilize only what is needed for suspension and/or stability, freeing the user from restrictive harnessing which can be uncomfortable and may lead to nerve damage.

Additional advantages of myoelectric control are that the terminal devices can be both voluntary opening and voluntary closing, the limb used for input is healthier due to increased circulation and muscle activity or tone, significant gross body movement is seldom required and prosthetic control more closely resembles natural body motions and/or functions.

The disadvantages are its initial and maintenance costs, weight and its distribution, limited feedback as described earlier, additional cognitive demands and battery maintenance issues (Fig. 7.12).

The final option to be discussed is the adaptive prosthesis, also referred to as recreational or, more correctly, activity-specific, as not all designs are intended for recreational use. This type of prosthesis is expressly designed for a particular activity, and pos-

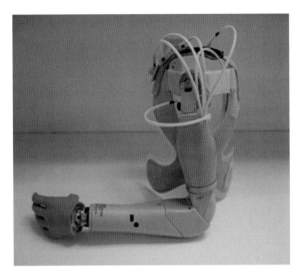

Figure 7.12

Myoelectric thoracic prosthesis with flexion wrist

sesses unique advantages and limitations. Where other options are incapable of or at least inadequate in fulfilling a particular role as a result of their more general functional scope, the adaptive prosthesis inherently provides the user with improved performance of the task it was intended for due to its specific nature. As well, this narrow scope results in the adaptive prosthesis often utilizing minimal componentry, as in a swimming prosthesis for example and this commonly results in reduced complexity and cost. It should be noted that this is certainly not always the case of course, as certain tasks may require an extremely complex terminal device or other component to achieve success, requiring many hours of specialized labor or extensive use of costly materials.

The principal disadvantage of the adaptive prosthesis is a direct result of its functional specificity, namely that adequate functional capability outside of its design specifications is greatly reduced or eliminated. In those countries where medical justification is required for provider reimbursement of costs associated with fabrication and delivery of such a device, it is often difficult to gain authorization or to be guaranteed payment.

---

* Recently, fully powered systems have been introduced by several manufacturers that allow simultaneous control of elbow and hand or wrist.

7.4 Components

7.4.1 Externally Powered Components for the Upper Limb Prosthesis

7.4.1.1 Hands and Work Hands (Terminal Devices)

It goes without saying that the primary function of the arm prosthesis is provided by the hand or, the more general term, the Terminal Device (TD), which encompasses any device attached at the hand position. The other joints of the prosthesis function, for the most part, to position the TD in space, for grasp, pushing or pulling, or even gesturing. Electric hands are available from several manufacturers at the present time and we shall describe the general features, without being specific to a particular manufacturer. A list of manufacturers is available at the end of the chapter, with sources for more information.

7.4.1.2 Pinch Force

The adult size electric hand offers the technical advantage of motorized drive of the fingers, which is capable in most versions, of producing very high pinch forces (20–25 lb. force at the finger tips) even higher than most natural hands are capable of generating. This gives the prosthetic hand the ability of gripping most objects very securely, even if they lack the compliance of a natural hand, i.e., the ability of the fingers to curl around an object. No prosthetic hand is available commercially which implements compliant gripping, as yet, although it has been the focus of several research hands in the past.

7.4.1.3 Weight

Unfortunately, the choice of a high-pinch force hand has, in the past, required a sacrifice in weight of the TD. The electric hands with 20+ lbs. pinch force weigh close to one pound, which is a heavy weight concentration at the end of the forearm. At the present time, lighter weight alternatives are beginning to be available, by configuring the drive of the hand in a smaller package, so the proximal quick disconnect can be eliminated, reducing the weight by approximately 30%. Other models of electric hands have been offered which simplify the drive unit, sacrificing the high pinch force for a lighter hand, reducing the weight of an adult hand to approximately 12 oz. but offering only 10 lb. of pinch force.

7.4.1.4 Work Hands

The use of a quick disconnect attachment system makes it possible for an electric arm wearer to use a variety of devices interchangeably. It is even possible for an electric arm wearer to use a body-powered TD, attaching a control cable with the rugged hook, to use in a dirty work situation, for instance. The electric work hands are available in several different varieties, some designed like a robot's end effector, some providing the same slender and lightweight shapes of a body-powered terminal device (see (Fig. 7.13)

7.4.1.5 Cosmetic/Protective Covers

The availability of highly realistic silicone and PVC covers has aided the adoption of electric prostheses, by allowing a natural looking hand. The cover complements the more naturally operated prosthesis, eliminating the external control cables and harness. The highest quality covers are typically made of silicone materials, which can be fabricated in layers, allowing natural coloring to simulate the opposite hand as well as the patient's skin tone and hair. The silicone materials also have the advantage that inks and fabric dyes do not stain the glove, as they do the more ordinary PVC materials. Silicone covers are becoming more widely available and at lower cost as time goes on. Improved PVC materials, which are stronger and less expensive than the silicone, are also being developed. New coatings for the PVC may offer a solution to their biggest drawback, the tendency to stain from contact with inks and newsprint.

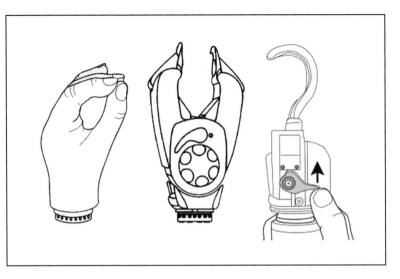

Figure 7.13

Interchangeable Terminal Device options allow the electric arm wearer to use the more natural-looking hand in public situations, and a mechanical-looking tool for more rugged tasks and hobbies

7.4.1.6 Electric Wrist Rotation

Since the advent of easily controlled and convenient control systems, electric wrist rotation is utilized in a high proportion of the electric arm prosthesis fittings in the U.S. and Canada (estimated 30–40% of myoelectric fittings). Surveys of electric wrist wearers show that the feature is highly utilized, by both unilateral and bilateral wearers. For bilateral prosthesis wearers, the added degree of freedom is important in a wide range of activities, for both prepositioning the TD for optimal gripping but also for actively turning an object after gripping in the TD. Unilateral amputees also utilize the wrist rotator a great deal more than expected, especially for prepositioning when the sound hand is being used to carry an object, or similar task. The wearer can easily reposition the TD using the electric wrist rotator, without requiring the sound hand (Fig. 7.14).

In transhumeral cases, the electric wrist has also been utilized a great deal, again due to greater convenience of recent control innovations. In a fully electric system, wrist rotation can be easily utilized by the high level amputee by means of a toggle switch which transfers control between hand and electric wrist with a bump switch or simple pull switch.

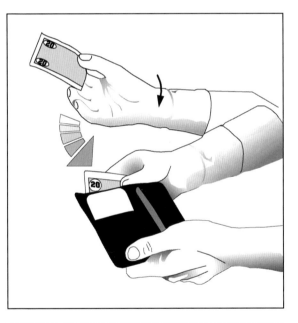

Figure 7.14

Electric wrist rotation is frequently utilized by unilateral as well as bilateral amputee's prostheses. The wearer can easily reposition the wrist, to preposition, or to actively rotate while performing a task

7.4.1.7 Wrist Flexion

Recently electric hands have become available which integrate wrist flexion into the hand mechanism, either with a lock (allowing prepositioning) or with a spring return (which does not allow prepositioning). Long recognized as an important degree of freedom in an arm prosthesis, flexion wrists allow greater ability to position the hand for optimal prehension. For example, carrying a tray at a horizontal position is awkward without the ability to flex the wrist. Also prehension close to the midline is made much less awkward with flexion integrated into the hand. Tying shoes, holding a clipboard, carrying loads in the hand more comfortably, are all tasks cited as more convenient with wrist flexion (Fig. 7.15).

7.4.1.8 Electronic Controllers

The actual electronic controller for the electric hand or TD may be installed in either of two locations: inside the hand, or outside of the hand. Typically, controllers installed inside the hand are supplied by the hand manufacturer. Suppliers of electric hands include Otto Bock, Motion Control, VASI, RSLSteeper Ltd., and Centri. The out of hand controller usually is an aftermarket product, chosen for features which are not found in the hand manufacturer's in hand product. Notable suppliers of aftermarket controllers are Motion Control, VASI, and Animated Systems, Inc.

To summarize the pros and cons of each: In-hand controllers are integrated with the manufacturers TD, so are more compact but may only control a single device, namely the TD. A price saving may also be had for the in-hand system. Out-of-hand controllers are capable of operating any of the interchangeable TD's as well as the electric wrist. In this case a cost saving may be had since only one controller is purchased for three or four devices. Special purpose controllers like these may offer greater versatility also, e.g., some can operate on a variety of battery voltages, giving the patient the capability of higher voltage supplies or the ability to use a disposable battery while traveling.

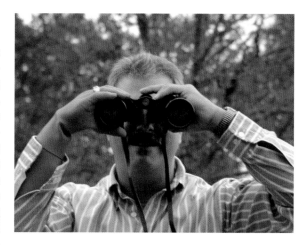

Figure 7.15

Wrist flexion allows the TD to be repositioned for optimal gripping. Holding binoculars is a good example of an ordinary task which would be awkward without the additional degree of freedom. Another type of wrist flexion is termed "FlexiWrist", which defines a compliant wrist joint, which can bend against a spring. This allows the wrist to reposition itself, in reaction to the forces pushing against the hand (or the object being held). This allows more optimal holding, although it does not allow prepositioning in flexion, as would units with a solid lock joint

7.4.1.9 Proportional Versus Digital Control

Early myoelectric control systems were capable of opening or closing the TD at only a single speed. This type of control has been called "digital control" because the TD is either fully on or off. The trans-radial wearer opens the hand by generating an EMG signal above threshold on the extensor muscle, or closes by generating an EMG signal on the flexor muscle.

Proportional controllers, now adopted by all manufacturers, allow the wearer to vary the speed of the TD (or other device) proportionate to the strength of the muscle contraction, as measured by the EMG. A proportional system also allows the wearer to vary the pinch force much more precisely than would be possible with the ON-OFF simplicity of the digital controller (Fig. 7.16).

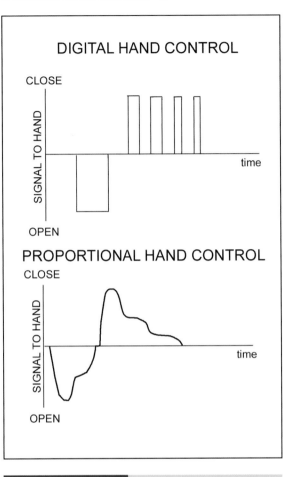

DIGITAL HAND CONTROL

CLOSE

SIGNAL TO HAND

time

OPEN

PROPORTIONAL HAND CONTROL

CLOSE

SIGNAL TO HAND

time

OPEN

Figure 7.16

Proportional controllers allow the power to the hand to be varied smoothly, proportionate to the EMG (or effort) generated by the opening or closing control muscle

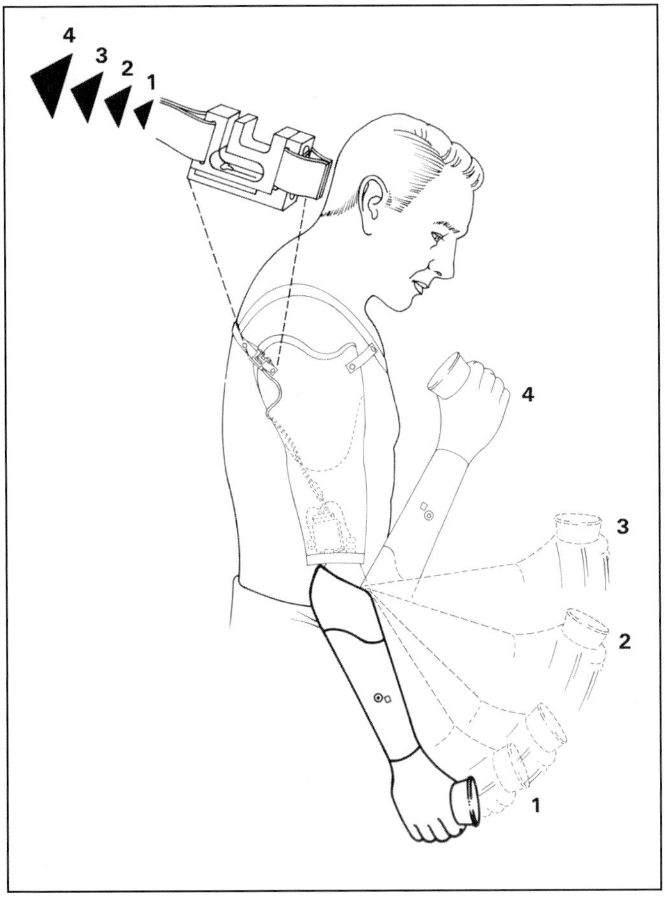

Figure 7.17

When muscle EMG signals are not available, a sensor may be installed in the harness, such as the Force Sensor pictured here, which provides hand power proportional to the level of force pulling on the sensor

Non-myoelectric control systems are also an option via most of these manufacturers. When a patient has not yet developed the muscle strength required for good EMG control, several options are available, including force sensors, linear potentiometers, touch pads (which all can control the TD proportionally) or, of course, a simple pull-switch or push-switch (which would only provide ON-OFF control, not proportional) (Fig. 7.17).

7.4.1.10 Elbow Components

Transhumeral (above the elbow) fittings with electric components may be thought of in two different basic types: Hybrid prostheses, or all electric components. Hybrid prostheses, by definition, would have some body powered components and some electric components, e.g., most commonly electric TD and body powered elbow but the combination of electric elbow with body-powered TD might also be clinically useful. To summarize pros and cons: Hybrid transhumeral prostheses would offer the advantages of somewhat lower cost and the appealing feature of simultaneous control of elbow and hand, so long as the wearer can coordinate the two control methods for the elbow and hand. In the most common hybrid, this would require control of the elbow control cable (usually by scapular abduction) simultaneous with control over biceps and triceps EMG signals. When loads must be held up by the forearm, the lock must also be actuated by pulling a separate cable, usually harnessed to shoulder depression.

Obviously, the disadvantage of the hybrid prosthesis at this level of amputation, is that two actions of the prosthesis must still be cable operated, thus limiting the work envelope within which the elbow controls will flex and lock. Also, there may be a comfort disadvantage for some wearers who find the harnessing required to be restrictive, hot and even painful.

7.4.1.11 All Electric Alternatives

The comfort disadvantages of the hybrid approach are exactly the advantages of an all-electric prosthesis, which would eliminate the need for control cables entirely. Some harness may still be required for suspension purposes, but pulling on the cable for control would be eliminated. The costs for an all electric system would nearly always be higher, using the premium components available. Control options are many with current electric components. Two muscle EMG could be used with any of the available electric elbows as well as servo controllers using force or pressure sensors in the harness and socket. Vendors include Motion Control, Hosmer and Liberating Tech-

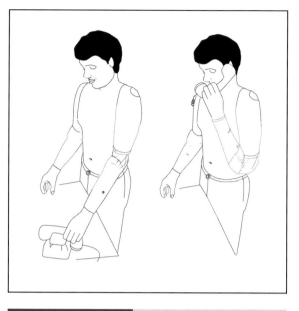

Figure 7.18

Simultaneous control of two functions is now possible with all electric systems. For high level amputees, or transhumeral amputees who prefer to eliminate control cables, the all electric system will now function much more naturally, without the need to lock the elbow when hand function is desired

nology Inc. Recent innovations will also allow the all electric systems to operate two functions simultaneously, one of the formerly unique advantages of hybrid systems. Simultaneous control of the electric elbow by a harness mounted sensor, along with myoelectric control of the TD by EMG sites is now a reality with the electric systems of several vendors (Fig. 7.18).

Reference

1. Sears HH, Shaperman J (1998) Electric wrist rotation in proportional-controlled systems. J Prosthet Orthot 10(4): 92–97

7.5 Control Systems

A comprehensive understanding of the different types of electric control available, and their advantages and limitations is also very important for the practitioner. A detailed discussion on myoelectric control has been given in another chapter and has been generally discussed earlier in the prosthetic options section of this chapter. Therefore, we will detail other types of electric control such as switch, touch pad and servo or force transducer control and end with a brief recap of myoelectric strategy.

Switch control as the primary input is often used when myoelectric control is not an option or when an individual who has worn or wears a cable-operated device habitually and prefers to utilize the gross body motions he or she is comfortable with, for control of the electric prosthesis. This is because, as a primary control, the switch behaves most like a cable operated strategy, the difference being that excursion and effort are typically far less. It still has similar limitations to cable operation, namely it requires gross body movement and therefore its functional envelope is similar, when used without the assistance of a controller it is not proportionally controlled. It does however provide increased pinch force if controlling an electric prehensor.

Switch control is most often used as a secondary input in addition to myoelectric or other types of electric control. A push or pull switch can be utilized to mode switch between a hand and wrist rotator for example or to unlock an electric elbow. While it can be used as an additional primary input, it is typically subject to gross body movement limitations and digital control and therefore seldom used in this manner.

A servo or force transducer can be used as a primary control strategy and is similar in some respects to cable operated and switch operated control, in that it relies on cable or strap tension for input. The major difference is that when used as a primary control, excursion is minimal (theoretically, it is zero, but soft tissue compression and minute elasticity in the control strap results in some gross body movement being required) (Fig. 7.19). The transducer simply reg-

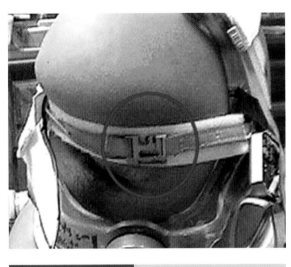

Figure 7.19

Close-up of force transducer

isters the force or tension applied and sends an appropriate signal to the system's controller. It can be adjusted for sensitivity, requiring extremely small amounts of tension for full control of the target component(s). The transducer's principal drawback is that it typically requires a "sleep" mode in order to prevent inadvertent activation of the hand or elbow. This sleep mode is required because it is cable tension which provides input to the transducer and if the tension is relaxed or tightened as might occur with shifting of body position in order to rest, for example, the hand or elbow or other component would respond accordingly. This is especially critical with respect to an object being grasped by the prehensor. In order to "wake up" the hand, slightly more tension must be applied to the transducer than was applied prior to the prehensor going into sleep mode. This can create situations in which the object can fall from the hand before the individual realizes the prehensor is activated. Still, with its greatly reduced requirement for excursion and energy expenditure, this type of control is a viable option.

A linear potentiometer is another control option that relies on excursion rather than force input and hence has the advantage of providing some feedback

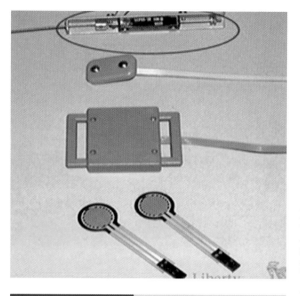

Figure 7.20

Linear potentiometer pictured at the *top*

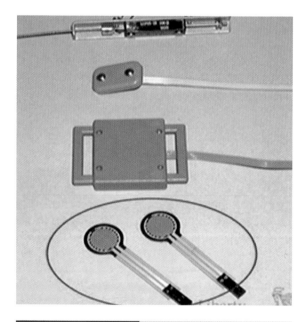

Figure 7.21

Touch pads (FSRs) at the *bottom*

to the user, similar in concept to cable operation. The required excursion is significantly less than that necessary in a cable driven system as the potentiometer is much more efficient. This control option can be used to control an entire prosthetic system from terminal device to wrist rotator to elbow or as a single input device for a specific component (Fig. 7.20).

Touch pads offer the individual freedom from a control cable while concurrently providing proportional control to a multitude of components. As the name implies, the touch pad relies on contact pressure for control input. For this reason, they can be placed wherever contact can be made, although it is usually important for the individual to have a fairly precise sensation of touch pad location and it helps to have adequate feedback at the point of contact. Mobile anatomical prominences such as remnant digits of the partial hand or the acromion in higher levels, typically provide good feedback and fairly precise control as do other areas devoid of large amounts of soft tissue. The primary drawback of current touch pad designs are their fragility and that if they are not mounted on an extremely flat and durable surface, they tend to fail. In addition, if there are inadequate anatomical sites with which to provide precise contact, then accurate control can be a problem (Fig. 7.21).

All of the above forms of control are commonly used and with great success, provided the prosthetist is well aware of the parameters pertaining to each method of input. Myoelectric control, however, is by far the most common method of primary input used when external power is indicated and adequate EMG signals have been identified. The advantages this type of input has are numerous and highly beneficial to the user. Chief among them are the myoelectric system's unique ability to significantly enlarge the user's functional envelope by eliminating the reliance on gross body movement required by other control methods that has so little association with human limb positioning and hand movement (Fig. 7.22). Like both the servo and touch pad inputs, it offers proportional control, again providing a much greater association with natural human movement than cable or switch inputs. Similar to the servo and touch pad systems, energy expenditure is minimal in most

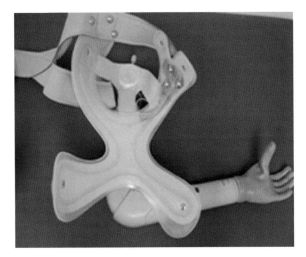

Figure 7.22

Definitive XFrame thoracic interface with myoelectric control

cases with respect to the effort required to utilize a harness. Maximum grip strength can be achieved with a myoelectric prehensor regardless of the user's strength. Myoelectric control promotes muscle tone and improved circulation as well as preventing atrophy due to muscle inactivity. Finally, with the elimination of gross body movement, myoelectric control exhibits the highest level of dynamic cosmesis, as intrinsic contractions are generally used for inputs and are hidden from view. The primary disadvantages myoelectric control shares with other forms of control are cost and fragility. An accurate tool that can determine the precise value of an enlarged functional envelope, healthy musculature and improved psychosocial integration has yet to be developed and, in the author's opinion, probably never will be as every individual subjectively holds the answer to this fundamental question within. However, it is probably fair to say that if an individual is a good candidate for electrical control for all the reasons stated previously and EMG signals are adequate, then myoelectric control should be the primary consideration.

7.6 Interface Designs

Being armed with an extensive knowledge of the prosthetic components, options and control systems available to individuals with limb loss or amelia, provides an excellent foundation with which to begin forming a successful rehabilitation strategy. However, it is also important to understand the critical interface and frame designs that ensure the suspension and stability of these prosthetic systems as well as the efficient transfer of user input, whatever form this may take, to component output. Because there exist designs unique to each level of limb deficiency, it is important to discuss them in adequate detail within the scope of this chapter. We will begin, however, by delineating certain aspects of interface design that are considered universal. Proper interface design should include optimum comfort, range of motion, stability, appropriate volume containment where required, adequate suspension if necessary (in situations when a suspensory strap alone is inadequate or inappropriate) and sufficient cosmesis. Though often ignored, the frame footprint, while sufficiently providing all of the above features, should be reduced to its absolute minimum whenever possible. To this end, many recent developments in frame design, particularly at the higher levels have occurred. A brief discussion of these new designs will follow a description of their predecessors and will entail a physical and biomechanical properties comparison with the more traditional styles (Fig. 7.23).

Restorations of partial hands using external power have begun to occur only recently, as length discrepancies, dubious functional advantage gained by the user and the elimination of tactile sensation have all retarded the development of electrically powered components for this level. With the advent of both the Otto Bock's Transcarpal Hand and Steeper's electric partial hand, much of the length discrepancy problem has been surmounted. For those individuals who require pinch force and prehension capability, these products address the issue of improved function. As products improve, tactile concerns may be offset with the advent of feedback mechanisms (Fig. 7.24).

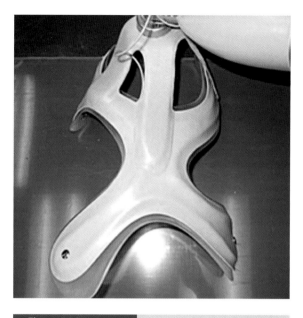

Figure 7.23

XFrame

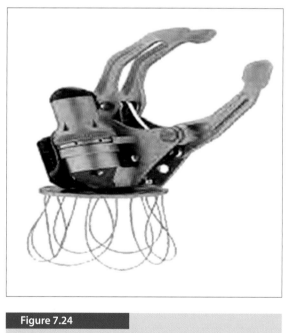

Figure 7.24

Transcarpal hand for electric fittings

As the shape and nature of partial hands vary so greatly, design characteristics of the interfaces for this level are hard to specifically define. Generally, because of the added weight of electric componentry and the need for maximum tactile sensation, minimal containment while providing maximum suspension, stability and range of motion must be provided. Critical areas which can be utilized for suspension and in the partial hand interface are the dorsum of the hand just distal to the wrist joint (as well as the medial and lateral surfaces just proximal to the wrist joint if wrist deviation or flexion and extension is either not present or desired), the hypothenar and thenar eminences and finally, the fleshy center of the palm.

As we progress more proximally, wrist disarticulation interface designs have not been radically altered to any significant degree, although technology for suspension and maintaining maximum range of motion has become available in the form of silicone inserts and sleeves, inflatable and other adjustable bladder technologies and negative pressure systems utilizing expulsion and other valve types. Major changes in interface design have occurred; however, at the radioulnar (trans-radial or below elbow) level which have greatly improved comfort, suspension and stability. When the Muenster design was introduced, it added significant improvements to the traditional interface. By suspending over the epicondyles, the design reduced and even eliminated the need for auxiliary suspension. However, its low profile proximal brim and compression over sensitive nerves and tendons resulted in only marginally improved stability, some loss in range of motion and discomfort for some individuals was exacerbated due to the location of the proximal modifications (Fig. 7.25). Improvements to the Muenster design were developed in the 1990s by Randall Alley which radically altered suspension and stability, achieving this while concurrently increasing patient comfort. This new design, referred to as the Anatomically Contoured and Controlled Interface (A.C.C.I.), incorporated many concepts introduced by William F. Sauter's three quarter design and NovaCare, Inc.'s Upper Extremity Prosthetic Program's (U.E.P.P.) Anatomically Contoured Socket (A.C.S.). Medial and lateral

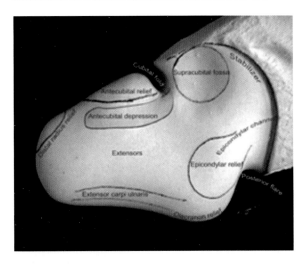

Figure 7.25

Anatomically Contoured and Controlled Interface (A.C.C.I.)

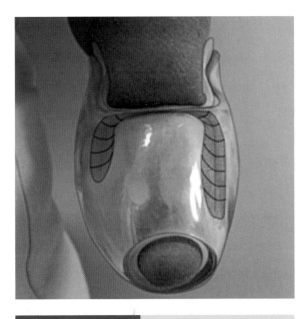

Figure 7.26

Medial and lateral antecubital depressions

stabilizers in the brim extend proximally much higher than either the traditional or Muenster designs. These stabilizers added much improved rotational stability. Areas of compression, positioned over the epicondyles in the Muenster socket, were transferred antero-proximally to areas of soft tissue not populated by critical nerves and tendons and were also increased in depth and scope, creating improved suspension and mediolateral (ML) stability while increasing comfort. The anterior-posterior dimension (AP) in both the A.C.S. and A.C.C.I. designs was drastically reduced, resulting in the creation of a new area for suspension previously underutilized. In addition, if the AP was reduced adequately, range of motion, while still marginally restricted, was improved over the Muenster socket. Furthermore, the olecranon relief was modified so that its neighboring distal and proximal regions were perpendicular to one another, greatly enhancing suspension and stability. Additionally, rather than reduce the proximal extent of the antero-proximal trim line to gain greater flexion as was traditionally done in both the Northwestern and Muenster styles, an area for expansion of the soft tissue just distal to the antecubital fold was provided. This relief enhanced range of motion and provided additional suspension, while preventing the building up over time of redundant tissue, which often occurs with the other designs.

The A.C.C.I. addressed a critical flaw in the A.C.S. by improving upon the lifting capacity of the interface by adding a modification which extended the trough of the antecubital fold distally along the medial and lateral aspects of the dorsal surface of the forearm. These medial and lateral antecubital depressions increase load bearing during initial flexion, reducing the pressure on the distal end and reducing the need for extra relief in this area. Rotational stability is also increased as a result (Fig. 7.26).

Improvements in elbow disarticulation designs have mimicked those at the wrist level, namely improved suspension technologies and short length sockets designed to maximize heat dissipation and general comfort.

The humeral (trans-humeral or above elbow) interfaces were improved significantly with the advent of Tom Andrews "Dynamic" socket design, utilizing some of the concepts introduced by Arnie Pentland and Albert Wasilies from British Columbia, which greatly decreased the mediolateral (ML) dimension and added stabilizers to the proximal brim of the socket. The lateral trim line of the socket was lowered significantly to allow for increased abduction capabilities. The reduced ML and added stabilizers offered vastly improved rotational stability, reducing the degree of contribution required of the harness in this role. The increased AP caused by reduced ML added room for muscle hypertrophy and contractile state. A more recent development in the humeral level interface, the Advanced Humeral Interface (A.H.I.) incorporates the stabilizers of the dynamic socket, albeit in modified form and reduces the degree of ML compression, returning to a more classic circumferential shape while providing distinct contouring for electrodes if used(Fig. 7.27). The flattened contour of the proximo-medial wall was maintained, though modified at the brim level to allow for easier donning and doffing. The modification of the anterior stabilizer which creates AP compression is shaped in similar fashion to the modifications made in the A.C.C.I. and ACC interfaces for ML stability and suspension. It is a fossa that is ovoid in shape and greatly reduces the AP dimension for enhanced stability and suspension over the soft tissues of the pectorals by producing a "triangular suspension" or "wedge effect." This results in a larger AP dimension distally, reducing the propensity for inferior migration of the socket.

As previously stated, the distal AP in the Andrews socket was enlarged in response to the reduction in volume caused by minimizing the ML. By reducing the amount of this ML compression, the cosmesis of the socket is greatly improved and by utilizing flexible interfaces within frames with appropriate cutouts, dynamic changes in bicep and tricep hypertrophy and contractile state can still be accommodated.

For simplicity, the author will combine very short humeral, humeral neck, shoulder disarticulation and interscapulothoracic levels into a single interface discussion, defined as a thoracic interface, as thorax-mounted designs for them are very similar. Obviously, if one can utilize a humeral style interface for an individual with a very short humeral or humeral neck amputation or humeral level amelia, then its at-

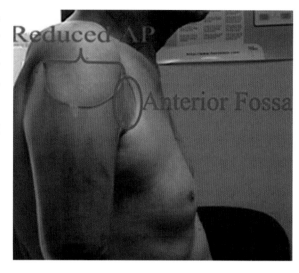

Figure 7.27

Example of wedge effect generated by AP compression

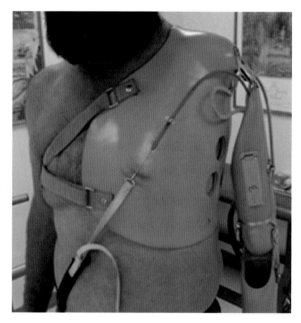

Figure 7.28

Encapsulatory style socket

tributes will be similar in scope and design to the humeral interfaces previously discussed, often with greater rotational control and suspension requirements.

Currently, encapsulatory "bucket-style" interfaces are still being taught in prosthetic schools and utilized in the field, much to the detriment of the user who has to endure poor heat dissipation, rotational instability, uncomfortable pressures, reduced mobility, added weight and poor static and dynamic cosmesis. One of the universal tenets of optimum interface design includes the minimization of socket footprint. Whenever possible, these interfaces should only contact the skin where support is required. This seemingly obvious aspect has been relatively ignored by some prosthetists in the field and attention was given only briefly to William Sauter's aluminum designs that featured window cutouts for heat dissipation and weight reduction back in the 1950s. This was in part due to difficult fabrication techniques required to produce the frame but also to a lack of available studies on the subject of interface tensile strength and general frame design. Although there still exists a dearth of information on this subject, advances have just recently begun to occur in spite of this (Fig. 7.28).

In the early 1990s, Randall Alley developed what is now known as the XFrame. Although similar in concept to Sauter's designs, it applied unique compression techniques and eliminated the rigid surface over the shoulder and trapezius found in previous designs. It was given its name by virtue of its appearance, which resembled the letter "X" with its ends rotated to correctly stabilize itself on the body. What is immediately recognized is how small of footprint is required in order to achieve stability and suspension.

The XFrame's key attributes are numerous. Perhaps most significant, it possesses a four point rotational control system. Its superior stabilizers resemble closely those of the most recent humeral interfaces, creating not only excellent rotational stability but also improved suspension. Its inferior stabilizers mimic its superior cousins in both structure and function, also providing rotational control and suspension. Secondly, it is characterized by a greatly reduced AP. As in the humeral interface, a triangular suspension effect is created in which the superior

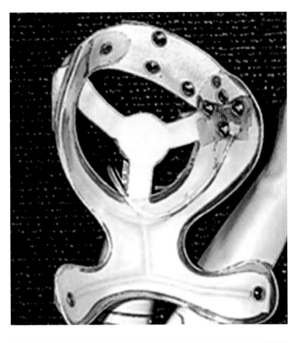

Figure 7.29

Fig. 7.29. XFrame design (medial view)

strut termini compress the areas over the pectoralis major anteriorly, while posteriorly compressing over both the teres major and minor as well as the infraspinatus.

The XFrame is "discontinuous", meaning that it does not pass over the trapezius as in other designs, preventing superior migration of the frame in response to gross body movements. Not only is this an important characteristic for cosmetic reasons as well as for electrode contact but it also allows the prosthetist to incorporate the trapezius as a control input without sacrificing dynamic cosmesis (Fig. 7.29).

The XFrame also incorporates scapulospinal suspension when the spine of the scapula is deemed prominent enough. This modification, which utilizes the terminus of the superoposterior stabilizer, greatly enhances suspension by preventing or reducing inferior migration of the frame. In addition, if contoured correctly, the frame is partially constrained from rotation along the frontal plane.

The XFrame is lighter, and due to its simplicity and smaller dimensions, it is extremely easy to modify and cost-effective to fabricate.

Finally, a distal thermoplastic or other flexible interface extends significantly beyond the frame at both inferior strut termini to allow for greater distribution and more gentle gradation of pressure caused by rotational and gravitational forces.

7.7 Indications and Contraindications

It is important to note that what may be considered a physical contraindication can be offset by other physical, psychological or psychosocial factors that, when taken as a whole, can overcome such an obstacle paving the way for a successful outcome despite preconceptions or anecdotal evidence to the contrary. With this in mind, we will discuss the physical attributes that may not necessarily be contraindicative for electrical use but may limit or simply challenge to some degree the overall success attained by the user.

Some indications and contraindications for powered use vary with the level of involvement and it is again outside the scope of this chapter to discuss each of these in detail. What follows is a brief discussion of the general issues that may indicate or challenge the use of electric power across all levels of amputation or amelia, again with the stipulation that these are merely contributors to the decision as a whole and not to be taken as an absolute.

One of the most commonly stated contraindications for the use of an electrically powered system in cases of lower level trauma (to be defined here as mid-length humeral level distally to partial finger loss or amelia) is the length of lever arm present in the involved limb. While this is certainly true when taken to the extreme, new interface designs (which will be discussed later in this chapter) and lighter prehensors for pediatric use (discussed in chapter 6), while not completely alleviating the issue of lever arm and its relation to weight tolerance, have effectively enhanced our ability to fit shorter limbs with electric componentry. In more proximal levels, shorter lever arms do not preclude the use of electrical

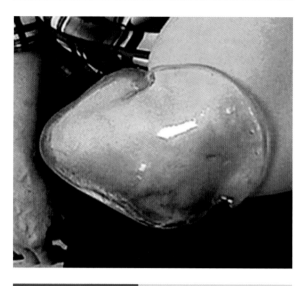

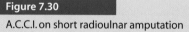

Figure 7.30

A.C.C.I. on short radioulnar amputation

power but rather require more stable interfaces with which to support these systems. This being said, one aspect that is often overlooked and which can be more critical than overall weight to an individual with a shortened lever arm is the distribution of this weight. In many instances, a myoelectric prosthesis, for example, may weigh less than two pounds, yet the predominance of mass occurs in the prehensor, creating a pendulum effect. Add to this terminal device a two pound object and it can be seen quickly that weight distribution becomes a critical factor (Fig. 7.30).

It is still important to recognize the effects of system weight; however, one of the most common difficulties in ensuring daily long-term wear is the effect this weight has on user tolerance throughout the wearing period. Very often the user must acclimate over an extended time frame, allowing the muscles and other soft tissue to grow accustomed to the constant stress of wearing a prosthesis.

Another commonly stated contraindication for the use of electric power is activity level and lifestyle. There are without doubt activities that preclude the persistent use of electrically powered prostheses.

However, similar in respect to limb length issues, advances in technology have greatly improved the durability and reliability of many electrical systems. While it used to be fact that cable operated systems were indeed more reliable than their electrically powered counterparts, it can now be argued that the incidence of repairs for both types of systems are nearly equal and the disparity now rests on the cost of repairs, rather than the frequency. This is extremely important to note, as proximity to a prosthetic facility was once a defining factor in deciding the use of a control system. As it is being discovered that cable operated systems break down frequently under heavy use and that even a minor failure will typically result in a visit to the local prosthetist, more of the focus should be on providing a secondary prosthesis in the advent of such an event, rather than confining an otherwise perfect candidate for electric power to an alternative control system. Of course, exposure to severe impact or immersion in water are to be avoided as with most electronic devices and electrical interference, although not as significant as in previous designs, still poses a problem in some cases.

Multilimb involvement is certainly important to consider when selecting a control system. In cases of contralateral upper extremity absence or loss of functional dexterity due to trauma, disease or congenital anomaly, donning and doffing issues, as well as battery removal and installation, for example, must be carefully weighed against prosthetic capability. An individual, who has contralateral limb loss or amelia in addition to suffering a brachial plexus injury, can still indicate the need for electric intervention, even if the trauma to the nerve bundle results in the inability to create volitional movement of the contralateral extremity (Fig. 7.31). In this case, although donning, doffing, and battery issues are severe, the critical prehensile capability afforded by an externally powered system may offset these significant obstacles. In addition, lower limb involvement can complicate the rehabilitation strategy, as specific balance and ambulation constraints can restrict the use of certain componentry or control systems. What is imperative to understand, however, is that many of these issues definitively require electrically powered intervention and it is paramount that the practitioner is aware of

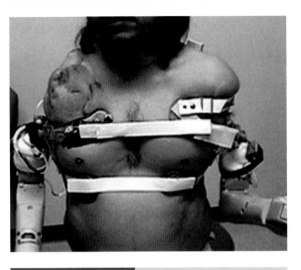

Figure 7.31

Individual with multiple limb loss

the relationships between the loss of extra limb function and prosthetic recommendation.

Cognitive ability is certainly an area of concern with the use of electrically powered prostheses, particularly with more complex systems incorporating strategies that require precise timing or strength of contractions, or that involve multiple contractions to achieve a desired result. Battery management is also an issue for the cognitively challenged and activities such as inserting and removing batteries (a challenge for most prosthetic users of externally mounted battery systems), safe and effective storage and charging and keeping track of a battery's charge state are all tasks that demand a certain level of cognition in order to assure a successful prosthetic outcome (Fig. 7.32). Unfortunately, there is no absolute standard or tool for objectively determining whether a particular individual has sufficient apperception to successfully utilize an electric prosthesis other than simple observation of specific tasks. Here again, however, the evaluator must assess the other factors, namely the strength of the individual's support system and/or the dynamic nature of his or her cognitive level. With training, failure to perform adequately in the initial stages can be overcome, but this is a judg-

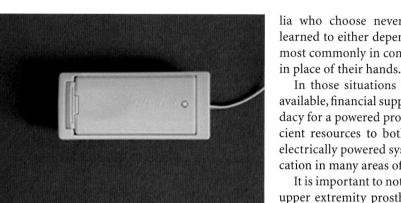

Figure 7.32

External Lithium Ion battery

ment call the rehabilitation team must make based on an overall assessment of relevant factors.

While lack of satisfactory electrode sites may rule out the use of a myoelectric control scheme, other options, which will be discussed later in this chapter such as switch or servo control, are viable alternatives and can provide a satisfactory solution to this problem.

Another instance of a situation, which in the past had been identified as a contraindication for the use of myoelectric control, is in the utilization of an immediate post-operative or early post-operative prosthesis (I.P.O.P. or E.P.O.P., respectively). Although volume reduction is inevitable, electrodes fitted to elastic membranes which retain contact at all times with the skin can be used effectively and predicate the use of this type of control system in those situations which involve rather dramatic volume fluctuations.

It has been shown that a "golden window" exists within which prosthetic acceptance is significantly greater than when the prosthesis is fitted outside this ninety day time frame. In unilateral cases, this window exists because the individual learns to become more self sufficient with their contralateral arm as time progresses. In bilateral cases, this golden window may not exist at all or is often greatly extended. Individuals with high level bilateral limb loss or ame-

lia who choose never to wear a prosthesis have learned to either depend on support from others or, most commonly in congenital cases, utilize their feet in place of their hands.

In those situations where funding is not readily available, financial support can also determine candidacy for a powered prosthetic solution. Lack of sufficient resources to both purchase and maintain an electrically powered system is a common contraindication in many areas of the world.

It is important to note that relatively few aspects in upper extremity prosthetics are absolute. When the big picture is not adequately assessed, individuals who may be strong candidates for a particular control scheme may be collectively classified into an alternative group. Although historical evidence may lead one to arrive at certain conclusions that have held true for many years, the advent of new technology or techniques may in fact render these assumptions invalid or at least only partially accurate. Thus, specific contraindications remain elusive and indeterminate and should simply be considered a point of additional reference when deciding whether or not to consider the use of electric power.

Indications for the use of electric power seem far easier to define; although ultimate success is never guaranteed, if a specific need is addressed or problem solved by its use, then the chances for a successful outcome are greatly increased.

Perhaps the ideal way to begin would be to discuss those aspects of external power capable of surmounting issues not readily resolved by the use of other control systems. Grip strength or pinch force is often desired at levels that demand the use of externally powered devices.** Indeed, this characteristic is one of the most common reasons for justifying or indicating the utilization of an electric hand or other type of prehensor. Whether this demand stems from voca-

---

** Voluntary closing prehensors can theoretically exceed pinch forces achieved with electric components, but these are not as commonly used and can cause tremendous stresses on both the cabling and harness system as well as the user. Voluntary closing TDs, however, have been used with great success from mid-length humeral level cases distally to wrist disarticulations.

tional or avocational requirements, pinch force remains one of the most significant attributes of electrically powered systems.

An enlarged functional envelope beyond that typically available to users of other types of prostheses is often required for activities of daily living as well as vocational and avocational activities. The most commonly referenced comparison made of functional envelopes is that between cable versus myoelectric operation. Because myoelectric control utilizes muscle activity rather than gross body movement, the theoretical envelope of adequate prehensile function is much larger than what is typically available with cable operated systems. While myoelectric control offers the largest envelope possible, it should be understood that other electric systems can often permit operation in a larger envelope than cable operated prostheses due to minimized requirements in terms of excursion and energy expenditure for operational and functional control.

The inability to wear a control harness for various reasons such as neck or back pain, shoulder strain, diabetes or nerve entrapment syndrome, for example, often indicates the use of electric power if active prehension is desired.

Diagnosed medical conditions such as diabetes, high blood pressure, a heart condition, contralateral carpal tunnel syndrome, overuse syndrome, tendonitis, neck, back and joint pain can all be strong indicators for the use of electrically powered prosthetic control, particularly when such conditions can be aggravated with the use of a cable operated system.

Prior successful and sustained use of an electrically powered system is often, though not always, a definitive indication for the use of a similar control strategy. Here again, one cannot evaluate in a vacuum and if changes have occurred in the patient's lifestyle, cognitive level or physical characteristics, for example, prior successful use serves only as a reference and not as an absolute indication for a repeat of the original rehabilitation strategy (Fig. 7.33).

Psychological issues can impede the acceptance of electrical power; however, some of the more common reasons precluding the use of electric power are the patient's refusal to wear such a device based on prior experience or the lack thereof, misconceptions about

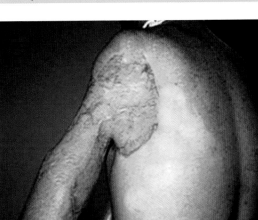

Figure 7.33

Scar tissue compounding harness design selection

the nature of such a control system or simply a refusal to wear an interface which is fitted more intimately. This is often the case when attempting to convert an individual from cable operation to myoelectric control, which requires consistent electrode contact to perform correctly. Similar to the problems experienced in assessing the appropriate level of cognition, psychological issues must be considered on a case by case basis, as there currently is no well defined tool for determining whether or not proceeding with an electrically powered system will be acceptable to the patient if given further education or reassurance. One of the greatest techniques to use during the initial evaluation is to have a successful wearer with similar limb involvement present, enabling the patient to not only become familiar with a prosthetic option but also to discourse with someone with whom they have something in common. In addition, it is important to have a variety of prosthetic demos on hand so the patient can see and feel the differences between control types. Sensitivity to patient psychology must include appropriate terminology. Words such as "stump" or "nubbins" convey a negative image to most individuals and adversely affect self-esteem.

While it is recognized that psychosocial concerns are numerous, perhaps the most significant are the degree of family and peer support available as well as prosthetic function and cosmesis. For adults, peer support may not be as significant as with young children and teens but it can still be an important factor in prosthetic acceptance. Family support, particularly in respect to individuals with recent amputations having close ties with their siblings and parents can be crucial and inquiries must be made by the practitioner in order to better understand the family situation. Finally, cosmesis should not be relegated exclusively to the physical appearance of the prosthesis itself. "Static cosmesis" is but one part of the equation. "Dynamic cosmesis", the visual characteristics observed when the individual operates the prosthesis, is also an extremely important aspect of how an individual integrates within his or her social environment. Dynamic cosmesis has not been recognized to the degree it should be when determining prosthetic control strategies and is one of the greatest advantages electrically controlled and in particular myoelectrically controlled prostheses offer. The desire to remain anonymous, to blend in with the crowd must be satisfied in both regards and it is imperative the patient understands dynamic cosmesis prior to the recommendation of a specific prosthetic control strategy.

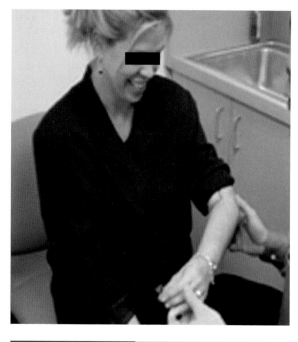

Figure 7.34

Post-delivery assessment

7.8 Therapy and Post-delivery Assessment

Both the utilization of occupational therapy and the post-delivery assessment phase are often just as critical to successful outcomes as the initial evaluation, the interface design incorporated or the type of prosthesis used. In many cases, whether or not therapy was integrated early enough or at all can determine success or failure (Fig. 7.34). An optimum rehabilitation strategy, particularly with new users of a prosthesis or users of a prosthesis that differs in control from their previous design, is one that includes the integration of an occupational therapist during the initial assessment phase and throughout the delivery process and beyond. This initial inclusion serves to expose all the members of the rehabilitation team to

other perspectives and helps to more clearly define a rehabilitation strategy at the earliest stage possible. It is rather remarkable how much can be learned from one another during this session and it serves prosthetists well to understand more clearly not only the role the therapist plays but the principles forming the foundation of rehabilitation from a therapist's point of view. Preprosthetic protocols should entail a focus on increasing or maintaining strength and range of motion, EMG training if applicable, muscle and limb strengthening and practicing the movements required for activation of secondary and tertiary inputs in addition to donning and doffing the prosthesis. A discussion on both operational as well as functional control should also be included, specifically in terms of performing activities of daily living (ADL). During the postprosthetic phase, the occupational therapist will better define these parameters as they pertain explicitly to the user's prosthesis. Patients sometimes may express their displeasure in being inadequately involved in their own rehabilitation. By including an occupational therapist early on, the specific needs of the individual can be addressed more comprehensively and the rehabilitation strategy can hence be tailored more appropriately to reflect this.

To cover the multitude of problems that can occur following prosthetic delivery would require a more comprehensive discussion than is possible in this chapter. It is best then, to develop a somewhat general procedure for assessing the prosthesis.

The post-delivery assessment phase should again, whenever possible, include the occupational therapist, for the reasons given previously. In following a general protocol, it is best to divide the approach into elemental sections in order to better quantify the approach taken. One example of this would be to segment the post-delivery assessment phase into personal, vocational and avocational components. The personal component can be described as how the prosthesis interfaces directly with the user. The vocational and avocational components pertain to how the prosthesis fulfills vocational and avocational requirements. Issues that fall under these headings are evaluations of fit, comfort, suspension, stability, operation or control, function, electronic efficiency, wearing time, cosmesis, reliability, durability and safety (Fig. 7.35).

If the prosthesis fits poorly or is simply uncomfortable, this will affect not only the other components but the very desire of the patient to wear, let alone use the prosthesis.

Adequate suspension and both static and dynamic stability are crucial to successful utilization of the prosthesis and play a significant role in the individual continuing to utilize the prosthesis. The lack of confidence that can ensue following an inadvertent loss of suspension can be a devastating blow to the success of the rehabilitation plan. Similar results can occur if the individual feels that the prosthesis is not stable. Instability can lead to significant problems in terms of efficiency of effort and even simple operation of a particular component or system. Operational control of the prosthesis should be carefully assessed and it should be noted and somewhat expected, that the dynamic nature of the human body as well as the sum of the components of the prosthetic

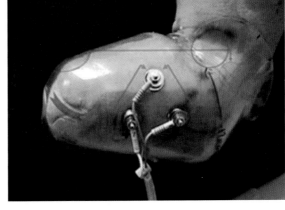

Figure 7.35

Intimate-fitting diagnostic interface

system themselves will have changed the operational outcome, whether it is positive or negative, to some degree. As the individual learns the various movements or contractions required for operation, control straps can stretch or alter their position. In a myoelectric control scheme that involves a precise balance between agonist and antagonist, for example, this balance can be offset by the strengthening of one muscle over another, resulting in the need for adjustment. When discussing electronic efficiency, this not only pertains to the level of effort required to produce movement or perform a task but also how many hours of operation are available. There is typically a compromise between battery life and individual energy expenditure, particularly with the use of myoelectric control.

All of these elements can affect functional range of motion, as it is the end result of these fundamental components working in concert with one another that determine the spatial limits of precision control. Wearing time should be sufficient to satisfy the individual's requirements, if possible and cosmesis should be assessed and evaluated in individual cases. One must keep in mind the importance of understanding that cosmesis comes in two flavors, as stated previously: static, which pertains to the physical appearance of the prosthesis and dynamic, which concerns the manifestation of the movements required to operate or function with the prosthesis.

All of the above elements are crucial to vocational and avocational pursuits as well; however, the priorities of each may change significantly or slightly, depending on the occupational or avocational environment. When considering vocational and avocational requirements, safety is a critical issue, as not only the individual can be affected but others, who may depend on the user for their own safety and well-being, can be adversely affected as well. While not to be ignored as simply a personal matter, it is common sense to recognize that risks are usually greater when working or playing around larger groups or with dangerous machinery or other dangerous objects. Reliability and durability are issues that must be carefully assessed in terms of their ability to fulfill not only personal needs and desires but occupational requirements and avocational pursuits for the reasons stated above. In order for the prosthesis to be effectively used in the workplace for example, it must perform the duties to which it is tasked reliably and must be able to perform them on a regular basis without repetitive failure.

In summary, it seems logical to approach the post-delivery assessment from a standpoint of how the prosthesis interfaces both with the individual and with his or her environment. Each of the three elements, personal, vocational and avocational, place differing demands on the prosthesis and determines how well it can be integrated into each. By following a standardized protocol, a prosthetist can efficiently quantify the issues to be addressed and convey his or her findings to the rest of the rehabilitation team.

7.9 Questions

1. What is wrong with judging outcome success solely on the type of control strategy used?
2. Why is the psychological impact typically more severe in upper extremity limb loss versus lower extremity limb loss?
3. What are three advantages of cable operated prostheses?
4. What are three advantages of electrically powered prostheses?
5. What does intrinsic muscular contraction mean in regard to prosthetic operation?
6. Define dynamic cosmesis and state how it differs from static cosmesis.
7. What is the most common configuration of a hybrid prosthesis?
8. What is simultaneous control in hybrid and electric prostheses?
9. Name the advanced interface designs for the radioulnar, humeral and thoracic levels.
10. Name two indications for electrically powered prostheses.
11. Name two fundamental aspects of interface design that affect functional range of motion.
12. In an optimum rehabilitation strategy, when should the occupational therapist be incorporated?

7.10 List of Hand Manufacturers

Motion Control, Inc., 1 888 MYO ARMS
Manufactures proportionally controlled myoelectric hands for adults.
2401 South 1070 West, Suite B
Salt Lake City
Utah 84119-1555
USA
Phone: 1.888.MYO.ARMS (696.2767) [in North America] or (801) 978.2622 Fax: (801) 978.0848.
Website: www.UtahArm.com
e-mail: info@UtahArm.com.
Listing of cosmetic cover suppliers available on website.

**Otto Bock Orthopedic Industry, Inc.,
MN 1-800 328 4058**
Manufactures proportionally controlled myoelectric hands for adults.
300 Xenium Lane North
Minneapolis, MN 55441
USA
Phone: 1(800) 328.4058
www.OttoBock.com.

VASI (Variety Ability Systems, Inc.) 1 800 891 4514
Manufactures hands and elbows for children from infancy to age 11.
2 Kelvin Ave., Unit 3
Toronto, Ontario
Canada M4C 5C8
Phone: 1(800) 891.4514 (North America) or (416) 698.1415
Fax: 1(416) 698.5860.
Website: www.vasi.on.ca
e-mail: ortc@oise.utoronto.ca
In U.S., VASI products available from L.T.I.

RSLSteeper, Ltd. 44-81-788-8165
Manufactures a powered gripper and electronic hand for both adults and children.
Queen Mary's University Hospital
Roehampton Lane
Roehampton, London, SW 15 5PL
England
Phone: 44-81-788-8165
Fax: 44-81-788-0137
In U.S., Steeper products available from L.T.I.

Liberating Technologies Inc (LTI)
Manufactures proportionally controlled myoelectric elbows for adults.
325 Hopping Brook Rd.
Ste. A, Holliston, MA 01746-1456
USA
Phone: (508) 893.6363
Fax: (508) 893.9966
www.liberatingtechnologies.com

Training

S. Hubbard · D. Stocker · H. Heger

Contents

Summary

The success of a powered prosthetic fitting is evident when a client is able to integrate the use of the prosthesis smoothly into meaningful daily living activities. A vital part of the fitting process, therefore, is the ongoing interaction between therapist and client. This chapter discusses training principles for children and for adults. Specific suggestions are provided for the various phases of training including pre-prosthetic preparation, site selection, signal or controls training, skill building, functional training and checkout. The chapter also includes a brief discussion of outcome evaluation.

8.1 Training for Children

8.1.1 Introduction

"A successful prosthetics program for the individual with a limb deficiency or loss is dependent upon a number of factors. It would be difficult to classify these in order of importance, for each is essential. An adequately fitted, comfortable, and well-functioning prosthesis is, of course, indispensable. The amount and kind of training the child receives is also of great importance. The age at which the child is fitted is highly significant...But perhaps the most essential single consideration is the attitude of the individual and family toward the disability and the idea of a prosthesis. If that attitude is not positive, not wholesome and constructive, then the prospects of failure are greatly increased and perhaps inevitable" [Brooks et al. 1965].

The key to success then is to recognize that both the parent(s) and the child are our clients (Fig. 8.1)!

There are a variety of developmental principles and theories that form the foundation of occupational therapy practice. Individual therapists, therefore, may follow different approaches. While working with children who have upper-extremity limb deficiencies or loss, the establishment of a therapeutic relationship with the child/family is the key to all treatment. Based on Weiss-Lambrou's guidelines for therapists working in upper-extremity prosthetics [18], the role of the occupational therapist in today's external-powered prosthetic practice may be defined as involving the responsibility to:

- Establish rapport and open communication with child and family to increase dialogue for choices/options ahead
- Evaluate the developmental status of the child and to monitor developmental progress
- Determine the child's readiness for myoelectric fitting and training
- Identify muscle sites, evaluate signals and assess the child's ability to operate a myoelectric control system
- Provide input to the team's evaluation, discussion and prescription decision process
- Provide muscle/component control training
- Evaluate the functional efficiency of the finished prosthesis
- In coordination with the prosthetist, instruct parents on the care and maintenance of the prosthesis, hygiene/skin care and the proper method of applying and removing the prosthesis
- Teach the child to operate the prosthesis and to use it functionally according to his or her chronological age and development
- Work closely with the family to help promote use of the device for home, school and community activities
- Provide follow-up evaluation of the child's tolerance, operational ability and functional use of the prosthesis
- Help the parents to understand their child's capabilities and limitations, and to provide them with continuous support and encouragement

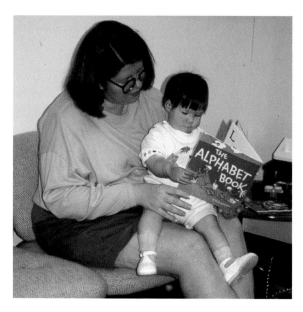

Figure 8.1

It is essential to establish a therapeutic relationship with child and family

- Foster the development of positive self-esteem and body image
- Communicate with the community therapist and/or child's teacher
- Communicate and consult with all members of the multidisciplinary team

8.1.2 Infants

8.1.2.1 Passive Prosthesis

Many centers begin the fitting process with a passive prosthesis between three to six months of age. This serves several purposes varying in importance for each child and family. The early fitting conditions the child to wearing a prosthesis and assists gross motor development. The prosthesis provides additional limb length that can assist the child in midline awareness and bilateral approach to tasks. It also helps to encourage the development of weight bearing and

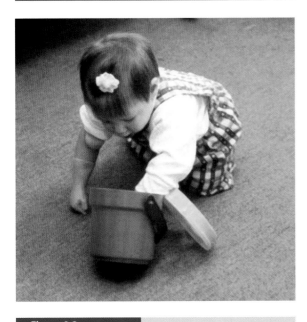

Figure 8.2

Passive prosthesis assists gross motor development

balance in sitting, crawling or pulling to stand. Not to be underestimated, the cosmetic appearance may also assist parents and extended family in coming to terms with the limb difference. Teams may utilize this phase of passive fitting as an opportunity to get to know the family and child, provide further education and support and offer other services (Fig. 8.2).

Therapy goals include facilitation of motor development and prosthetic use, monitoring growth and development and the provision of reassurance and psychosocial support to parents. Specific treatment suggestions include:

- Showing the parent how to position the affected limb when carrying, feeding, washing and playing with the child
- Teaching and facilitating positioning of the limb with and without the prosthesis as the child begins to roll, prone prop, crawl, pull to stand and walk
- Guidance in choice of toys to encourage prosthetic awareness and use such as busy boxes, activity

centers on the floor and positioned in crib, large balls or cuddly toys, rattles forced into passive hand or attached by velcro to wrist, and toys that wobble or move in place when pushed.

Equal time should be devoted to both limbs to encourage bilateral awareness. This may include placement of toys or person to one side or the other or in front, placement of toys just out of range to encourage movement, washing both hands after meals or snacks and holding either limb when the child begins to walk. Frequent follow-up with the family is essential at this stage to provide reassurance, monitor growth changes and guide parents in developmental progression.

8.1.2.2 The First Powered Prosthesis

Practices vary as to when clinics begin to provide powered prostheses to children. Some centers proceed directly to a myoelectric prosthesis after a period of passive fitting, whereas others prefer to switch from passive to body powered before considering a powered limb. Different practices are also evident with the criteria used to determine the readiness for activation of a prosthetic terminal device. For example, in California at the Child Amputee Prosthetics Project (CAPP), a device is activated when the child shows a readiness to learn to open the terminal device and a readiness to relate the opening to purposeful play. Criteria include: ability to follow simple two-step directions, interest in bimanual prehension, reasonable attention span of 10 minutes, willingness to be handled and awareness of the prehensile potential of the terminal device [9]. Other facilities use age-based criteria. For example, myoelectric prostheses are generally not provided in the United Kingdom before the age of 3 1/2 years [5] and 2 1/2 to 4 years in Sweden [15]. In some cases, financial support systems dictate team practices and fittings may be delayed to an older age to reduce expenditures.

Centers taking a developmental approach to myoelectric fitting, recognize that hand use begins very early, and believe that the younger the age of fitting, the more likely the child is to integrate the use of the

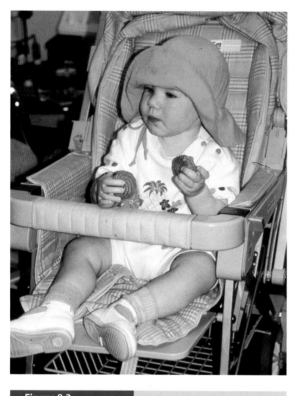

Figure 8.3

Use of "cookie-crusher" control system for infants

and place toys or objects in it. The child is then encouraged to try to open the hand to release the grasped object (Fig. 8.3).

Site Selection

The electrode is placed on the forearm extensors, as close as possible to the lateral epicondyle to ensure good electrode contact and to provide some growth allowance.

Obtaining an adequate signal is not usually difficult due to the fact that the electrode is very large in size in relation to the infant's small residual limb.

To begin with, the electrode sensitivity is set high (for easy activation) to attract the child's attention to the hand movement. As the child becomes accustomed to wearing the prosthesis and more conscious of the control strategy, the electrode level can be reduced gradually and voluntary grasp/release encouraged in play activity [7] (Fig. 8.4).

Training

In training a child to use a myoelectric prosthesis, it is important to keep in mind both the functional benefit and the limitations afforded. A properly designed prosthesis should provide symmetry of limb length for midline activity. The prosthesis may be used in a passive manner to stabilize items or it may be used actively to grasp an object. The child-sized electric hands provide a three-point pinch between the tip of the thumb and the first two fingers. A cylindrical grasp may be possible in some cases if the object to be grasped fits within the hand shape adequately. The grip force and the amount of hand opening vary between hands according to their size and design. Once the hand has been closed, no ongoing effort is required to keep it closed. The child does, however, need to be taught to keep the control muscles at rest to prevent the hand from opening unintentionally. In general, individuals with unilateral limb loss will use the prostheses in a non-dominant capacity, as a holder or stabilizer to the item that is actively manipulated by the dominant, non-prosthetic hand.

prosthesis. They therefore transfer an infant from a passive fitting to a myoelectric prosthesis at a point when the child has outgrown the passive socket and growth and development permit myoelectric fitting. This may occur as early as before the child's first birthday [2, 7, 8, 14, 16]. Factors considered include the physical size of the child, developmental readiness, cognitive growth and family readiness.

From the age of 10–12 months, toddlers are able to master the simple control strategy of a single-site, one-function "cookie crusher" quite easily. Although the hand is activated only inadvertently at first, the noise and activity attracts attention and the child very quickly figures out how to open it intentionally. A "parental access" switch, located on the forearm, assists the training process as it enables the clinician or parent to open the hand independently of the child

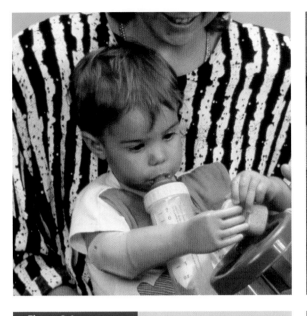

Figure 8.4

A toddler is able to master cookie crusher system quite easily

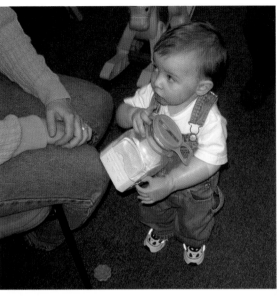

Figure 8.5

While passively holding the milk jug, one can observe hand opening inadvertently

Initial reactions to the newly fitted powered prosthesis may be mixed. A parent may inappropriately suggest that the child try to pinch their finger or nose, or reach down and pick up an object from the floor. Education is paramount at this stage to provide families with specific suggestions for encouraging child awareness of the hand's action and appropriate use of it. Caregivers need to be reminded that the infant may not immediately understand the cause and effect relationship of the hand's operation and therefore might not be able to immediately open and close it intentionally when asked.

When the prosthesis is first fitted, it is important to give the child some time to adjust to the added size, weight and sound of the powered device before drawing a lot of attention to the hand's operation. While encouraging the child to use the prosthesis passively in play activity, the therapist can assess the degree of inadvertent opening of the hand and adjust the electrode sensitivity level accordingly (Fig. 8.5). Initially, one may observe that the use of the new powered prosthesis is less than that of the previously fitted passive one.

Activities such as carrying large balls or stuffed animals, crawling games, climbing up a slide ladder, catching balls or balloons, pushing play putty into a ball and supporting a doll to dress or remove clothing, can be used to encourage passive use of the powered prosthesis. During passive play the child may notice the noise of the hand if it opens or closes. Reactions vary from curiosity, to fear and even hitting the hand in annoyance.

Children need to be allowed to discover how the electric hands work in their own time. This process can be facilitated through play activity. It has been observed that children tend to become aware of the hand opening first before any closing or holding action. Some do not want to hold anything in the hand and will immediately try to pull objects out. In doing so, they generally activate the control muscles and cause the hands to open. The therapist or parent can use the control access switch to open the hand, place

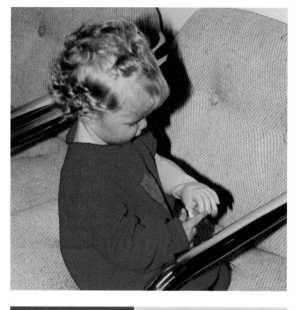

Figure 8.6

"Self-discovery"

Training Suggestions

- Placing a bracelet or toy watch on the wrist of the prosthesis to attract the child's attention to the hand
- Holding the prosthetic hand when walking with the child
- Use of the parental access switch for grasp/release play activity i.e. dropping toys in a bucket
- Filling a small film container of food treats (cheerios, teddy grahams, animal crackers) and having the child hold it while eating the treats
- Placing a kleenex in the hand and letting the child shred it with the sound hand
- Holding a non-spill bubble jar while blowing the wand held in the dominant hand
- Holding the handle of ride-on toys
- Holding the rope of a swing
- Rolling out play putty
- Grasping the handles of push toys
- Carrying objects from one person to another
- Carrying pieces of laundry to the laundry basket.

a toy in it and then encourage the child to drop it in much the same way as children enjoy dropping things from a highchair or out of a playpen (Fig. 8.6).

Development of any skill takes place over time and simultaneously as the child develops, not just in a few sessions with a therapist. As an infant, much of the *training* to use the prosthesis occurs within the home setting. Parents need to be given appropriate expectations for prosthetic wear and function as well as specific ideas for encouragement of use at home or with other caregivers. In addition to written suggestions, frequent contact in person or by telephone, will help to build on successes achieved. Parents can be shown how to progressively change training expectations so that i) the child realizes that the hand opens and closes, ii) the child can open and hold at the parent's request, iii) the child can place toys in the hand alone, and iv) that the child eventually has the confidence to hold objects, carry them about and release them at will. Through ongoing dialogue problems can be averted, suggestions made and progress acknowledged.

At first, children may not want to hold or have toys in the hand and may pull away when the parental access switch is being used. More time may need to be spent in non- focussed play or passive use activities, to allow adjustment to the new prosthesis before proceeding further. Parents, too, should be reminded that attention span is limited in young children and that frequent short sessions playing games is best. Once reliable open and hold operations are achieved, then other activities such as carrying items without dropping them while moving about, threading beads and paper tearing can be introduced according to the developmental readiness of the child (Fig. 8.7).

It is important for parents to be aware of the need to pre-position the wrist effectively for maximum functional benefit. If the hand is not positioned properly, the child will begin to use awkward, compensatory shoulder/trunk motion or be discouraged from trying to use it at all. For example, when the wrist is placed in some positions, the fingers of the hand can occlude the vision of a toy in the hand and this may diminish the child's awareness of the finger function.

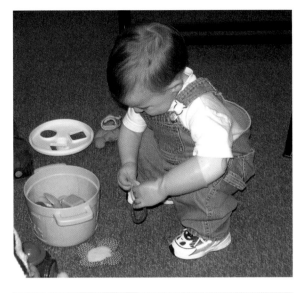

Figure 8.7
Infant training

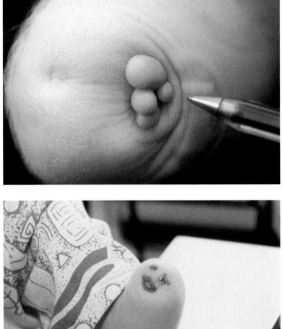

a

b

Figure 8.8 a, b
Use of nubbins for control purposes

Therapists should design treatment programs with developmental considerations in mind.

For example, children two years of age need frustration kept to a minimum. Short training periods requiring concentration mixed with frequent breaks for free play can maximize the productivity of a session. Because this age group loves messy play, blowing bubbles, finger painting (water-based paint) and play putty are good activities. Some therapists will include supervised water/sand play, while teaching parents and the child to check for cracks in the cosmetic glove and taking care not to allow the limb to be immersed above the glove covering. Riding toys and rhythm band instruments, with rhymes and music, also interest this age group.

Children at the age of three love to paint and draw, make believe and play outdoors. They are more cooperative and become frustrated less easily. At three years of age, fine motor skills improve rapidly, ability to problem-solve has expanded and they are very bilateral in their approach to tasks [4]. They usually enjoy construction toys, lacing cards, cut and paste, riding toys and playground equipment. It is also possible to begin to introduce some basic self-care activities.

8.1.3 Pre-school Age

By three to four years of age, children have developed improved communication skills and longer attention spans. The youngsters will have become familiar with the members of the prosthetic team and have learned to trust them. They can now cooperate more easily and be effectively evaluated and trained to use more advanced control strategies. Procedures used are the same as those employed for an older child or adult.* If the child is already a myoelectric wearer and accus-

* Acknowledgement: Portions of this section were extracted from previous work by the author and reproduced with the permission of the publisher, Variety Abilities Systems Inc. [8].

tomed to using a single-site voluntary opening system he or she should be evaluated for two-site control. To be successful, the antagonist muscle group must be trained to contract independently in order to close the hand. It is often helpful to paint a face on the distal residual limb in order to encourage the child to wriggle the soft tissue to make the nose wriggle or eyes blink. Many congenital amputees have nubbins or mobile soft tissue at the distal end that they can learn to move to attain the desired muscle response (Fig. 8.8a,b).

If more than one control site is required, the muscles chosen must be capable of contracting and relaxing independently. Therefore, it is advisable to work with one muscle group at a time until the child is able to obtain and sustain a consistent and repeatable signal that is independent of other movements. Once this is achieved with each individual muscle group, electrodes can be applied to the two muscle sites and the child trained to contract, hold and relax each muscle group independently (Fig. 8.9).

System Selection

Control system selection is dependent on:

- The number of muscle sites which the amputee is able to control independently
- The number and nature of the electrical components to be used in the prosthesis
- The characteristics of the EMG signals generated
- The degree of complexity that the child is able to manage.

For a trans-radial amputee it is usual to start control training with a two-muscle system. An elastic cuff is used to hold the electrodes on the surface of the forearm flexor and extensor groups and the child is trained to contract and relax each of the muscle groups. If co-contraction is observed continually and it does not appear possible to train the muscles to operate independently, the strongest muscle group is chosen and a one-muscle system is considered. Selection of the most appropriate one-muscle system is then based on the ease of operation for the child and prosthetic design/space considerations.

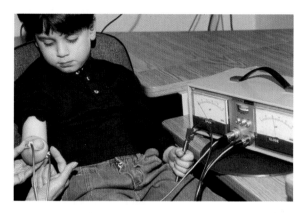

Figure 8.9

Training – second muscle site

If a 2-site system is selected, the choice has to be made between proportional and digital controls. The proportional system gives the person the ability to vary the speed and force of the terminal device, if that is desired. Proportional control is of more advantage when used with a larger hand (greater opening distance) and used for refined grasp of more delicate objects.

At the trans-humeral and forequarter level in particular, the selection process will be limited by the number of muscle sites available for use. Combinations of myoelectric control with electric switches or body-powered control may be required to meet the individual's need to operate more than one component.

Electric switch control is often preferred over myoelectric control for amputations at the shoulder disarticulation level. The child can use bony prominences (clavicle or acromion) to activate small contact switches installed in the socket. The number of switches used and their complexity will depend on the child's age, needs and abilities.

If this is the first experience with myoelectric fitting, it will be necessary to teach the child how to use his or her muscles for control purposes. It is usually advisable to begin this instruction on the non-affected limb. The therapist palpates the appropriate muscle group and allows the child to feel and observe the desired muscle contraction during lightly resisted wrist or elbow motion. A myo-tester can then be attached to display the resultant EMG response during contraction and relaxation. Once the child has become successful with the sound limb, it is then possible to teach them to parallel the same action with the residual limb muscles.

For further detail on the processes of site and system selection for new clients, please refer to the corresponding **Sect. 8.3.1** for adults.

Control Training

Once the basic operation of the new control system has been mastered, some time is spent training the child: to open and close the hand as needed, to grip with light or strong pinch, to maintain grip on an object while moving it from one place to another and to open the hand while reaching to grasp an object. Control training can be started early on with the use of a training toy or electric hand, refined during the check socket and/or temporary prosthesis stage(s) and checked again at the final stage of check out with a completed prosthesis. Activities such as stacking blocks, puzzles, simple board games or picking up and throwing bean-bags can help teach the child how to close and hold objects. Refining the ability to open and close the hand to varying degrees can be accomplished with tasks such as picking up and placing wet sponges without squeezing the water out, picking up cereal pieces, and moving various sizes and weights of objects (Fig. 8.10).

After the child is fitted with the completed prosthesis, further control training is practiced before proceeding on to functional training. Games like Simon Says can add fun to a drill and allow the therapist to check for accidental opening/closing of the hand. For example Simon may ask the child to pick-up a blue block and move it to a blue cup placed on the opposite side of the room, to wave his or her arms like a bird, or to hop like a bunny. Observing inadvertent opening or closing of the hand at this phase and then determining the cause of the accidental motion (usually unwanted contraction of a muscle or electrode lifting) and remedying the situation imme-

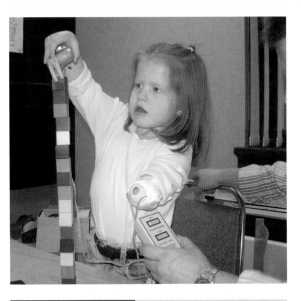

Figure 8.10

Control system training

diately can prevent frustration when practicing functional tasks.

Proper positioning of the wrist and elbow is introduced when the child has achieved successful control of the hand. Until this point, the parent or therapist may have been placing the hand and elbow in an effective position for functional activities. If the child's prosthesis includes an elbow component, positioning and/or locking of the elbow can be taught as a drill by again, using adaptations of various children's games. For example, stickers can be placed at various positions on a wall and the child asked to practice adjusting the position of the elbow in order to reach and touch them.

A sequence of specific activities can be used to teach proper positioning of the wrist and hand. As an example, carrying a plate, holding down a paper or stencil and carrying a jar without spilling would require the child to position the wrist to supinate the hand, pronate the hand and then adjust the hand to a mid position.

For the child with a prosthetic elbow joint, the task may be made more complicated by asking the child to

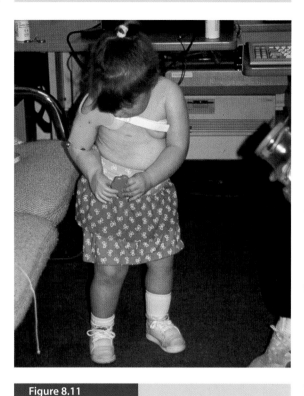

Figure 8.11

Elbow positioning

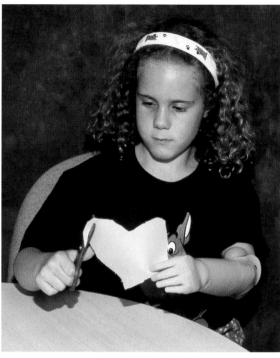

Figure 8.12

Cut and paste activity

move from sit to stand to grasp an object. This would require repositioning of the elbow, hand positioning and then opening and closing of the hand (Fig. 8.11).

Functional Use Training

Functional-use training with pre-school age children is directed towards further refinement of control and use of the prosthesis. As the child continues to practice with the prosthesis, spontaneity and skill of prosthetic use should gradually develop. By age four, many activities enjoyed by this group are bimanual in nature. Using a play-based approach, children can be guided through various daily tasks to prepare them for school entry. The child will continue to use the prosthesis passively as a stabilizer for table-top tasks such as holding down a paper while drawing or writ-

ing. Imaginative play, including dress up activity, can be used to ensure that the child can zip a jacket, initiate tying laces and use the prosthesis to stabilize items against the body. Children can learn to tie laces by wrapping parcels, or making paper and cardboard toys that require the use of lacing and tying. This age group also loves to experiment with paper and pencil tasks, markers, glue and scotch tape. Projects involving the use of scissors will help ready the child for school craft activities (Fig. 8.12).

Functional use of the prosthesis may be compromised by the limited size of the hand opening. Monkey bars, handle bars for bikes, and many toys (for safety) are designed with a grip circumference that is larger than the opening width of the electric hands. Juice bottles, pop cans, some jars of bubble fluid and other items tend to be too large to fit into the hands. Parents need to be advised when looking at toys and

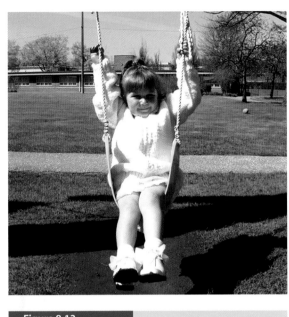

Figure 8.13

Outdoor play

tions for check-out activities that require different functional ranges of motion or different categories of use include:

Passive use: Stabilizing paper while writing, using a ruler or stencils, folding

Maintained grasp: Grasp a toothbrush to apply toothpaste, hold jar or bottle to open, hold fork while cutting meat, push shopping carts, connect plug of appliance to extension cord, open pencil case/wallet, grasp swing, tricycle riding

Maintained grasp while arms in motion: Hang clothes on hanger, blow dry hair, use rolling pin, spread table cloth, grasp bowl to stir, sweep floor, Zoom Ball, hold skipping rope to skip

Repetitive grasp and release of various sized objects (at desk or waist): Open makeup jars, open and apply band-aid, wash/dry dishes, slice, grate, peel, potatoes, carrots etc., thread beads, wrap parcel, hold paper to cut, assemble models

tasks to realistically evaluate the hand opening width and not expect gripping where it is not possible (Fig. 8.13).

Activities used with this age group should vary from table top to gross motor or standing. By kindergarten, children may be working in various play centers which require a variety of play positions, standing, sitting, kneeling, climbing etc (Fig. 8.13).

Grasp and release in any position: Tie shoelaces, tie scarf or necktie, fasten necklace, fold clothes, hang laundry on clothesline

Grasp of delicate objects: Grasp toothpaste tube to open, take Kleenex from wallet size container, spread jam on crackers, open individual jam, creamers, crackers, hold playing cards, hold badminton bird or table tennis ball to serve

8.1.4 School Age

Site selection and controls training procedures with school-age children do not vary much from those used for younger children. Table-top activities or board games such as checkers, chess, tic-tac- toe or Connect Four can be used as cognitive and play skills allow. Computer games have great appeal to this age group and can be used effectively to strengthen muscles and refine control system operation.

A variety of functional tasks will be required to maintain motivation and interest (Fig. 8.14). Sugges-

Grasp of heavy objects: Carry grocery or garbage bags, push loaded wheelbarrow, climb monkey bars or rope ladder, carry bucket or pail, carry briefcase/book bag, carry cafeteria tray

To keep a child's interest, yet achieve performance in different activities, two different "games" can be used with the activities above. Activities from the different categories of use can be written on small pieces of paper and placed in a hat or box. The child then picks a piece of paper and completes the task indicated. It has been found that children will stick with a non-

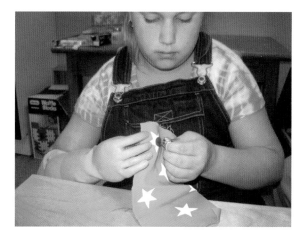

Figure 8.14

This pre-teen is learning to sew and would like to make her own clothes

preferred task to completion with the knowledge of something more interesting in the box. Another approach is to wrap a parcel with a prize in various layers of paper. On each layer is written a task that must be completed before opening the next layer. Eventually, the child reaches the prize and is rewarded.

Behavior management techniques have also proven to be useful with children who have learning difficulties or concentration problems. For example, the use of a timer to specify the amount of time a child must be actively engaged in specific treatment activities before a break for free play is allowed, is one technique that has been found to be quite successful in maintaining interest.

8.1.5 Teens

Teens' attitudes and motivations can be a mixture of those typical of both children and of adults. Treatment interventions that have proven to be successful for a child in the past may need to be reviewed and revamped. The needs, feelings and interests of the adolescent usually begin to change at this point in their

life. Some may even elect to discontinue use of their myoelectric limb. Approaches to treatment may include the need to refer to other support systems or counselor to assist the young person in coping with their feelings. If the adolescent has been a long-term client of a treatment team, the team members must be sensitive to the changes and allow for choice of expression and consideration that all the adolescent's concerns are valid.

As adolescents become engaged in different activities of daily living, their prosthetic needs change as well. Self-care activity, in particular, will assume greater importance for most. Team members must interact with the adolescent to determine if there are new recreational or vocational interests that require specific prosthetic design considerations. It is vital to consider these needs when developing functional training programs (Fig. 8.15). Teens, ultimately make their own choices, so it is important to consider them as partners and provide them with the appropriate information and options. Within the parameters of functional range of motion training, teens need to choose training tasks that are relevant to their needs and lifestyles. Some teens may have difficulty defining what is important to them, in which case, limiting choices may make decision-making easier.

Site selection and myoelectric control training procedures require exposure of the affected limb. Since their bodies are changing and growing, teens will be self-conscious of their body image. It is essential to ensure that the teen has maximum privacy during all fitting stages.

Adolescents who have experienced a traumatic amputation or an amputation for medical reasons will require a lengthier, more inclusive rehabilitation. As well as adapting to the amputation, the teen will also be dealing with ongoing psychosocial issues typical of the age. Wound healing, stump care and wrapping and desensitization during post- operative care will offer the opportunity to discuss body changes and appearances that are often vital to teens. The choice to use a myoelectric prosthesis can be driven by the appearance, linked with function. Some teens are actually willing to spend more time learning to operate the prosthesis so that the motions of using the prosthesis will appear smooth and natural.

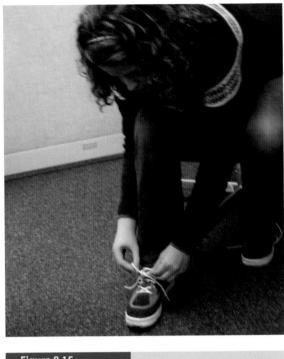

Figure 8.15

Activities of daily living

The process of being fitted with a myoelectric prosthesis including stump care, location of signal sites and signal or controls training will be similar to those used for adults with amputations (see Sect. 8.3.1). Adolescents need to become familiar with the choices of prosthetic components since they need to be part of the decision- making processes. Likewise, teens need to be able to choose functional activities that are relevant to their needs.

Teens may require extra understanding and assistance in returning to school and their communities. Meeting other teens that have a limb loss can often be of benefit in providing support. Programs such as the War Amputations of Canada [17] and the Amputee Coalition of America [1] provide a variety of programs, resources and contacts that may be helpful.

8.2 Outcome Measurement

Outcome measurement involves the use of scientific methods to determine results of interventions. Ideally, standardized, valid and reliable measurement instruments are needed to link outcomes to the services provided. A good outcome measure should be easy to administer, relevant to the interests of the clients and service providers and have proven psychometric properties.

Occupational therapists are specifically concerned with the measurement of functional outcome of upper-extremity prosthetic fitting and training. Functional benefit should be assessed according to the value and use of the prosthesis in daily life, not simply the number of hours the device is worn. Functional tests may take the form of *observational assessments* scored by a therapist or *self-report* questionnaires completed by the client and/or parent. Observational assessments demonstrate the person's capabilities while self-report questionnaires elicit subjective responses about the person's typical day to day performance.

8.2.1 Observational Assessments

The UNB Test [13] is an observational test and training tool designed specifically for use with children who are upper-extremity prosthetic users. The UNB Test enables therapists to assess prosthetic performance with developmentally-based daily life activities. The therapist has the option of using any of three different sub-tests (10 tasks each) for each of the four age groups: 2–4 years, 5–7 years, 8–10 years and 11–13 years. Ranking scales are used to evaluate the spontaneity of use of the prosthesis and the skill of prosthetic function. It has been evaluated for inter-rater reliability and the rating system was proven able to differentiate between the skill and spontaneity aspects.

The Skill Index Ranking Scale (SIRS) was designed by Hermansson [6] to measure the acquisition of myoelectric control capacity in daily activities. According to this scale, the child's accomplishments with the prosthesis can be assessed according to 14 different levels of function when using an electric hand prosthesis. Each step puts a higher demand on the child, compared to the previous one. The SIRS can also be used to plan training sessions as the therapist can use it to progressively increase the demands presented to the child.

Both the UNB Test and the Skill Index Ranking Scale can be used effectively by therapists in clinical practice to assess a child's skill and progress in training. The main drawback with observational assessments for outcome measurement is that there may not be a strong relationship between the individual's ability to use the prosthesis when asked and actual use in daily life.

8.2.2 Self Report/Parent Report Functional Questionnaires

Self-report functional measures have the potential to evaluate a greater number and diversity of tasks than is possible with an observational functional assessment. Theoretically, responses should also reflect what individuals do within their usual environment. For amputees, responses should reflect actual use of the prosthesis rather than just capability or simply wear pattern so that results are meaningful in evaluating effectiveness and cost-benefits. Self-report functional questionnaires carry the assumption that reporting of abilities and actual performance are in close agreement. However, studies conducted with several diagnostic groups and using different functional measures are somewhat discrepant in their findings, varying in degree of agreement between observation and self-report. It is likely that the three main determinants of agreement are the population being studied, and the format and properties of the questionnaire [19].

The Child Amputee Prosthetics Projects- Functional Status Instrument (CAPP-FSI), was designed to measure the physical functional health outcomes for children 8–17 years with upper or lower limb deficiency [10]. There are 34 upper extremity items in this parent-report questionnaire and 6 lower extremity items. The child's behaviour is reported on two scales: the child does the activity (frequency of performance of the task) and child's use of the prosthesis (frequency with which the child uses a prosthesis to perform the task).

Use of the instrument was then extended to preschool age children [11] and a second, similar measure developed to assess functional abilities of toddlers one to four years of age [12]. The authors reported that the new scales had good discriminant validity and that the instruments had shown internal consistency. Further work on reliability and validity has not yet been reported.

The Prosthetic Upper Extremity Functional Index (PUFI) is a parent or older child, self-report instrument designed to evaluate the extent to which a child uses a prosthesis (conventional or powered) for common bimanual activities, the ease of task performance with and without the prosthesis and the perceived usefulness of the prosthesis. Two versions were developed to allow use and evaluate progression through the developing years. The younger-child PUFI (children 3–6 years) contains 26 functional items and the older child version (children 7–18 years) has 38 items. All of the tasks are bimanual activities that require either the use of the prosthesis (active or passive) or the use of the residual limb if the child is not wearing the prosthetic device.

Reliability and validity testing [19, 20] have been conducted. Results indicate that the PUFI achieved acceptable discriminant, construct and criterion validity with the sample that was evaluated and shows strong promise in identifying prosthetic skill and use patterns between children and across functional activities. A new computer software package version, the PUFI-PC, contains graphics and animation to attract and maintain interest of the child or parent respondent. It also provides instantaneous scoring and data summaries on completion thereby allowing the therapist to discuss results with the client/family and assess the need for additional training. The PUFI-PC is currently being used in a two-year project designed to establish an international registry of paediatric upper-extremity prosthetic clients. This new partnership should permit a longitudinal investigation of the functional abilities of young children with upper-extremity prostheses and will encourage systematic

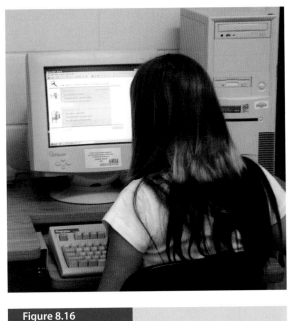

Figure 8.16

Follow-up evaluation

follow-up of this cohort as they progress from childhood to adolescence.

In order to obtain meaningful data, it is essential that outcome measures be used with larger populations. Collective investigation and collaboration are needed in order to identify problems with current tools, establish psychometrically sound instruments and to compare results across groups. Clinicians and their respective institutions must recognize that systematic implementation of measurement, data collection and analysis as routine procedures are just as integral to their care as the interventions themselves. Evidence-based practice is essential for survival and development of future best practices (Fig. 8.16).

8.3 Myoelectric Prosthetic Training for Adults

8.3.1 Introduction

Myoelectric prostheses are sophisticated devices that can provide enhanced function for individuals with an arm amputation, particularly when the amputation is of a higher level. However, these individuals may have high expectations of what a myoelectric prosthesis will do for them based on inaccurate media and internet information, perception of technological magic and the hope of restoring a lost limb. Working with these expectations/dynamics can be a challenge for the prosthetic team.

A thorough assessment by the multidisciplinary team, sharing of relevant information throughout the rehabilitation process and inclusion of the individual in decision making processes are necessary to promote realistic expectations, design a prosthesis that meets the functional and cosmetic needs of the individual and train him or her in the use of the device. The training program focuses on assisting the individual in understanding the potential and limitations of the prosthesis and in learning to control and use it effectively. Achieving significant gain in function combined with cosmesis facilitates the integration of the prosthesis as a useful tool into the person's daily functions.

8.3.2 Training Program

The training program includes:
- Initial assessment of the condition and needs of the individual
- The pre-prosthetic program to prepare him or her for prosthetic fitting
- Assessment of myoelectric signals and selection of control sites
- Selection of the system and components to be used in the prosthesis
- Training in the control of the myoelectric signal
- Orientation to the prosthesis
- Training in the control and functional use of the device

- Evaluation
- Follow-up

8.3.2.1 Initial Assessment

In the initial assessment, relevant information is obtained regarding

- The person's history
- The physical status of the residual limb and the general condition of the person
- Functional and psychosocial needs
- Previous/current use of a prosthesis
- The individual's expectation of a myoelectric prosthesis

Information gathered from the person's history includes personal data, the medical history, cause of amputation, surgical records relating to the amputation, x-ray reports, current state of health, emotional highs and lows since the amputation, family and other social supports, current living situation, family plans for the future, previous exposure to another person with an arm amputation, hand dominance, education and funding issues.

The residual limb is examined for length, size, range of motion, strength, sensation, scar placement, soft tissue coverage over the end of the limb, skin graft, voluntary control of muscles, fatigue, cramps, painful areas, phantom sensation, phantom pain and factors that may influence the control of the prosthesis, such as a tendency for profuse perspiration. The examination also includes joint range of motion, strength and sensation of the sound arm.

Inquiry into the functional needs includes areas of self care and daily activities, previous and/or prospective vocation and recreation. Of importance are the type of activities to be performed, including the tools, objects and weights to be handled and the characteristics of the environment (i.e., clean or dirty, wet or dusty, contact with materials that may stain or damage the prosthesis or the presence of a strong transformer that may interfere with the control of the prosthesis).

Psychosocial issues to consider include the degree of acceptance of the amputation, identity and the need for cosmesis, the level of motivation to learn to use the prosthesis and the person's learning style.

If the individual has been or still is a prosthetic user it is essential to know the type of prosthesis, tolerance to wearing and using it, pattern of use in activities of daily living, vocation, recreation and social events, likes and dislikes, problems encountered with the present device and unmet needs or possible problems with the sound arm due to overuse syndrome. This information is valuable in determining if the myoelectric prosthesis would be suitable for the intended functions and more advantageous than the previous prosthesis for specific tasks.

The person's extent of knowledge and particular expectations about the myoelectric prosthesis need to be clarified to avoid disillusionment and subsequent rejection. Education is provided regarding the components and functions of the prosthesis, advantages and disadvantages, fitting procedure, training program, cost and maintenance of the device, follow-up regime and service (see Appendix A).

The initial assessment defines the extent of the pre-prosthetic program necessary to prepare the individual for prosthetic fitting. In the case of an individual with a recent amputation, all aspects of the program need to be included. If the amputation is of longer standing and the person has already worn a prosthesis, relevant aspects of the program need to be selected.

8.3.2.2 Pre-prosthetic Program

The pre-prosthetic program consists of:
- Providing psychological support and education
- Preparing the residual limb for prosthetic fitting, improving the person's general condition
- Maximising function in self care, general activities and leisure
- Vocational liaison
- Determining prosthetic prescription

The individual receives support in coping with the loss of the limb and the necessary adaptation process through individual and family counselling and group therapy. Peer interaction with other individuals with amputations at various stages of rehabilitation is often helpful. General and specific information is provided by the respective team members in relation to the program and prosthesis, exploration of needs and interests, setting and reviewing of goals and physical and psychological issues arising at varying times.

The residual limb is prepared for prosthetic fitting through wound management, instruction in hygiene and care, pain control, oedema control and shaping of the limb with tubular elastic or use of ace bandage and intermittent positive pressure pump. Scar management is carried out through massage, vibration and compression. A graduated program of passive, active-assisted, active and resisted exercises optimises mobility and muscle strength in the limb. This also aids in desensitisation of the limb with additional modalities of massage, tapping and vibration added. An individually designed exercise program and pool therapy can be used to address strength and mobility of the remaining limb and the shoulder girdle, as well as the general physical condition of the individual.

Function is improved and daily frustrations are reduced through learning adaptive techniques for performing ADL tasks and, if necessary, providing assistive devices. The bilateral work pattern is maintained through use of the residual limb for stabilizing objects, if possible. When the dominant hand is amputated, a dominance transfer program consisting of strength and dexterity exercises and one-handed writing/typing programs improves the skill of the remaining hand.

Liaison with the pre-accident or prospective employer assists in clarifying job demands and work conditions. An on-site work visit is useful for analysing vocational tasks and exploring ergonomic concerns.

Criteria for readiness of the residual limb for prosthetic fitting are: complete healing of the wound, satisfactory control of pain, reduction of oedema and consistent circumferential measurements of the residual limb, reduction and elimination of flexion contractures, maximum range of motion and adequate muscle endurance for myoelectric control. The time required to achieve sufficient reduction of the oede-

ma varies with each individual. The intimate fit necessary to ensure dependable control of a myoelectric prosthesis requires maximum stability of the size of the limb. In a person with a recent amputation, early fitting of a prosthesis is encouraged to avoid a one-handed work habit and to facilitate acceptance of the prosthesis. It has proven useful to fit and train these individuals with a temporary, body powered prosthesis that can be adapted more easily to the gradual decreasing size of the limb and help to maintain bilateral patterns of function.

8.3.2.3 Myoelectric Assessment

A myoelectric tester is used to identify suitable muscles and the optimal sites for electrode placement. The prosthetist and therapist collaborate in identifying the most suitable control system in discussion with the individual, based on the results of the assessment and the identified needs.

Site Selection

The characteristics of an optimal control site are:

- The superficial location of the muscle to access the EMG signal, related to normal movements if possible, e.g., wrist flexors and extensors for closing and opening of the hand in a trans-radial amputation
- Sufficient strength to activate the control system with ease and without undue fatigue
- Voluntary control of muscle contraction and relaxation independent of other muscles or movement of the limb
- Voluntary control of rate or level of contraction if only one muscle can be used for one powered unit, or 2 muscles are to be used for 2 powered units
- Appropriate voluntary co-contraction, if required to change the mode of operation from one powered unit to another
- Location within the constraints of the socket design

System Selection

The selection of the appropriate system depends on:
- The characteristics of the EMG signal the individual is able to generate
- The number of muscle sites the person is able to control independently
- The individual's ability to cope with the complexity of a system and the weight of the prosthesis
- The number and type of myoelectric components to be used, based on the level of amputation, the individual's specific functional and cosmetic needs and the cost/funding factors

A variety of systems are available to match the individual's abilities and needs. The most common system uses two muscles where one muscle is used for each direction of a powered unit, e.g., opening and closing the hand in a trans-radial amputation. If only one muscle is available for control, a rate sensitive or a level sensitive system can be used for controlling the two movements of the hand. If control of two motors is required, two of the latter systems could be used, i.e., hand function and wrist rotation in a trans-radial amputation and hand and elbow control in a trans-humeral amputation.

The change from one powered unit to the other can also be achieved through activation of a switch such as a harness pull switch, a mounted push switch or a nudge switch. A quick co-contraction of both muscles is another option that can be used to change from the hand to the wrist rotator or to unlock the elbow unit. The prehensile force of the hand or the speed of a powered unit can be varied with the intensity or rate of the EMG signal for refined control of the components (Fig. 8.17).

Force sensing resistors (FSR's) are useful for a shoulder-disarticulation prosthesis if optimal muscle sites cannot be found or trunk movements interfere too much with the EMG signals. The individual may find shoulder movements easier to use for control than isolating muscles that are still used for trunk movements.

Programmable systems allow exploration of the various control schemes, single or in combinations and the setting of specific signal thresholds for each

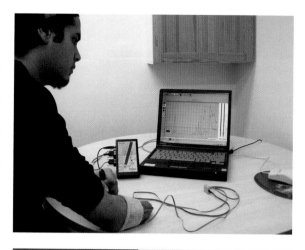

Figure 8.17

Control system selection

function. A combination of myoelectric components with body powered components may be chosen for control or weight issues or functional needs of the individual requiring a more robust prosthesis. Examples include use of a myoelectric hand and cable-operated elbow unit or vice versa for a trans-humeral prosthesis, or a myoelectric hand and a passive elbow unit for a shoulder-disarticulation prosthesis.

Test Procedure

The nature and use of the myoelectric signal is explained to the individual and demonstrated by the therapist on the myoelectric tester through muscle contraction and skin contact of the electrode. Demonstration on the non-affected limb of the person follows. The appropriate muscles are palpated and contractions are demonstrated through the specific movements. The skin is prepared through cleaning and moistening with water or electrode gel to ensure optimum pick up of the EMG signal. The test electrodes are placed longitudinally along the flexor and extensor muscles. The contractions, strength of signals and relaxation is observed on the tester.

The muscles in the residual limb are palpated, the skin is prepared and the electrodes are placed over the area of strongest contraction. The individual is instructed to contract one muscle group first and observe the signal and subsequent relaxation. The antagonist is observed for possible co-contraction. Attempting to move the phantom limb or contracting the muscle simultaneously with the movement of the contra-lateral arm can be helpful in achieving the desired muscle contraction. The optimal signal is identified by moving the test electrode in the medial-lateral plane and then the proximal-distal plane while observing the effects on the signal. When the signal of the first muscle can be repeated consistently the procedure is repeated with the antagonistic muscle group. After achieving sufficient signals with both muscles, independent control and relaxation of each muscle is practised.

Co-contraction should be reduced to a minimum level to achieve optimum control of the prosthetic components. The likely cause of co-contraction needs to be assessed by checking the cues the individual uses to generate the signals e.g., an isolated signal in a transradial amputation is usually generated with wrist flexion and extension of the phantom limb rather than opening and closing of the phantom hand. Contracting the muscles in conjunction with the appropriate movement of the sound limb or relocating the electrode site slightly away from a stronger antagonist may be helpful. If co-contraction cannot be eliminated sufficiently through training, appropriate calibration of the electrodes may achieve adequate separation of signal levels or a one-muscle system may be considered more appropriate for the individual.

Muscle signals may vary or be activated inadvertently during arm movements. Therefore the signals and relaxation of each muscle are checked in all planes of arm movement and with and without resistance applied to the residual limb (see Appendix B).

The ability to generate independent signals and to relax is eventually checked by eliminating visual feedback for the individual from the myotester while the therapist observes the effect on the tester. Some individuals are able to generate strong independent EMG signals sufficient for the effective control of a myoelectric prosthesis during the test. Others demonstrate muscle weakness and/or co-contraction and

require further testing and training. For most individuals, the ability to generate myoelectric signals seems to bear little relationship to the time elapsed since the amputation. However, atrophy of the muscles in the residual limb within a few months after the amputation has been noted in a few cases and seems to be more prevalent in women. Early testing and training is advisable to preserve their potential for controlling a myoelectric prosthesis. The length of testing/training sessions depends on the amputee's tolerance. An average is one-half hour, two to three times a day.

8.3.2.4 Control Training of Myoelectric Signal

The control training is aimed at improving the accuracy and strength of the signals, increasing the tolerance to repetitive muscle contraction and achieving appropriate muscle relaxation. Refining the voluntary control of signals builds a good basis for the effective control of the prosthesis and leads to a more immediate and successful prosthetic use.

The equipment used is a myotrainer matched to the control system, a set-up of myoelectric components (consisting of a hand, electrodes, battery) and objects of different sizes, shapes, density, weight and peg boards. Computer programs are also available to evaluate and practice control of signals and components. The amputee practices control of the signals with the myotrainer until the signals are sufficiently strong and isolated and the characteristics of the particular system, such as level or rate for proportional control, are achieved.

He or she progresses to the use of the myoelectric hand set-up for more realistic feedback. Practice in varying the amount of opening and closing of the hand is followed by grasping, placing and releasing hard objects at different heights e.g., stacking blocks while the myoelectric hand is held with the sound hand. Attention is paid to smooth control and efficient grasping pattern. Control of grip force is practised through grasping and releasing crushable objects such as foam cups (Fig. 8.18).

The control system is calibrated to accommodate the changes in the signals and achieve maximum ef-

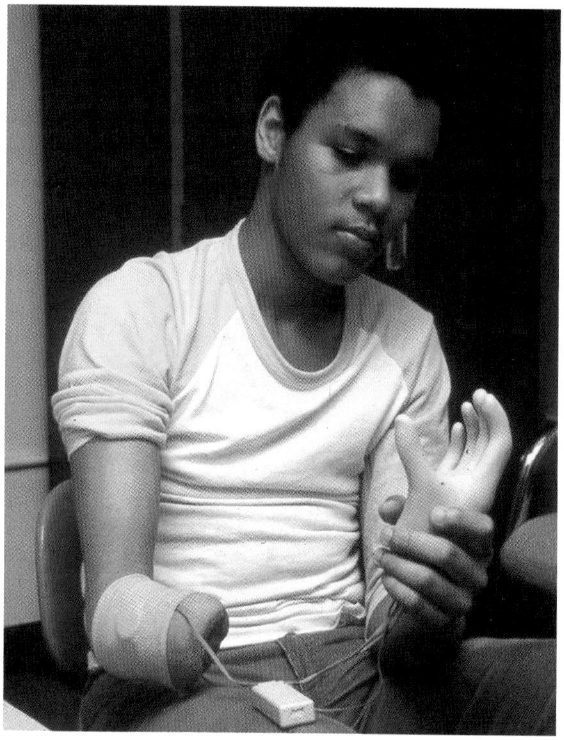

Figure 8.18

Control training

feedback to the prosthetist and the individual. A test socket with temporarily attached electrodes and myoelectric components will permit assessment of fitting and control issues, selection of components and even the start of control training with a prosthetic set-up.

8.3.2.5 Training with the Prosthesis

Following the fitting of the myoelectric prosthesis, the individual participates in a training program consisting of orientation to the prosthesis, control training and training in functional tasks. The aim is to increase the individual's understanding of the prosthesis and to develop good habits of use, care and maintenance.

Orientation to the prosthesis includes familiarizing the client with the components and the terminology used by the prosthetist and the therapist. The individual practices donning and doffing of the prosthesis and receives information about the care of the residual limb and the care of prosthesis and batteries. An appropriate wearing schedule is developed based on the tolerance of the individual.

Control Training

During the control training, the individual practices basic control motions to achieve proficiency in the operation of the prosthesis and progress from cognitive control efforts to a more automatic control for higher level functional skills. Length and frequency of training sessions are adjusted to the individual's tolerance. Initially, frequent rest periods are indicated to avoid fatigue of muscles and subsequent pain and control problems.

Control practice starts with opening and closing of the hand and relaxation between movements, first at waist level and then at various arm positions. If the prosthesis has more than one powered unit, control of each unit is practised separately. The wrist is rotated in varying increments in each direction. Control of the elbow unit starts with elbow flexion and extension, following a target and then locking the elbow at

ficiency by adjustment of the electrode gains, using feedback from the amputee, analysis of the EMG signals and evaluation of control problems. These may be caused by muscle imbalance, pain in the residual limb or the phantom limb, cramps, fatigue, anxiety, tension, high expectations, concentration or motivation.

The training time necessary to achieve good control varies and depends on the person's neuromuscular control and state of relaxation. Most individuals are able to generate and isolate the signals in one to a few sessions. During the construction of the prosthesis re-testing of myoelectric signals and location of signal sites in the test socket may be advisable.

If there is a concern about the individual's ability to tolerate the weight of a myoelectric prosthesis, a test socket with the correct weight added will provide

different positions. Co-contraction for switching between hand and wrist or for unlocking the elbow usually requires extra practice and fine-tuning of the electrode gains. Finally sequences of control are practised.

This is followed by practice in grasping and releasing objects of varying sizes, shapes, density and weight at different positions. The performance is checked for accurate control and efficient grasp/release and positioning pattern. Pre-positioning of components is performed as required.

Controlling the high pinch force of the myoelectric hand effectively to avoid damage of fragile objects requires practice. This can be achieved through grasping crushable objects such as foam cups, wet sponges or aiming for different levels of pinch force on a pinch gauge. If the person wishes to experience the pinch force of the hand, they can grasp their own sound forearm and feel the pressure. He or she should be warned not to use the prosthesis for shaking another person's hand until they have mastered their control ability. When smooth control of all units is achieved, repetitive tasks requiring additional focus such as strategy for board games (tic-tac-toe, chess etc.) are introduced.

If problems in the control of the components occur, the prosthetist and/or therapist determine the possible causes and remedial actions. Control problems may be related to socket fit (insufficient or excessive electrode contact) or inefficient calibration of the electrode gain, insufficient battery charge, switch in the "OFF" position or mechanical failure of components. The individual may experience pain, fatigue and muscle cramps interfering with muscle contractions. He or she may co-contract muscles inadvertently. Excess perspiration may increase the pick-up of the EMG signal inappropriately. Psychological factors of tension, anxiety, pressure from competition or high performance expectations may also cause poor performance. Reassessment of myoelectric signals on the myotester may be helpful.

Functional Training

When satisfactory control of the prosthesis is achieved, the training shifts to performance of bimanual tasks of gradually increasing complexity. The tasks have to be meaningful to the individual and address the identified needs in activities of daily living, vocation, recreation and social use.

The practice starts with simple grasping of various objects such as blocks, cups, utensils and other daily use items. The wrist and elbow are positioned as needed. Tasks that require holding an object with the prosthesis for manipulation with the sound hand are added e.g., removing the lid from a jar, pulling on a glove. The best way to grasp an object securely is explored. Electric elbow units allow some live-lift. This is practised by grasping an object at one level and moving it to a new level using elbow flexion and locking at each position.

The complexity of the two-handed tasks should be increased gradually as the individual masters each task. In many activities the prosthesis is most useful as a tool to assist the sound hand. The tasks provide opportunity to encourage good work habits and conscientious use of the prosthesis. The individual is instructed in measures to avoid staining or damage of the glove and damage of the prosthesis through water, dirt, vibration etc. A variety of tasks are presented in the therapy session to broaden the experience and demonstrate the usefulness of the prosthesis for personal care, meal preparation, household tasks, clerical tasks, use of tools, vocational and leisure tasks and handling weighted objects. The individual is encouraged to use the prosthesis at home and report on his or her success, need for specific training or problem solving (Fig. 8.19, 8.20, 8.22).

Choosing the appropriate sequence of tasks assists in dealing with initial awkwardness, frustration or a one-handed work habit and increases skill and tolerance in using the prosthesis. Facilitating a sense of success in accomplishing a variety of activities increases self-confidence. This is particularly important in social settings where observation by others can cause anxiety and subsequent control problems. Practising relevant tasks e.g., cutting meat, carrying a tray, filling a plate at a buffet build the necessary confidence.

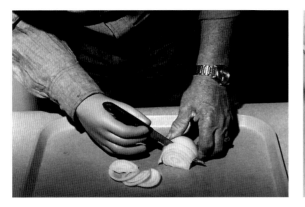

Figure 8.19

Functional training

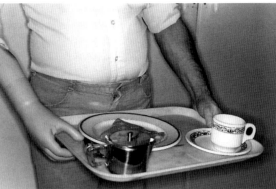

Figure 8.21

Functional use

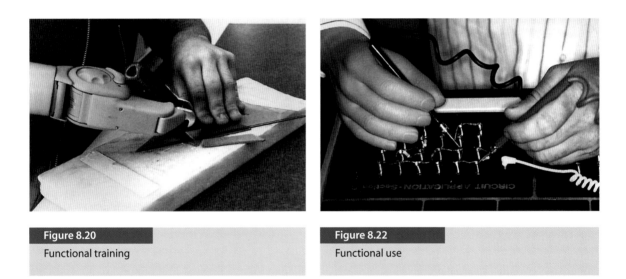

Figure 8.20

Functional training

Figure 8.22

Functional use

Throughout the training a problem solving approach is used and the individual is guided in trouble shooting to determine possible causes of malfunction of the prosthesis (see Appendix C). The training is completed when the individual demonstrates effective use of the prosthesis in activities of daily living tasks and the vocational and recreational needs have been addressed satisfactorily (Figs. 8.21, 8.23).

8.3.2.6 Evaluation

The prosthesis is evaluated at the beginning of the functional training session regarding fit and comfort of the socket, function of the components, calibration of the electrodes and cosmesis. All aspects are monitored during the training and checked again at the completion of the training program. Modifications and adjustments are carried out as necessary.

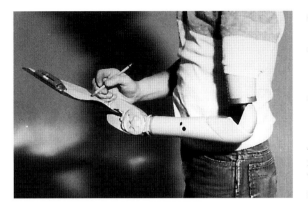

Figure 8.23
Functional use

The individual is assessed in his or her ability to control the prosthesis and use it effectively in activities of daily living, vocational and recreational tasks as well as tolerance to wearing the prosthesis and using it actively. He or she is observed for spontaneous incorporation of the prosthesis during task performance.

8.3.2.7 Follow-up

The fit and function of the prosthesis and the individual's ability to use it for required tasks needs to be evaluated on an ongoing basis. Identifying and eliminating problems, ideally in their early stages, will improve the acceptance and use of the prosthesis.

Issues to be addressed include:
- Medical/physical status of the individual and the condition of the residual limb, as well as the sound limb
- Pain management, psychosocial and emotional needs, acceptance of the amputation and the prosthesis by the individual and the social environment

- Fit, function, cosmesis and maintenance of the prosthesis
- Tolerance to wearing the prosthesis, pattern of using it and integration into the lifestyle of the individual
- Level of functional independence, vocational and recreational needs

A useful protocol for follow-up is three months, six months, annually and then, on an "as needed" basis. This assists in providing necessary modifications and servicing of the prosthesis.

The training program provides the foundation for functional use of the prosthesis. Full integration into the person's daily life requires motivation and practice. The myoelectric prosthesis will more likely be used when sufficient functional gains outweigh the disadvantages the person experiences. Individuals who are provided with myoelectric as well as conventional and/or cosmetic prostheses benefit from being able to choose the prosthesis most useful for the required function or situation.

8.4 Questions

1. Identify the major roles of an occupational therapist in myoprosthetic practice.
2. Describe several appropriate uses of a myolectric prosthesis for a toddler and for a preschool child.
3. When choosing a control system for an older child, what four factors influence the final decision?
4. Give some examples of activities that require the user of a prosthesis to use different ranges of motion or types of grasps/uses. Example: an activity requiring a heavy load.
5. Describe the components of a training program for adult myoelectric users.
6. Describe how to select appropriate signal sites for a client to be fitted with a myoelectric trans-radial prosthesis.

Appendix A

Advantages of a Myoelectric Prosthesis

Function:	Stronger prehension force
	More secure grasp
	Graded grip strength through proportional control
	Greater span for terminal device or hand opening
	Greifer has wrist deviation for better approach to work, fine pinch, safety release
	Control requires minimal body movement and effort
	Ease of operation and use in all spatial planes
Comfort:	Lack of harness for a transradial prosthesis
	Lack of control cables
	Freedom of movement
Cosmesis:	More natural appearance of hand
	No harness and cables for a trans-radial prosthesis
	No obvious control motions required
Convenience:	Easy to don/doff

Disadvantages of a Myoelectric Prosthesis

Cost:	Initial purchase and repairs are higher
Fragility:	Gloves are easily stained by grease, ink, newsprint, carbon paper, fabric and leather, dyes, vegetable colors, egg yolk, mustard, ketchup, tobacco smoke, shoe polish etc. or damaged by sharp objects
	Components are damaged by dirt, sand, water, vibration, dropping, excessive weight
	Batteries require proper maintenance regime

Disadvantages (continued)

Function:	Decreased by cold temperatures (battery function, glove stiffness)
	Control is influenced by excess perspiration and external interference (transformers) and fit of socket (body weight increase/decrease)
	Control may be complex
	Decreased proprioception
Comfort:	Greater weight
	Heat build up from the socket
	Intimate fit may cause discomfort (Muenster) or be harsh on fragile skin
	Greater care in hygiene is required
Cosmesis:	Glove is easily soiled or torn
	Hand size may be too small or too large in comparison to sound hand
	Noise from motor
	Increased space requirements for elbow unit

Vocational Use

Myoelectric prosthesis	Cable-operated prosthesis:
Office work	Manual labour
Supervisory work	Skilled work
Contact with public	Office work
Skilled work	Supervisory work (hands on)
Manual labour	
Workplace	
Fairly clean	Unclean
Lifting	
Light objects	Heavy objects

Appendix B

Myoelectric Test for Transradial Amputation

Name_____

Date_____

Age_____ Date of Amputation_____ Type_____ Dominance_____
M/F

Length of residual limb_____

Length of sound limb _____

Placement of Electrodes:

Flexors: from epicondyle to flexor electrode_____

Flexors: from ulna medial to electrode _____

Extensors: from epicondyle to extensor electrode _____

Extensors: from ulna lateral to electrode

Signal Strength:

Flexors   _____

Co-contraction?_____

Extensors   _____

Co-contraction?_____

Movement of the phantom hand to generate signal:

Flexors

_____

Extensors

_____

Can the amputee

sustain the signals for 1 second

_____

alternate the signals

_____

co-contract purposely

_____

relax while moving arm through full

range_____

generate signals in all spatial

planes_____

relax while resistance is applied to

limb_____

generate signals while resistance is applied to

limb_____

generate accurate signals without visual

feedback_____

Does pro/supination influence

signals_____

Comments: (condition of residual limb, tolerance, learning ability, motivation,

functional needs in activities of daily living, vocation, avocation, use of cable-

operated prosthesis etc.)

_____
_____
_____
_____
_____
_____
_____
_____

Appendix C

Trouble Shooting

If prosthesis does not work or control problems occur check:

- Switch: "OFF"
- Terminal device properly inserted in wrist unit
- Battery charge
- Electrode contact
- Excess perspiration
- Muscle fatigue
- Muscle cramps
- Pain
- Signal strength
- Co-contraction
- Electrode calibration
- External interference (transformer, TV, ham radio etc.)
- Wires disconnected, wrong connection
- Corrosion of battery terminal, wire connections
- Component malfunction (clutch, transmission etc.)

References

1. Amputee Coalition of America, 900 E. Hill Ave. Ste.285, Knoxville, TN 37915–2568
2. Brenner CD (1992) Electronic limbs for infants and pre-school children. J Prosthet Orthot 4:24–30
3. Brooks B, Setoguchi Y, Thue J, Beal L, Tom D (1965) Crisis intervention. Inter-Clinic Information Bull 4(11):7–15
4. Clarke S (1987) Prehension and developmental theory: review of normal skills acquisition. In: Krebs D (ed) Prehension assessment. SLACK Inc., Thorofare, NJ, pp 1–11
5. Datta D, Ibbotson V (1998) Powered prosthetic hands in very young children. Prosthet Orthot Int 22:150–154
6. Hermansson L (1991). Structured training of children fitted with myoelectric prostheses. Prosthet Orthot Int 15: 88–92
7. Hubbard S (1995) Myo-prosthetic management of the upper limb amputee. Rehabilitation of the hand: surgery and therapy vol. 2, 4th edn. CV Mosby Company, St Louis, pp 1241–1252
8. Hubbard S (1991) Prosthetic considerations: pre and school age children. In: VASI manual, Variety Ability Systems Inc., Toronto, Canada, Sects. 2.1–2.2
9. Patton J (1989) Developmental approach to pediatric prosthetic evaluation and training. In: Atkins DJ, Meier RH (eds) Comprehensive management of the upper limb amputee. Springer, Berlin Heidelberg New York, pp 137–149
10. Pruitt S, Varni J, Setoguchi Y (1996) Functional status in children with limb deficiency: development and initial validation of an outcome measure. Arch Phys Med Rehabil 77:1233–1238
11. Pruitt S, Varni J, Setoguchi Y (1998) Functional status in limb deficiency: development of an outcome measure for preschool children. Arch Phys Med Rehabil 79: 405–411
12. Pruitt S, Seid M, Varni J, Setoguchi Y (1999) Toddlers with limb deficiency: conceptual basis and initial application of a functional status outcome measure. Arch Phys Med Rehabil 80:819–823
13. Sanderson ER, Scott RN (1985) UNB Test of Prosthetics Function: a test for unilateral upper extremity amputees, ages 2–13. Bio-Engineering Institute, University of New Brunswick, Fredericton, New Brunswick
14. Schuch M (1998) Prosthetic principles in fitting myoelectric prostheses in children. In: Herring J, Birch J (eds) AAOS/Shrine Symposium: the limb deficient child. American Academy of Orthopaedic Surgeons, Rosemont, IL, pp 405–416
15. Sorbye R (1989) Upper extremity amputees: Swedish experience concerning children. In: Atkins DJ, Meier RH (eds) Comprehensive management of the upper limb amputee. Springer, Berlin Heidelberg New York, pp 227–239

16. Stocker D, Caldwell R, Wedderburn Z (1995) Review of infant fittings at the Institute of Biomedical Engineering: 13 years of service. Conference Proceedings, MEC '95, UNB's Myoelectric Controls/Powered Prosthetics Symposium, Fredericton, NB, Canada, pp 23–27

17. War Amps of Canada, 2827 Riverside Drive, Ottawa, ON K1V 0C4, Canada

18. Weiss-Lambrou R (1980) A manual for the congenital below-elbow child amputee. University of Montreal, Quebec

19. Wright V, Hubbard S, Jutai J, Naumann S (2001) The prosthetic upper extremity functional index: development and reliability of a new functional status questionnaire for children who use upper extremity prostheses. J Hand Ther 14: 91–104

20. Wright V, Hubbard S (2003) Evaluation of the validity of the prosthetic upper-extremity functional index (PUFI). Arch Phys Med Rehabil 84(4): 518–527

Research and the Future of Myoelectric Prosthetics

P. J. Kyberd · D. Gow · P. H. Chappell

Contents

Summary

The design of an artificial limb must encompass many features involving both anthropomorphic constraints and practical engineering. A study of human physiology and anatomy gives some clues to a design, which is both acceptable to the user and meets engineering standards. A discussion is given of the engineering components such as actuators, electronics and materials. This chapter explores new control methods including pattern recognition of EMG signals, hierarchical organisation and extended physiological proprioception.

9.1 Introduction

The advancement of prosthetics relies on several different approaches. Notable of these is a study of the physiology of the natural system with a view to replicate an engineered solution and the investigation of novel methods, which to some extent have no connection with human function and are rooted firmly in engineering.

A study of the natural hand shows that the index and middle fingers are used for prehensile tasks with the opposing thumb. The ring and little finger provide strength during grasping with the thumb providing a critical component for the secure grip of any object. An adaptable and compliant palm completes the form of a natural hand. So future development of artificial hands must encompass independent digits, a mobile thumb and their integration into a palm. This leads to a design that has multiple degrees of freedom and incorporates a number of actuators to allow independent flexion and extension of the fingers and at least two independent movements of the thumb.

9.2 Design Constraints

Any replacement of the upper limb by an artificial device is constrained by physical limits of the natural system and by the available technology.

The following is a list of constraints imposed by a consideration of the physical dimensions of a human.

9.2.1 Appearance

It is critical that the prosthesis should be acceptable for the users. This does not necessarily mean that the device is anthropomorphic in shape and action. For some this is the overriding function of their prosthesis. Others are supremely indifferent to the appearance and a number believe to have a naturalistic device is dishonest, as it would mean that they would be pretending to be that which they are not. The result of needing to provide the two broadly divergent requirements means that the manufacturers generally provide different prostheses maximised for appearance, where the hand has five digits and the colour can be matched to the user's skin (to a limited extent) or one with manipulative function. What is less often considered is a non-anthropomorphic device that is functional whilst being aesthetically pleasing, which is possible, but it is likely that very non-anthropomorphic motions will not be liked or used often (such as a continuously rotating wrist or an elbow that bends backwards) as it may attract unwanted attention, or have limited additional utility.

9.2.2 Weight

The constraints on the attachment methods mean that the mass of any device must be as low as possible. A target weight of 500 grams (or less) is desirable for a hand while the rest of the upper limb should be less than 1500 grams. For a powered device this target is hard to achieve. However, it is becoming more practical as new technologies become available.

9.2.3 Power Consumption

Components must make efficient use of energy. It is desirable that an artificial limb should operate for a minimum of one day without the need to replace the power source (i.e. battery). Additionally a high energy density (joules per kilogram) for the storage medium is required in order to minimise the weight. Newer forms of battery have greater capacities and are significantly lighter, however the rate at which they can deliver the power (current in an electrical battery) still limits their usage in the upper joints of the arm.

9.2.4 Modularity

Since every device has to meet the specific requirements of an individual user it makes the provision of the device simpler if it is made up from a small kit of basic parts. For example, designing a device that is symmetrically neutral or having only one design of fingers for both left and right hands. This also has the added benefit of reducing costs in the design, construction and fitting phases on the life of the prosthesis.

9.2.5 Size

As above it should be possible to match the physical dimensions of a prosthesis and its components to an individual. This means either that the basic parts can be smaller with spacers to allow expansion, or that the devices are manufactured in different sizes.

9.2.6 Speed

The perception of the performance of a device partially relies on the user not feeling they have to wait for the prosthesis to react. Additionally, the illusion of life-like movements requires the prosthesis to be able to flex and extend at the appropriate speeds. For example, a finger should cover its full range of flexion in around one second, similarly for the wrist and elbow (longer for the shoulder). However it may not be possible to control the joints at these speeds; this is a consideration for the design and use of the control format.

This also introduces the concept of "dynamic cosmesis". Conventional prostheses can be statically attractive and thoroughly anthropomorphic in appearance but move in ways that are too clearly artificial in appearance. The human brain is extremely good at detecting aberrant motion. It has strong survival advantages and so mechanical motions are easily spotted, smoother, more anthropomorphic motions are therefore more desirable.

9.2.7 Sound

Users generally do not want to attract attention to themselves, thus a prosthesis that makes noise is not one that is valued by them. All sounds are unacceptable, electric motion generally produces some noise but it is the sound of the gear train in such systems that makes the majority of the noise and so the design and construction of the gears have the biggest effect on the total noise output. Different forms of power generation may have different performances in this area (i.e. quieter but slower).

9.2.8 Reliability

It is natural that most users wish to have a device that allows them to conduct their lives with the minimum of outside attention or help. The loss of one hand is generally not so disabling that most individuals can cope without specific aids. Thus a hand/arm they cannot rely on is not one they will choose to use. For those with a bilateral loss their need is so acute that they will only employ devices that give them a positive benefit, thus an unreliable prosthesis will rapidly be rejected.

9.2.9 Price

The majority of health care is becoming very price sensitive. Prosthetics is no exception. Thus the cost of a device is always an important consideration.

9.3 Actuators

9.3.1 Electrical Motors

For many years the preferred method of actuation has been the brushed dc electric motor. This device affords the best compromise in terms of reliability, weight, control and cost. These devices continue to improve and in particular the power output per unit weight, which is of considerable importance to the designer of artificial hands. Despite the developments in motor technology, with brushless devices becoming widely available they will probably not see use in prosthetics due to the increased power requirements and the greater amount of digital electronic components required for their operation. Although switched reluctance motors offer some weight savings they again require considerable electronics and have yet to be exploited commercially at the lower power levels.

9.3.2 Pneumatic

Pneumatics has always been an option that was considered for more flexible prostheses. As a means of moving joints it has many apparent advantages, particularly in the past when electric motion was less efficient than it is at the present time. It has the high energy density required, the actuators can be made small, powerful and fast, thus it is popular in some areas of industrial robotics. An example of one of the more anthropomorphic forms of actuation is the McKibben muscle. This uses an inflatable tube operating inside an outer sleeve which shortens when the tube is pressurised. The device thus becomes shorter and wider, mimicking the action of muscle and is thus seen as a good bio-mechanical analogue. It is however, hard to control precisely and suffers from the problems associated with all pneumatic sources.

A more innovative use of compressed air uses the small carbon dioxide containers, such as those used in soda siphons, as they are small and readily available. They were applied to a child's hand, resulting in an expensive means to drive a prosthesis. Other designs of arm that were gas powered include the early Simpson arms. The problems of replenishing the gas became a significant drawback since the cylinders cannot be refilled at home (unlike electrical batteries) and so a distribution system has to be established. Additionally, compressed gas containers are not allowed on board aircraft making transportation of gas supplies or limbs using them difficult in certain countries. The operation of gas cylinders is also hindered by the feeling of sponginess due to the compliance of the gas. Finally most pneumatic systems create significant noise when actuated although the Simpson's team perfected a reasonably efficient and simple silencer for their devices.

9.3.3 Hydraulic

These actuators are very reliable, can produce large forces and previously have required bulky power sources. They are not as efficient in their use of electrical energy needed to pump the hydraulic fluid. This is beginning to change and there are some groups looking into the application of hydraulic systems. A major advantage of these systems is that they are silent in operation. Even if their pump makes a noise it will be a constant noise as the pump motor acts all the time. As a result the designers can optimise the structure to reduce the noise to a minimum. However, the remaining problems with hydraulics are that they are prone to the fluid leaking from the cylinders and also that safety constraints may require the cylinder to be made especially strong and thus heavy.

9.3.4 Piezoelectric Motors

These are much newer means of obtaining motion from electricity. They have a high torque at low speeds which is ideally suited to prosthetics, conventional electric motors should run at high speeds to be efficient users of the energy supplied.

The devices work by employing a material that is a piezoelectric ceramic, this means that it changes dimension when an electric field is applied. When it is excited by an alternating voltage, a disc of this material vibrates and can be designed to generate rotary or linear motion of a rotor. They have no need for a gearbox unlike conventional electric motors. This reduces the weight and size considerably. Secondly they will only turn when the power is supplied, so the rotor is locked when the device is not powered and thus does not need braking systems. Currently these devices are too new to have achieved the level of commercial exploitation which would prove their usefulness in prosthetics.

9.3.5 Artificial Muscles

An electrical or chemical trigger activates polymer hydrogels to produce a device with a 'muscle' characteristic. Laboratory experiments have demonstrated their potential but further development is required before they can be evaluated as a suitable prosthetic actuator.

9.3.6 Shape Memory Alloys

Recent studies of the use of shape memory alloys to prosthetics and robotics have investigated their potential due to a high power to weight ratio. They have a two-phase characteristic with different thermal, electrical and mechanical properties in each phase. At room (low) temperature (the martensitic phase) the material is easily deformed and electrically conductive. The second phase (austentic) is reached by heating the alloy where it will recover its shape, which has been set initially by heat treatment methods. The actuator effect is produced by lengthening the mate-

Table 9.1. Actuator systems

Actuator	Advantage	Disadvantage
DC motors	Small, robust, high efficiency	Gearbox required, limit on the smallest size
Pneumatic	Fast, high power/weight ratio	Acoustic noise, large power source
Hydraulic	High force, low acoustic noise	Heavy, fluid leaks
Piezoelectric motors	High torque, low speed, passively static	Not widely and commercially available
Artificial muscles	Micro-scale size	Laboratory based
Shape memory alloys	High power/weight ratio, silent operation, inherent position feedback	Needs cooling, low speed

rial at low temperature, heating it to the second phase, causing the device to shorten and return to its original shape. Hence a tension can be produced in a manner reminiscent of the way a natural muscle produces force when it contracts. The wire made of SMA can be thought of as a wire with two different spring tensions; soft at low temperature and stiff at high temperature. Useful work is obtained by the combination of the differential force times the movement obtained between the two thermal conditions.

Ideally, the wire has the properties of high power to weight ratio which suggests that it is an ideal candidate for actuators. There is a linear relationship between electrical resistance and extension, which should be useful in a feedback control loop. It is silent in operation and does not require any additional mechanics and so is a popular suggestion by engineers. However, the characteristic of the metal is hard to control and easy to destroy if it is over stretched, so that it has no shape memory effect at all. Also, when the wire is used it needs quite a high temperature, which means the heat must be removed from the wire before it can relax making it quite slow to react. Thus despite considerable interest in this material it has not so far been used effectively in external prostheses (Table 9.1).

9.3.7 Electric Power Sources

Battery technology has a wide range of application for use in portable devices (for example personal communication) and the need to have 'clean' transport. In this application, an acceptable source is one that has enough energy for normal use of the prosthesis during one day. The energy density (in Watt hours kg^{-1}) of a power source is the most important parameter and should be as high as possible since it is proportional to the time that a prosthesis can be used before the battery needs to be replaced or recharged. The power density is an indication of how rapidly power can be drawn from the source and therefore the potential force that can be produced from the actuators. A wide range of operating temperature is desirable as a prosthesis can be used in winter and summer conditions. In terms of cost of operation then the cycle lifetime is an important parameter to consider.

In general, primary (non-rechargeable) batteries have higher energy densities than secondary (rechargeable) types and therefore are smaller in size for a given energy capacity. However, over the life of the battery, a rechargeable type is cheaper and so it is generally the type used in prosthetics.

Lead-Acid batteries, in general, have good parameters except for their low energy density and the presence of acid which makes then unsuitable for use in upper limb devices. Nickel-Cadmium batteries have been used in prosthetic devices but are being replaced by types that have better energy densities

Table 9.2. Battery parameters

Battery	Energy density (W hours kg^{-1})	Power density (W kg^{-1})	Temperature (°C)	Cycle life
Lead-acid	35	100	−49–55	1,000
Nickel-cadmium	60	110	−40–60	2,000
Nickel-metal hydride	70	175	Ambient	1,550
Lithium	150	300	Ambient	300

(Table 9.2). Also a major disadvantage of this battery is that the cadmium is highly toxic. They cannot be discarded but require disposal where the cadmium can be recovered. Additionally incomplete discharging of the battery leads to a change in the crystalline structure of the battery, reducing the amount of the stored charge that is available to the user (the so-called *memory* of the battery). The observed change is that the life of the battery from fully charged to flat is reduced. More recent technologies based on Lithium or Nickel Metal Hydride do not suffer from these problems, however the prosthetics industry was slow to adopt them in the 1990s, when they were already widely used in many domestic consumer products, with many of the major prosthetics manufacturers finally beginning to incorporate this mature technology into their product lines by 2000.

Neither of these forms has the same life-span as Nickel-Cadmium, (numbers of complete charge/discharge cycles) and Lithium tends not to be able to deliver as large a current to the motors. Since the power that the motor can develop and so the overall power of the prosthesis depends on the current in the motors, this has had a detrimental effect on the speed and power of the action of the prosthesis. So they tend to be used for hands rather than arm joints.

Future electric power sources are being developed that do not rely on chemical reactions. Notable is the flywheel energy storage system where rotational kinetic energy is stored in a spinning flywheel. High energy and power densities can be achieved. If a small device can be produced at a low cost then this device has the potential to replace conventional batteries for prosthetics.

9.4 Prosthesis Control

The manner by which a prosthesis is controlled has an effect on the way that the device is used. The conventional control format of electric prostheses has been to use simple electronics, this meant that the type of control performed by the user and the ease by which it was changed was very limited. Originally the myoelectric signal was used as a switch input. If the amplified signal exceeded a set threshold the motor was turned on at a fixed speed in a set direction. Although it was shown that a continuous signal could be used to control a prosthesis it took a great deal longer before it was adopted by the commercial prosthesis manufacturers.

If the prosthesis is controlled proportionally, then some action gets larger when the command signal does. The action most commonly used is motor speed. As the muscle tension increases so does the amplified signal and the rotation speed of the motors (and so joint) increases. So the user can control the position more precisely and quickly, it is most commonly used to control electric elbow action. The position of the joint can be made proportional to the myo signal, then the hand opens as wide as the command is large and then closes again as the user relaxes (this is termed Voluntary Opening Involuntary Closing – VOIC).

Work at Southampton in the 1980s showed that the application of microprocessors would allow much more sophisticated control actions, a fact which is now generally recognised. Microprocessors are the heart of all computers, thus the advantages of using one in a prosthesis are the same as using a computer in many other machines, it simply takes a change in the program. So with a microprocessor controlled prosthesis the prosthetist can simply change the way the hand is controlled and indeed potentially customise the way it is controlled to suit the individual user. One of the earliest sophisticated systems based on this idea was produced in Toronto at Bloorview Macmillan Children's Centre and marketed by VASI. Through a graphical user interface the prosthetist can change every aspect of the control format. Originally, the professional prosthetists did not want to have such control over the programming. While their concern is justified, ultimately it is to be hoped that they will take to the computer packages that help them program the controllers as it is *they* (in conjunction with the users) and not the engineers or manufacturers who should have the final word over the control format.

Originally, different control formats needed different electronics packages built into the hands, meaning each type was a different product. The first commercial microprocessors were used to reduce the number of different electronics packages that were needed for a particular device so that one microprocessor circuit could serve for every different type, needing only a simple switch between control formats. Now the companies are beginning to appreciate the real possibilities of using these devices, for example simple and easy change of the control, customisation to the user etcetera. However, the most advanced devices are currently still part of the research field. This chapter will outline the most advanced or sophisticated devices currently in development.

9.4.1 Intelligent Control

9.4.1.1 Hierarchical Control of the Limbs

The movement of our limbs is something that is broadly effortless. Generally we do not need to think about how we control individual joints. When babies are born they do not have fine control of their limbs. Initially they have little control over their arms and they wave them with little purpose or precision. Rap-

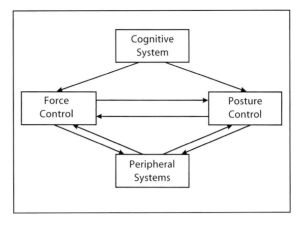

Figure 9.1

A simple model of the human central nervous system. The control is arranged in an hierarchical fashion with the lower levels co-ordinating so the conscious levels do not need to devote attention to grasping an object

idly their control is refined and as they learn to concentrate, can be seen moving one hand under visual control leaving the other to wave aimlessly. Then even this control is improved so that they can hold objects while they concentrate on other tasks. This process takes many months and a lot of effort on a baby's part. We go through a similar process when we learn to drive. Initially too much happens all at once, but quite soon we can see all that is going on around us, listen to music, talk to the passengers or navigate.

This is because the operations are hierarchical. We are aware of the simplest actions or desires and the rest is looked after by other parts of our central nervous system barely supervised. Conventional myoelectric control is difficult because the contraction of the command muscles is more voluntary as the new user has to learn the new actions and so they are generally kept to a very simple level. Hierarchical control resembles a simple model of the central nervous system where the perceived action of the natural hand by the user is above the lower levels of control (Fig. 9.1). At an intermediate level there are the position and force reflexes of the fingers. Lower down the system, information is gathered from peripheral sensors while neural loops co-ordinate the hand's posture and grip force. Force and posture control is supervised by electronics using data from sensors mounted on the prosthesis. The contact area is generally maximised so that the contact forces can be spread over as wide an area as possible and the effort is kept to a minimum. Most forces are less than 12 N while most prostheses cannot adjust their grip shape and wrap around the object, their points of contact are small, thus they are often seen to be too weak to be used in any important tasks.

When an arm is lost or absent these structures are hard to access. The direct myoelectric control of a prosthesis links the top conscious control box down to the reflex layer. So the user must concentrate quite hard and use other senses, such as sight to be sure that the operation is successful.

A second problem with myoelectric control is that as the actions often used by a wearer to generate the signal are unnatural and hard to learn, then there is little scope for simultaneous control of more than one motion (joint). This would need the co-ordinated contraction of many different muscles at once or in a specific sequence. It is a skilled task, each action is separate and has to be done in the right sequence to get the performance right. For example a pianist playing a tune, with different actions and timings for each and every finger. We are all aware that it needs enormous amounts of practice and concentration to be a pianist. Few users would wish to, or may be capable of, that level of practice and skill. What the user needs is a simple task that they can learn quickly to control the prosthesis. Thus in general the tasks and types of prosthesis control is limited. A number of research groups have attempted to overcome this. They either try to leave as much of the control of the prosthesis to a computer, or they attempt to use the structures that exist in the human CNS as efficiently as possible.

9.4.1.2 Pattern Recognition Techniques

One route is to use the patterns of muscle activity that are associated with motion. As muscle action is tied to a particular limb motion it is possible that the motion of the limb is related to the pattern of contractions in the surface muscles in the arm. This un-

derstanding has fed the desire to use such complex signals in controllers that can drive multiple axes prostheses easily and intuitively. This would allow the internal feedback from the muscles and all the practice that already exists to control the prosthesis. This is focusing on the Phantom Limb Phenomenon (PLP). Groups have recorded the patterns of signals from the multiple electrodes on the forearms of users and extracted the underlying information.

The most successful of these was that in Sweden in the 1970s. It formed part of the Sven Hand project, which produced a hand with flexion and extension of the fingers and thumb and then pro-supination and flexion/extension of the wrist. They then captured the signals from 2 electrodes on the forearm while the user performed six specific tasks. The critical elements of the signal were then extracted and built into an electronic controller that drove the hand with ease and fluidity. A number of users were fitted with the device and it was used in domestic and work settings. The research led onto the semi-commercial ES hand.

While the work has been investigated further no other group has fitted a multi motion hand with a controller based on these principles. However Hudgins, Parker and Scott have shown that at the initial stage of contraction there is information in the myoelectric signal from single electrodes that allows more than one state to be selected from a *single* electrode. An electronics package has been developed that allows it to control conventional hands.

All other research groups so far have addressed the signal processing ideas without clinical use or application to a prosthesis. There are two major problems associated with this technique. The first is that it requires a usable phantom the user can control and the intact musculature to drive it. For example it would seem that only persons with a loss acquired later in life would have the phantom to drive it. Paradoxically this does not seem to be entirely true. There seem to be some users with congenital absences that have something they can use. This indicates that the science behind what the phantom is, is far from completely explored.

The second problem is a more practical consideration: If the detection of the control signals is a subtle matter of the timing and strength between different muscles then the physical location of the electrodes becomes critical. As the myoelectric signal depends on the location of the electrodes and the strength and activity of the muscle it is clear that the complex signal needed for pattern recognition will change from day to day, (even minute to minute) as the prosthesis shifts on the arm and the sweat and other confounding factors change with wearing.

Often the suggested solution is to make the electronics learn the changes in the signal, perhaps with a calibration step first thing in the morning and then at other times of day. Not only would this level of interaction seem unacceptable to many users, the Sven team realised that having the system adapt to the user is flawed. The users themselves adapt. To have the arm attempting to adapt while the wearers do, means that it will never settle and will not be easy to use. The user's perception will be that the arm always needs them to adjust to it.

A better way to interact with the device is using electrodes fixed in place. Buried subcutaneous electrodes have been developed for other purposes. Their casual usage in prosthetics is currently unacceptable, however with techniques like osseointegration this is becoming a more practical possibility.

9.4.1.3 Extended Physiological Proprioception

A different method of using the existing control structures in the CNS is to feed information about the hand back to the operator, in a manner like the original arm. This generally requires connections back to the nerves of the person. Direct neural connection is something the researchers have talked about for the past 50 years, without clinical success. Although experimental neural connections now do exist they are still in their infancy as far as casual use is concerned and may be something that will occur any time in the *next* 50 years.

A different approach is to feed the signals back to the skin surface. The problem is that they must use the correct form of information, otherwise the user must concentrate on changing (say) vibration into information about the force the hand is gripping.

It has been suggested that a person will accept a prosthesis as a replacement of a natural limb as part of their overall body, if the feedback is of the right form and at the point of application. This concept is called extended physiological proprioception (epp) and was first coined by Simpson and his co-workers during their work with Thalidomide affected children in Edinburgh in the 1960s and 1970s. Simpson's work eventually realised hundreds of fittings of gas powered prostheses controlled by epp which demonstrably had improved control of multi degrees of freedom. Four spatial co-ordinates could be controlled in parallel by experienced users who had cable linkages present between their residual shoulder joint movements and the equivalent prosthetic joints. Further evidence for the usefulness of this control strategy is based on experiments with normal subjects and those fitted with artificial devices carrying out tracking tasks. This takes the force on a commanding lever as the input but the position of the lever is related to the position of the arm (force feed forward and position feedback). This is similar to the manner in which natural limbs are controlled and so the hierarchy is used to its fullest extent.

9.4.2 Advanced Controllers

9.4.2.1 Slip Detection

Salisbury and Coleman pointed out that if the hand system detected the sliding motion of any held object directly it could be used to correct insufficient grip forces applied by the hand. This formed one of the central points of the control philosophy referred to as the *Southampton Hand*. More recently it has also been applied by other groups and was finally adopted by the Otto Bock corporation in their *Sensorhand*.

The basic principles remain the same, that if the hand detects the motion of the held object within the grasp of the prosthesis then it automatically increases the grip until the chance of slipping ceases. This motion can be detected by means of one of three ways:

The first detects the fact that when an object starts to move the forces between the object and the fingers change. There are more sideways forces (or shear). If this is detected by measuring the direction of the forces at the tips of the fingers this can decode slip. The advantage of this method is that it can detect slip before there is any relative motion between the hand and object, unfortunately it can also detect changes in forces that will not give rise to any slippage, for example if an object is inverted while in the hand, the measured shear will change from one direction to the opposite.

A second means is to study the pattern of forces at the surface between the hand and object. As slip begins the disposition of forces and their shape changes. This is sometimes referred to as *partial slip*. The disadvantage of this method is that it requires any computer based controller to spot patterns in the forces and control the hand's response. This has required powerful computers to react in time or simpler methods (algorithms) to react faster.

A final method is to record the vibrations set up when the object begins to slip. The noise created under such conditions is familiar to everyone in one form or another. The quality of the signal depends on the surfaces in contact. It might then mean that rougher, noisier surfaces are more likely to give rise to a big signal that will be detected and reacted to. A prosthesis controller needs to be consistent and predictable so reacting to different surface textures differently is undesirable. However, studies of the signals generated show that the low frequencies generated are common to the majority of surfaces in contact, so that a narrowly filtered signal will give rise to a consistent response. A second criticism of this method is that it can only operate when the slide has started. While this is true it is possible to make the detection sensitive and specific to slip while shear can pick up other non-slip motions. Additionally, as stated above, it is possible to observe slip between parts of the surface (partial slip), this will give rise to a slip signal even when the bulk of the object is stationary relative to the hand so that the amount of motion is small.

All three methods have some failings but then the human system is also fallible, (for example a straight sided glass covered in condensation). The human system is less prone than others as it tends to use a combination of all three techniques, indeed the human methods combine all systems with experience to detect motion, including other methods like knowledge of the slipperiness of the target, weight, shape and, if it is colder or hotter than the hand, the change in the sensed temperature. When used separately each method must compromise to obtain a satisfactory response. For example, a system may have a high minimum grip force of 15 N, to ensure that the shear forces are large enough to be detected. However, this force is fifty percent larger than the typical grip force used by the human hand. This is because the hand does not adapt to the shape of the held object and has rigid fingers. The result is that even with a maximum grip force of over 120 N the hand is still seen as weak and it is hard to pick up delicate objects.

The best strategy is like the natural system to combine two or more of the means to measure slip so that only when the correct signals are generated across the range will the slide be detected.

9.4.2.2 Southampton Hand

As it is difficult to feed the information back to the operator, the alternative approach is to leave most of the control to the prosthesis itself. For this reason the Southampton Adaptive Manipulation Scheme (SAMS) was developed. The user generates a proportional two-site myoelectric signal, while a microprocessor and sensors control the prehensile movement and grip force. This arrangement allows the user to simply instruct the prosthesis to *open, close, hold, squeeze* or *release* an object. So that there is only a limited conscious input from the user but the prosthesis maintains a natural co-ordination of the fingers. Hence a stable grip is kept on an object without the disadvantage of constant visual feedback which would otherwise place an additional control burden on the user.

While in the *position* state, extensor muscle activity causes the hand to open in proportion to the processed myoelectric signal using position sensors. Removal of the signal causes involuntary closure of the hand until the object makes contact with touch sensors on the fingers and palm. At this point, the actua-

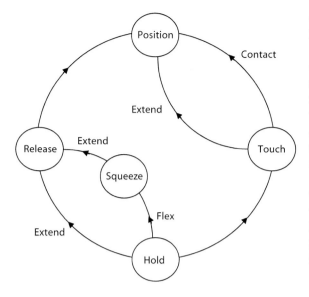

Figure 9.2

The basic control states of *position, touch, hold, squeeze and release*. Movement from one state to the next is achieved either by the user generating EMG signals above set thresholds or by information from the sensors

object begin to move from the hand's grasp (see Fig. 9.2).

Should the user wish to exert greater force on the object then the *squeeze* state causes force to be generated in proportion to the flexor activity. An important feature of the control scheme is that the person has total command over the hand so during *hold* and *squeeze* an extensor signal causes the controller to enter a *release* state followed by a return to the *position* state.

With the control scheme there is minimal intervention by the user and a stable grip is maintained without the use of visual feedback. This format has been used to control hands with one, two, four and five independent motions of the fingers. The control input from the users has been the same.

9.4.2.3 Electronics

An obvious aim of the electronic design is to make it as small as possible and to consume as little power as possible. It has the two main functions of input and output of signals (Table 9.3) and implementing control algorithms. Information is gathered from the sensors and is processed. The controller executes algorithms outputs control signals to the actuators and produces any alarms such as a small beeper to warn the user of a malfunction or low battery state. Engineers design complex systems and there is a trade-off between this complexity and size, thus limiting the number of functions performed by any controller.

The circuits for the input signals need to be as compact as possible. For example, an EMG signal can be processed using operational amplifier circuits but

tors stop and the controller moves to the *touch* state causing a minimal grip force to be exerted on the object.

A natural progression is to request that an object be held automatically in a similar manner to the low-level autonomic system. This is achieved by the generation of a flexor signal. In the *hold* state slip sensors allow for the automatic increase in force should an

Table 9.3. Types of input and output signals for the Southampton Hands

	Type	Electronic requirement
Input signals	Touch	Analogue to digital conversion
	Digit position	Analogue to digital conversion
	EMG	Analogue to digital conversion
	Object slip	Threshold and detect
Output signals	Motor	Pulse width modulation
	Alarm	Digital to analogue conversion

a better solution is to convert it into a digital form and then process it in a single integrated circuit. This device should have as many features as possible and will contain analogue to digital converters, digital to analogue converters, memory, timers, digital ports, interrupt control and a fast instruction time, to name but a few. Typical of these devices is a Digital Signal Processor (DSP). An electronic solution is produced which contains a minimum of support circuits with the signal processing and control performed digitally.

9.4.3 Modular Systems

Since the industrial revolution the standardisation of parts and systems has lead to simpler and cheaper application of engineered products. While this has been carried through in the raw componentry of the products, the advent of computer controllers has allowed this to be spread into the prosthetics field.

Prosthetist Chris Lake pointed out that the prostheses controllers have moved through multiple generations of increasing sophistication: The First generation were very simple controllers. They relied on discrete electronics and simple packages. They were the On-Off controllers, with the motors either running in one direction as fast as possible, or the other, or stopped (confusingly called "digital" controllers).

Second generation added simple proportional control with the speed of some joints being proportional to the myo level input. Later on they were controlled using microprocessors with fixed programs that meant that the prosthetist could only change the program by changing the module. By this time groups such as those at Southampton and Oxford in the UK and Toronto in Canada were applying microprocessors to perform reconfigurable tasks, ones where the controller can be rapidly changed to suit the user's needs or even learn from the interactions with the user. These are third generation microprocessor based controllers. Previously, all the functions that were offered by the manufacturers on their older controllers used a different electronics package for each controller. The adaptability of a microprocessor means that *the same* package could perform all these

functions on a single device. The manufacturers then responded with a series of self contained add-on microprocessor packages. These can control existing prostheses with greater flexibility and add some interchangeability.

This leads to the logical extension of this progression, that manufacturers should be presenting a fully integrated approach to prosthesis design. The current systems have tended to grow up as the market or technology could provide, starting with hands and then adding wrists or elbows as they could be powered. Although the lower reaches of the devices *are* modular plugs, cabling and mechanical connectors, the higher parts of the systems remain disparate. The ideal is that an arm should be as modular as possible. That the connectors, electronics, mechanisms are all sufficiently similar that they can be interchanged. One leading example of this philosophy is the Edinburgh Modular Arm System (EMAS). This uses the same drive system (ProDigits) which is based round a worm and wheel gearing system. The size of the motor and gearbox dictates its position in the arm, so that a child's shoulder could be a small adult's elbow. This keeps the stock of parts low, allows the system to be mechanically customised to the user and results in a modular electronics system, where each motor/joint has its own electronics controller so that the communications to each joint is simple and all the local control is made at the joint. Then the control format, myo processing and any feedback system can be decided at fitting and altered as the user becomes accustomed to their device. Estimates in 2003 were that about 1000 MPU prostheses were now fitted annually.

9.4.4 Materials

Transitional lightweight materials are aluminium alloys, which are easily machined and readily available. However the development of other materials such as carbon fibre composites enable the construction of a hand which has a considerable saving in weight (Fig. 9.3). Further weight saving can be made using polymer thermoplastics, especially those that have good bearing surface properties as these can be used

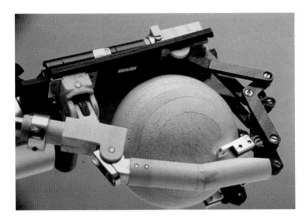

Figure 9.3

The Southampton-Remedi Hand, the sixth multiple axis Southampton Hand to be produced. Individual fingers flex when the hand closes and a microprocessor selects the most appropriate grip to hold the object, in this case it is a power grip

Figure 9.4 ▼

SHAP classification of prehensile patterns

for gearbox housings and therefore remove the need for shaft bearings. Once again manufacturer's have been slow to adopt newer materials due to their considerable investments in existing designs.

9.5 Assessment of Hand Function

It is the desire of engineers to improve prosthetic hand designs through objective testing. Components can be either individually or collectively tested for their reliability and modes of failure using standard methods. A more difficult evaluation is comparing one device to another in terms of its function. For this reason the Southampton Hand Assessment Procedure (SHAP) was developed. It is a broad-based method of assessing hand function irrespective of the disability, thereby allowing assessment of both natural and prosthetic function. The outcome measure is an index of functionality, which is determined with respect to normal hand function.

All ranges of grip need to be included in any rigorous test of hand functionality. For SHAP the classifi-

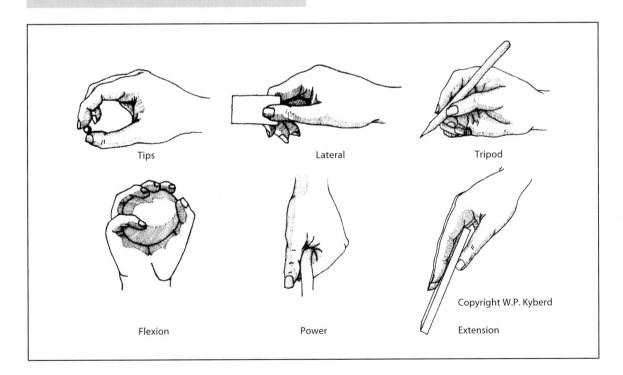

Tips   Lateral   Tripod

Flexion   Power   Extension

Copyright W.P. Kyberd

cation of grips is defined in terms of six prehensile patterns (Fig. 9.4). The procedure is based on timed measurements using twelve 'abstract tasks' and fourteen activities of daily living (ADL). The former is divided into six tests using lightweight objects (made from balsa wood) and a similar set made from aluminium. The ADL includes tasks such as picking up coins and pouring water from a jug.

9.6 Conclusions

The evolution of electronic devices will continue to have a significant impact on the control of upper limb prostheses. This is manifested in the packaging of more features and processing into a single device. Sensors are becoming smaller, which allows for better integration into hand and arm designs. Research into composite and plastic materials will result in less heavy devices. Perhaps it is in the area of actuators that the most advances are needed in order to improve the power to weight and torque to weight ratios.

9.7 Questions

1. Compare and contrast suitable actuators for use in prosthetic devices.
2. Discuss the design constraints of upper limb prosthetics.
3. A designer considers using the EMG signals from four muscles to control a powered prosthesis. Describe why this proposal is not a practical solution and discuss suitable methods.
4. Explain the concept of hierarchical control and its advantages to the user of a prosthesis.
5. Discuss the Southampton and Edinburgh control philosophies, compare them with more conventional styles.
6. Discuss the use of a state driven controller, which allows the user of a prosthesis to not rely on visual feedback whilst maintaining a stable grip on an object.
7. Draw a block diagram to illustrate the digital requirements for the signal processing in an artificial hand.
8. The mass of an artificial hand is 500grams when made out of aluminium (density 2.7 gcm^{-3}). Calculate the reduction in mass if the fingers are made from carbon fibre composite (density 1.9 gcm^{-3}) and the gearboxes from thermoplastic materials (density 1.6 gcm^{-3}). Assume the volumes of the fingers, gearboxes and rest of the components are constant and in the ratio of 3 to 2 to 5.
9. Calculate if a 1000mAh battery has enough charge to allow for the use of a prototype hand during one day. The charge required for a power grip is 0.48mAh, for a precision grip is 0.45mAh and for a lateral grip is 0.26mAh. A power grip is used 30% of the time, the precision grip 50% and the lateral grip 20%. The number of grips required each day is 2000.

Suggested Reading

Almstrom and Herberts (1981) Experience with Swedish multifunctional prosthetic hands controlled by pattern recognition of multiple myoelectric signals. Int Orthop (SICOT) 5:15–21

Bergman et al. (1992) M Functional benefit of an adaptive myoelectric prosthetic hand compared to a conventional myoelectric hand. Prosth Orthot Int 16:32–37

Burroughs and Brook (1985) Patterns of acceptance and rejection of upper limb prostheses. Orthot Prosthet 39(2):40–47

Branemark (2000) Osseointegration in amputee rehabilitation. Second International Conference Advances in Osseointegration, University of Surrey, 16–17th June, 2000

Codd (1975) Development and evaluation of adaptive control for a hand prosthesis. PhD thesis, University of Southampton

Doubler and Childress (1984) An analysis of extended physiological proprioception as a prosthesis-control technique. J Rehab Res Dev 21(1):5–31

Escher et al. (1994) A gripper based on NiTi-silicone-composite materials with reversible shape memory effect. Trans Mat Res Soc Japan 18B:1167–1170

Fraser (1993) A survey of users of upper limb prostheses. Br J Occupat Ther 56(5):166–168

Gasson, Hutt, Goodhew, Kyberd, and Warwick (2002) Bi-directional human machine interface via direct neural connection. Proceedings of IEEE International Conference on Robot and Human Interactive Communication, 25–27 September, Berlin, pp 265–270

Gow (1999) The development of the Edinburgh modular arm system In: MEC'99 Symposium upper limb prosthetic research and consumer needs: narrowing the gap. 25–27 August 1999, Fredericton, NB, Canada, pp 64–66

Gow et al. (2001) The development of the edinburgh modular arm system. Proc Instit Mechan Eng Vol 215-H:291–298

Gregory-Dean (1991) Amputations: statistics and trends. Ann Royal Coll Surg Engl 73:137–142

Hasselbach and Stork (1994) Electrically controlled shape memory actuators for use in handling systems. In Proc 1st Int Conf on Shape Memory and Superelastic Technologies

Haslinger (1997) The Grip-stabilising sensor. An Example for integrating miniaturized sensors into a myo-electric hand. In: MEC'97 UNB's MyoElectric Contyrols/Powered Prosthetics Symposium: Issues in Upper limb prosthetics. 23–25 July 1997, Fredericton, NB, Canada, pp 44–45

Herberts et al. (1978) Clinical application study of multifunctional prosthetic hands. J Bone Joint Surg 60B(4)

Hudgins et al. (1993) A new strategy for multifunction myoelectric control. IEEE Trans Biomed Eng 40(1)82–94

Kurtz (1999) Programmable control: clinical experience at Bloorview MacMillan Centre, In: MEC'99 Symposium Upper limb prosthetic research and consumer needs: narrowing the gap. 25–27 August 1999, Fredericton, NB, Canada, pp 130–133

Kyberd (1990) The algorithmic control of a multifunction hand prosthesis. PhD thesis, University of Southampton

Kyberd and Chappell (1992) Object-slip detection during manipulation using a derived force vector. Mechatronics 2(1): 1–14

Kyberd and Chappell (1994) The Southampton Hand. An intelligent myoelectric prosthesis. J Rehab Res Dev 31(4): 326–334

Kyberd and Chappell (1993) A Force sensor for automatic manipulation based on the Hall effect. Measure Sci Technol 4:281–287

Kyberd et al. (1998) A Survey of upper limb prostheses users in Oxfordshire. J Prosthet Orthot 10(4):85–91

Lake (2001) Microprocessors in upper-limb prosthetics. 10th Triennial World Congress of the International Society of Prosthetics and Orthotics. 1–6 July 2001, Glasgow, Scotland

Light, Chappell and Kyberd (1999) Quantifying impaired hand function in the clinical environment. In: MEC'99 Symposium Upper limb prosthetic research and consumer needs: narrowing the gap. 25–27 August 1999, Fredericton, NB, Canada, pp 43–48

Light and Chappell (2000) Development of a lightweight and adaptable multiple-axis hand prosthesis. Med Eng Phys 22(10):679–684

Light, Chappell and Kyberd (2002) Establishing a standardized clinical assessment tool of pathologic and prosthetic hand function: normative data, reliability, and validity. Arch Phys Med Rehab 83:776–783

Lippold and Cogdell (1991) Physiology illustrated. Edward Arnold, London

McDonnell et al. (1988) Incidence of congenital upper-limb deficiencies. J Assoc Child Prosthet-Orthot Clin 23(1): 8–14

Plettenburg (1989) Electric versus pneumatic power in hand prosthesis for children. J Med Eng Technol 13:124–128

Popovic, Keller, Morari, and Dietz (1998) Neural prosthesis for spinal cord injured subjects. J BioWorld 1:6–9

Rogala et al. (1974) Congenital limb anomalies: frequency and aetiological factors. J Med Genet 11:221–233

Rood (1860) On the contraction of muscles, induced by contact with bodies in vibration. Am J Sci Arts 24:499

Salisbury and Coleman (1967) A mechanical hand with automatic proportional control of prehension. Med Biol Eng 5:505–511

Schultz and Pylatiuck (2001) Lightweight bionic hand prosthesis. 10th Triennial World Congress of the International Society of Prosthetics and Orthotics. 1–6 July 2001, Glasgow, Scotland

Senski (1980) A consumer's guide to "bionic arms". Br Med J 12:126–127

Silcox et al. (1993) Myoelectric prostheses – A long term follow and a study of the use of alternate prostheses. J Bone Joint Surg. 75A(12):1781–1789

Soares (1997) Shape memory alloy actuators for upper limb prostheses. PhD Thesis, University of Edinburgh

Taffler and Kyberd (1999) The use of the Hilbert transform in EMG analysis. In: MEC'99 Symposium Upper limb prosthetic research and consumer needs: narrowing the gap. 25–27 August 1999, Fredericton, NB, Canada, pp 94–99

Taffler and Kyberd (1999) The use of fuzzy logic in the processing of myoelectric signals. In:In: MEC'99 Symposium Upper limb prosthetic research and consumer needs: narrowing the gap. 25–27 August 1999, Fredericton, NB, Canada, pp 100–105

Throndsen (1996) Characterisation of shape memory alloys for use as an actuator. Master's Thesis, University of Oxford

Weir et al. (2003) Design of artificial arms and hands for prosthetic applications. In: Myer Kutz (ed) Standard handbook of biomedical engineering design. McGraw-Hill, New York, pp 32.1–32.61

A Bibliography on Myoelectric Control of Upper Limb Prostheses

H. Smart

10.1 Introduction

This bibliography has been compiled using the RE-CAL Bibliographic Database and the resources of the Library of the National Centre for Training and Education in Prosthetics and Orthotics, University of Strathclyde, Glasgow, Scotland, UK.

References are drawn primarily from the relevant journal literature reflecting the strength of the journal collection held at the National Centre.

Some coverage of textbook and conference literature is given but is in no way exhaustive.

All the relevant papers are listed alphabetically by the first author.

Bibliography

Aaron SL, Stein RB. Comparison of an EMG-controlled prosthesis and the normal human biceps brachii muscle. Am J Phys Med 1976 55, 1–14

Abul-Haj CJ, Hogan N. Functional assessment of control systems for cybernetic elbow prostheses – Part I: description of the technique. IEEE Trans Biomed Eng 1990 37, 1025–1036

Abul-Haj CJ, Hogan N. Functional assessment of control systems for cybernetic elbow prostheses – Part II: application of the technique. IEEE Trans Biomed Eng 1990 37, 1037–1047

Aghili F, Haghpanahi M. Use of a pattern recognition technique to control a multifunctional prosthesis. Med Biol Eng Comput 1995 33, 504–508

Agnew PJ. Functional effectiveness of a myo-electric prosthesis compared with a functional split-hook prosthesis: a single subject experiment. Prosthet Orthot Int 1981 5, 92–96

Agnew PJ. Training for myoelectric prosthesis with sensory feedback. Br J Occup Ther 1979 42, 286–288

Agnew PJ, Shannon GF. Training program for a myo-electrically controlled prosthesis with sensory feedback system (myo-electric prosthesis, functional training). Am J Occup Ther 1981 35, 722–727

Almstrom C ... (et al.) Electrical stimulation and myoelectric control. A theoretical and applied study relevant to prosthesis sensory feedback. Med Biol Eng Comput 1981 19, 645–653

Alstrom VC, Herberts P, Caine K. Klinische erprobung einer myoelektrische gesteurten multifunktionshand (clinical evaluation of a myoelectrically controlled multifunctional hand). Orthop Tech 1978 29, 77–79*. (9000187)

Almstrom C, Herberts P, Korner L. Experience with Swedish multifunctional prosthetic hands controlled by pattern recognition of multiple myoelectric signals. Int Orthop 1981 5, 15–21

Al-Temen I, Mifsud M, Spencer J ... (et al.) New variety Village electromechanical elbow and forearm for juvenile amputees (abstract). J Assoc Child Prosthet Orthot Clin 1986 21, 53

American Academy of Orthopaedic Surgeons. Atlas of limb prosthetics: surgical and prosthetic principles. - St Louis: CV Mosby, 1981

American Academy of Orthopaedic Surgeons. Atlas of limb prosthetics: surgical, prosthetic and rehabilitation principles. Edited by IH Bowker, IW Michael. 2nd edition. - St Louis: Mosby-Year Book, 1992

Anani AB, Korner LM. Afferent electrical nerve stimulation: human tracking performance relevant to prosthesis sensory feedback. Med Biol Eng Comput 1979 17, 425–434

An artificial hand with a sense of touch. Acta Chir Plast (Prague) 1979 21, 260–262*. (23740)

Artificial hand. Design Council, 1986. single page leaflet*. (05232)

Artificial hands are getting better. MBEC News 1988 6, N5*. (20732)

Aspects techniques d'une nouvelle main myoelectrique pour enfants (technical details of a new myoelectric hand for children). Ortho-Scop 1982 7, 79–83

Atkins DJ. Comprehensive management of the upper limb amputee. /edited by DJ Atkins, RH Meier. - New York: Springer-Verlag, 1989

Atkins DJ, Donovan WH, Heard DCY ... (et al.) Current trends in fitting the child with an upper limb deficiency and implications for future research (abstract). Orthop Trans 1995 19, 123

Atkins DJ, Meier RH, Muilenburg A. The upper-limb prosthetic prescription: conventional or electric components? (abstract). J Assoc Child Prosthet Orthot Clin 1985 20, 37

Bailon H, Vuskovic MI, Ivankovic B. Force interface for the multifingered robotic hand. In: IEEE International Conference on Systems, Man and Cybernetics; intelligent systems for the 21st century, Vancouver, B.C., October 22–25, 1995.- Piscataway, N.J.: IEEE, 1995. p96–102*. (9615940)

Ballance R, Wilson BN, Harder JA. Factors affecting myoelectric prosthetic use and wearing patterns in the juvenile unilateral below-elbow amputee. Can J Occup Ther 1989 56, 132–137

Ballance R. Review of prosthesis-wearing patterns and use in congenital unilateral below-elbow child amputees wearing a myoelectric prosthesis (abstract). J Assoc Child Prosthet Orthot Clin 1987 22, 19

Banziger E. Wrist rotation activation in myoelectric prosthetics – an innovative approach. O & P Business News 1996 15 July, 14–15, 17*. (9617483)

Banziger E, Hewitt C. Partial hand external powered myoelectric controlled fitting, a case presentation (abstract). Orthop Trans 1998/99 22, 1205

Basha T, Scott RN, Parker PA ... (et al.) Deterministic components in the myoelectric signal. Med Biol Eng Comput 1994 32, 233–235

Battye CK, Nightingale A, Whillis J. The use of myoelectric currents in the operation of prostheses. J Bone Joint Surg 1955 37B, 506–510

Baumgartner R, Ploger J. Die kanalplastik nach Sauerbruch: spatergerbnisse und verleich mit myoelektrischer versor-gung (the cineplasty according to Sauerbruch: long term results in comparison to myoelectric fitting). Orthop Tech 1989 40, 5–8

Becker FF. Optimierung der pro- und supinationsbewegung von myoelektrisch gesteuerten unterarmprothesen (optimization of the forearm rotation in myoelectric below-elbow prostheses). Orthop Tech 1978 29, 131–134

Becker FF. Untersuchungen uber die benutzungshaufigkeit von eigen-und fremdkraftbetriebenen armprothesensystemen (an examination of the frequency of use of manually and externally powered upper limb prostheses). Biomed Tech 1978 23, 185*. (01878)

Bender LF. Prostheses and rehabilitation after arm amputation.- Springfield: CC Thomas, 1974

Berger N, Edelstein JE. Children's performance with myoelectrically controlled and body-powered hands (abstract). J Assoc Child Prosthet Orthot Clin 1989 24(2/3), 34

Bergman K, Ornholmer L, Zackrisson K ... (et al.) Functional benefit of an adaptive myoelectric prosthetic hand compared to a conventional myoelectric hand. Prosthet Orthot Int 1992 16, 32–37

Berke GM, Nielsen CC. Establishing parameters affecting the use of myoelectric prostheses in children: a preliminary investigation. J Prosthet Orthot 1991 3, 162–167

Bierwirth W. Konzept fur myoelektrische armprothesen bei hohen amputationsniveaus (a concept for myoelectric prostheses for high amputation levels). Orthop Tech 1989 40, 441–445

Bierwirth W. Orthopadie-technische konzepte zur myoelektrischen armversorgung (orthopaedic-technological programmes for myoelectric arm fitting). Orthop Tech 2002 53, 291–297

Bierwirth W. Schafttechnik bei unterarmprotheses und eine anmerkung zur definierung von myosignalen (socket-design of below-elbow-prostheses and a comment on the definition of myo-signals. Orthop Tech 1992 43, 720–724

Bierwirth W, Fitzlaff G, Winkler W. Die versorgung mit myo-elektricschen armprosthesen in der rehabilitationsklinik Bellikon (myoelectric arm prostheses fitting at the rehabilitation hospital Bellikon). Orthop Tech 1985 36, 735–738

Bierwirth W, Winkler W. Bis zu welcher amputationshohe kann mit eigenkraft-ellenbogen versorgt werden? Ein grenzfall am beispiel einer beidseitigen oberarm-prothesenversorgung (up to what amputation level can the body-powered elbow prosthesis be used? A boundary case exemplified through bilateral above elbow prostheses). Med Orthop Tech 1992 112, 24–28

Blair A. Inclusion of a battery level meter in a standard myoelectric prosthesis. Prosthet Orthot Int 2001 25, 154–155

Boenick U, Becker FF. Der derzeitige entwicklungsstand adaptiver kunsthande mit elektromechnischem antrieb (tiel 1) (the present state of development of electromechanically driven adaptive hands). Orthop Tech 1980 31, 85–87

Boenick U, Becker FF. Der derzeitige entwicklungsstand adaptiver kunsthande mit elektromechnischem antrieb (tiel 2) (the present state of development of electromechanically driven adaptive hands, part 2). Orthop Tech 1980 30, 97–100*. (23729)

Boivin G. Nothing like the human hand. ICIB 1968 7(4), 17–19, 22

Bonivento C, Davalli A, Fantuzzi C ... (et al.) Automatic tuning of myoelectric prostheses. J Rehabil Res Dev 1998 35, 294–304

Bottomley AH. The control of the upper limb. In: Modern trends in biomechanics-I./ edited by DC Simpson.- London: Butterworth, 1970. p1–24*. (9207504)

Bottomley AH. Myo-electric control of powered prostheses. J Bone Joint Surg 1965 47B, 411–415

Bottomley A, Wilson ABK, Nightingale A. Muscle substitutes and myoelectric control. J Br Inst Radio Eng 1963, 439–448*. (16548)

Bousso D, Ishai G. A study of myoelectric signals for arm prosthesis control. Biomed Eng 1971 6, 509–517

Bousso D, Ishai G. Reports on the use of myoelectric signals for multiple degree-of-freedom arm prosthesis control. - Haifa: Technion-Israel Institute of Technology, 1969 (v.p.)* (22695)

Bouzigues B, Chaluleau C, Bernardini R ... (et al.) Le medicin-conseil et l'appareillage du membre superieur (national health service and orthoses and prostheses of the upper limb). Probl Med Reed 1989 16, 13–17*. (22579)

Brenner CD. Electronic limbs for infants and pre-school children. J Prosthet Orthot 1992 4, 184–190

Brinkley L. Development of a prosthetic system for an adolescent with congenital trimembral limb deficiency (abstract). Phys Ther 1997 77, S45

Brittain RH, Sauter WF, Gibson DA. Sensory feedback in a myoelectric upper limb prosthesis: a preliminary report. Can J Surg 1979 22, 481–482*. (02271)

Brody G, Balasubramanian R, Scott RN. A model for myoelectric signal generation. Med Biol Eng 1974 12, 29–41*. (03951)

Brohmke F. Travel report of a German delegation of experts, on the bioelectric below-elbow prosthesis in the USSR (abstract). ICIB 1965 4(9), 15–19

Broomfield MS, Hepburn PL. A clinical trial of the "Reach" electric hand (abstract). ISPO UK Newsletter 1993 Winter, 19

Bruckner L. Betrachtungen zur veroffentlichung versorgung mit myoelektrischer armprothese bei Sauerbruch-oberarmmyoplastik (comments on: myoelectric prosthesis for an above elbow amputee with a Sauerbruch cineplasty – by E Castenholz in issue 1/90). Med Orthop Tech 1990 110, 148–149

Bush G, Young W, Olive M ... (et al.) Powered partial hand prosthesis – a case report (abstract). Orthop Trans 1998/99 22, 460

Caldwell RR. A new myoelectric below elbow prosthesis for infants. Orthot Prosthet 1985–86 39(2), 72–74

Canty TJ. New cineplastic prosthesis. J Bone Joint Surg 1951 33A, 612–617

Carrozza MC, Micera S, Massa B ... (et al.) The development of a novel biomechatronic hand – ongoing research and primary results. In: 2002 IEEE/ASME International Conference on Advanced Intelligent Mechantronic Proceedings, 8–12 July 2001.- Coma, Italy, 2001. p249–254*. (2237024)

Castenholz E. Versorgung mit myoelektrischer Armprothese bei Sauerbruch-oberarmmyo-plastik (myoelectric prosthesis for an above elbow amputee with a Sauerbruch cineplasty). Med Orthop Tech 1990 110, 30–32

Cavrini R. Myoelektrische prothesen und spezielle schaftkonstruktionen fur kinder (myoelectric prostheses and specific socket designs for children). Orthop Tech 1992 43, 740–745

Chappell PH, Kyberd PJ. Prehensile control of a hand prosthesis by a microcontroller. J Biomed Eng 1991 13, 363–369

The child with an acquired amputation: a symposium held in Toronto, June 9–11, 1970./ edited by GT Aitken. - Washington: National Academy of Sciences, 1972

Childress DS. Myoelectric control: brief history, signal origins and signal processing. Capabilities 1995 4(2), 6–7*. (9514842)

Childress DS. Myoelectric control of powered prostheses. IEEE Eng Med Biol Mag 1982 1(4), 23–25

Childress DS. Myoelectrically controlled NYU-hosmer prehension actator and Michigan hook (abstract). J Assoc Child Prosthet Orthot Clin 1986 21, 31

Childress DS. Neural organization and myoelectric control. In: Neural organisation and its relevance to prosthetics./ edited by Fields WS. – New York: Intercontinental Book Corp., 1973. p117–130*. (9205729)

Childress DS. Powered prostheses with "boosted" cable activation. Capabilities 1991 1(2), 1, 4*. (9105191)

Childress DS, Billock JN. Self-containment and self-suspension of externally powered prostheses for the forearm. Bull Prosthet Res 1970 10(14), 4–21

Childress DS, Hampton FL, Lambert CN ... (et al.) Myoelectric immediate postsurgical procedure: a concept for fitting the upper-extremity amputee. Artificial Limbs 1969 13(2), 55–60

Chitore DS, Rahmatallah SF, Albakry KS. Digital electronic controller for above knee prostheses. Int J Electronics 1988 64, 649–656*. (19937)

Clancy EA, Bouchard S, Rancourt D. Estimation and application of EMG amplitude during dynamic contractions: processing nonstationary EMG for applications in prosthesis control, biofeedback, and joint torque estimation. IEEE Eng Med Biol Mag 2001 20(6), 47–54

Clark RR, Hoyt WA. Prosthetic pollicization. ICIB 1968 7(11), 1–7

Clarke SD, Patton JG. Occupational therapy for the limb deficient child: a developmental approach to treatment planning and selection of prostheses for infants and young children with unilateral upper extremity limb deficiencies. Clin Orthop 1980 148, 47–54

Computerized prosthesis adapts to patients as they gain strength and skills. O & P Business World 1999 2(3), 66–68

Cooper R. New amps for old. BAPOMAG 2000 No. 3, 18

Crandall RC, Tomhave W. Pediatric unilateral below-elbow amputees: retrospective analysis of 34 patients given multiple prosthetic options. J Pediatr Orthop 2002 22, 380–383

Crane S, Mcmillan P, Rodriguez R. Non-dominant hand function in elementary school-aged children (abstract). J Assoc Child Prosthet Orthot Clin 1993 28, 9–10

Curran B, Hambrey R. The prosthetic treatment of upper limb deficiency. Prosthet Orthot Int 1991 15, 82–87

Daley TL, Scott RN, Parker PA ... (et al.) Operator performance in myoelectric control of a malfunction prosthesis stimulator. J Rehabil Res Dev 1989 27(1), 9–20

Dalsey R, Gomez W, Seitz WH ... (et al.) Myoelectric prosthetic replacement in the upper-extremity amputee. Orthop Rev 1989 18, 697–702*. (9513258)

Daly W. Upper extremity socket design options. Phys Med Rehabil Clin North Am 2000 11, 627–638

Datta D, Brain ND. Clinical applications of myoelctrically-controlled prosthese. Crit Rev Phys Rehabil Med 1992 4, 215–239*. (9307678)

Datta D, Ibbotson V. Prosthetic rehabilitation of upper limb amputees: a five year review. Clin Rehabil 1991 5, 311–316

Datta D, Kingston JE. Myoelectric prostheses in the management of Poland's syndrome. J Hand Surg 1994 19B, 659–661

Datta D, Kingston J, Ronald J. Myoelectric prostheses for below-elbow amputees: the Trent experience. Int Disabil Studies 1989 11, 167–170

Davidson L. Survey shows benefit from myoelectric prosthesis. Therapy Weekly 1988 7 April, 3*. (17670)

De Luca CJ. Control of upper-limb prostheses: a case for neuroelectric control. J Med Eng Technol 1978 2, 57–61

De Luca CJ. Physiology and mathematics of myolectric signals. IEEE Trans Biomed Eng 1979 26, 313–325*. (9411683)

Debear P. Functional use of myoelectric and cable-driven prostheses. J Assoc Child Prosthet Orthot Clin 1988 23, 60–61

Debear PC. Functional use of myoelectric prosthesis and standard cable driven prostheses (abstract). Arch Phys Med Rehabil 1987 68, 592

Derhaag MMC, Schoorl PM, Derhaag PJFM. Personality development in one-handed children treated with a myoelectrically controlled prosthesis. J Rehabil 1990 56(3), 25–29*. (9513577)

Desoutter E, Peyrard O, Rivera S ... (et al.) L'appareillage myoelectrique des enfants: aide our contrainte?: experience d'un service de reeducation fonctionnelle infantile (the myoelectric apparatus in children: aid or constraint?: experience of a functional rehabilitation service for children). J Ergother 1992 14, 94–98*. (9307944)

Dorcas DS, Dunfield VA, O'Shea BJ. A myoelectric prosthesis for a forequarter amputation. ICIB 1968 7(11), 15–20

Dorcas DS, Dunfield VA, Scott RN. Improved myo-electric control system. Med Biol Eng 1970 8, 333–341*. (03948)

Dorcas DS, Scott RN. A three-state myo-electric control. Med Biol Eng 1966 4, 367–370

Dunfield V, Shwedyk E. Digital EMG processor. Med Biol Eng Comput 1978 16, 745–751

Dupont A-C, Morin EL. A myoelectric control evaluation and trainer system. IEEE Trans Rehabil Eng 1994 2, 100–107

Edelstein JE, Berger N. Performance comparison among children fitted with myolectric and body-powered hands. Arch Phys Med Rehabil 1993 74, 376–380

Electronic technology aids UE amputees. O & P Business World 1999 2(1), 42–46

Englehart K, Hudgins B, Parker PA ... (et al.) Classification of the myoelectric signal using time-frequency based presentations. Med Eng Phys 1999 21, 431–438

Englehart K, Hudgins B, Parker PA. A wavelet-based continuous classification scheme for multifunctional myoelectric control. IEEE Trans Biomed Eng 2001 48, 302–311

Epps CH. Clinical report: a functionally advanced juvenile above-elbow prosthesis (abstract). J Assoc Child Prosthet Orthot Clin 1987 22, 18

Epps CH. Externally powered prostheses for children – 1984. Clin Prosthet Orthot 1985 9(1), 17–18

Epps CH. Special prostheses enhance rehabilitation. Clin Prosthet Orthot 1982 6(4), 5–6

Esquenazi A, Leonard JA, Meier RH ... (et al.) Prosthetics, orthotics and assistive devices: 3. Prosthetics. Arch Phys Med Rehabil 1989 70(Suppl 5-S), S206-S209

Ey MC. Experiences with myoelectric prostheses: a preliminary report. ICIB 1978 17(3), 15–17

Feron J. New process will help amputee to control limb with thought. ICIB 1965 5(2), 22

Fielden RHN, Fisher S. Electronic prostheses for children: use and abuse (abstract). J Assoc Child Prosthet Orthot Clin 1988 23, 32

Fleming LL ... (et al.) Management of upper extremity amputation with myoelectric prostheses (abstract). Orthop Trans 1983 7, 506

Gaber TA-ZK, Gardner CM, Kirker SGB. Silicone roll-on suspension for upper limb prostheses: users' views. Prosthet Orthot Int 2001 25, 113–118

Galway HR, Hubbard S, Dakpa R. Myoelectrics for the achiria and partial hand amputee (abstract). J Assoc Child Prosthet Orthot Clin 1987 22, 19

Gassinger LA. Technische moglichkeiten der armversorgung mit myoelektrischen und schaltergesteuerten modulsystem (technical possibilities of upper extremity supply with myoelectric and switch controlled modul systemsar). Orthop Tech 1978 29, 129–131

German research gives a helping hand to the disabled. New Scientist 1982 18 November, 424*. (23735)

Godfrey SB. Workers with prostheses. J Hand Ther 1990 3, 101–110

Godin DT, Parker PA, Scott RN. Noise characteristics of stainless-steel surface electrodes. Med Biol Eng Comput 1991 29, 585–590

Goenaga-Alecki M. Presentation de la prothese myoelectrique pour enfant et place de l'ergotherapie (presentation of a myoelectric prosthesis for a child and the role of ergotherapy). J Ergother 1986 13, 42–49*. (14333)

Gozna ER, Scott RN. The UNB "three state" myoelectric control system (abstract). J Bone Joint Surg 1982 64B, 260

Graupe D, Cline WK. Functional separation of EMG signals via ARMA identification methods for prosthesis control purposes. IEEE Trans Syst Man Cybern 1975 5, 252–259*. (9105339)

Graupe D, Salahi J, Kohn KH. Multifunctional prosthesis and orthosis control via microcomputer identification of temporal differences in single-site myoelectric signals. J Biomed Eng 1982 4, 17–22

Graupe D, Salahi J, Zhang D. Stochastic analysis of myoelectric temporal signatures for multifunctional single-site activation of prostheses and orthoses. J Biomed Eng 1985 7, 18–29

Greatting MD, Hill JJ. Myoelectric prostheses in upper extremity amputees: cost, mechanical reliability and long term wear rate (abstract). Orthop Trans 1991 15, 783

Greshik J, Andrew JT, Doolan K. Toddlers and myoelectrics – do they go together (abstract). J Assoc Child Prosthet Orthot Clin 1993 28, 25–26

GROCH J. Advances in artificial hands. Med Trial Technique Q 1974 21, 171–177*. (9513563)

Groth H, Weltman G, Lyman J. An exploratory investigation of functional muscle isolation for coordinated arm prosthesis control. (Biotechnology Laboratory Technical Report No. 15). - Los Angeles: University of California, 1962. 8 pp*. (22689)

Hambrey RA, Withinshaw G. Electrically powered upper limb prostheses: their development and application. Br J Occup Ther 1990 53, 7–11

Hartman HH, Hobart DC, Waring W ... (et al.) A myoelectrically controlled powered elbow. Artificial Limbs 1969 13(2), 61–63

Hean CC, Heidinger B, Bourhis G ... (et al.) Les electrodes myoelectriques en technologie hybride pour la commande des protheses motorisees des membres superieurs (myoelectric sensor in hybrid technology for the upper limb electric prosthesis control). Innov Tech Biol Med 1987 8, 485–492*. (17502)

Heckathorne CW, Philipson L. Cable-actuated position control of children's electric elbows: a joint U.S.-Sweden evaluation. Capabilities 1992 2(2), 4–5*. (9206863)

Hedstrom L, Holmquist T, Randstrom S ... (et al.) Technische aspekte einer neuen myoelektrische gesteuerten hand fur kinder (technical aspects of a new myoelectrically controlled hand for children). Orthop Tech 1980 31, 23–25*. (23730)

Heger H, Millstein S, Hunter GA. Electrically powered prostheses for the adult with an upper limb amputation. J Bone Joint Surg 1985 67B, 278–281

Hell C. Das DMC-system: ein universell einsetzbares steuerungskonzept (the DMC control: a control system for universal application). Orthop Tech 1998 49, 182–190

Herberts P. Myoelectric signals in control of prostheses: studies on arm amputees and normal individuals. Acta Orthop Scand (Suppl) 1969 40 (Suppl 124), 83pp*. (14596)

Herberts P, Almstrom C, Caine K. Clinical application of multifunctional prosthetic hands. J Bone Joint Surg 1978 60B, 552–560

Herberts P, Almstrom C, Kadefors R ... (et al.) Hand prosthesis control via myoelectric patterns. Acta Orthop Scand 1973 44, 389–409

Herberts P, Kadefors R, Kaiser E ... (et al.) Implantation of micro-circuits for myoelectric controls of prostheses. J Bone Joint Surg 1997 50B, 780–791

Herberts P, Kaiser E, Magnusson R ... (et al.) Power spectra of myoelectric signals in muscles of arm amputees and healthy normal controls. Acta Orthop Scand 1973 44, 161–193

Herberts P, Korner L. Clinical evaluation of myoelectric prostheses in below-elbow amputees. Int J Rehabil Res 1982 5, 62–63

Herberts P, Korner L. Ideas on sensory feedback in hand prostheses. Prosthet Orthot Int 1979 3, 157–162

Herberts P, Korner L, Caine K ... (et al.) Rehabilitation of unilateral below-elbow amputees with myoelectric prostheses. Scand J Rehabil Med 1980 12, 123–128

Hermansson L, Eliasson A-C, Bernspang B. Development of an evaluation tool for children's control of myoelectric hand prostheses (abstract). Dev Med Child Neurol 2001 43(Suppl 89), 19–20

Hermansson LM. Structured training of children fitted with myoelectric prstheses. Prosthet Orthot Int 1991 15, 88–92

Herment JP. Reeducation et problems professionnels des amputes du membre superieur appareilles par prostheses myoelectriques (rehabilitation and vocational problems for upper limb amputees with myoelectrical prostheses). Rev Readapt 1983 11, 51–54

Hierton T ... (et al.) The application of myoelectric hand prosthesis at different amputation levels below the elbow. Scand J Rehabil Med 1970 2, 23–26*. (02361)

Hirsch C, Kaiser E, Petersen I. Bioelectrical control in a servosystem: analysis and application of muscle action potentials in an experimental hand prosthesis. Acta Orthop Scand 1964 35, 1–15

Hodgins J, Curtin M. Silicone elastomers – diverse application for upper limb prosthetics (abstract). J Assoc Child Prosthet Orthot Clin 1993 28, 6

Hoek J. A temporary prosthesis for the forearm. ISPO Bull 1975 No. 13, 6–7

Hogan N, Mann RW. Myoelectric signal processing: optimal estimation applied to electromyography – Part II: experimental demonstration of optimal myoprocessor performance. IEEE Trans Biomed Eng 1980 27, 396–410*. (02036)

Holland OE, Kyberd PJ, Tregidgo R ... (et al.) Erfahrungen mit einer hierarchisch kontraollierten myoelektrischen hand (experiences with a hierarchically controlled myoelectric hand). Orthop Tech 1996 47, 968–974

Hortensius P, Onyshko S, Quanbury A. A microcomputer-based prosthetic limb controller: design and implementation. Ann Biomed Eng 1987 15, 51–65

Hortensius P, Onyshko S, Quanbury A. Low power multichannel electromyographic data acquisition system. J Biomed Eng 1986 8, 364

Hortensius P, Quanbury A, Onyshko S. A low-powered multichannel electromyographic signal data acquisition system. J Med Eng Technol 1987 11, 11–16

Horvath W. Neue elektrohand fur kinder (a new electric hand for children). Orthop Tech 1992 43, 732–739

Hubbard J, Bebko JM, Jutai J. The self-concept of children with congenital upper-limb deficiencies (abstract). Orthop Trans 1998/99 22, 457–458

Hubbard S. The Toronto experience with pediatric myoelectric training. In: Comprehensive management of the upper-limb amputee./ edited by DJ Atkins, RH Meier.- New York: Springer-Verlag, 1988. p190–193*. (9927083)

Hubbard S, Bush G, Kurtz I ... (et al.) Myoelectric prostheses for the limb-deficient child. Phys Med Rehabil Clin North Am 1991 2, 847–866

Hubbard S, Galway HR, Milner M. Myolectric training methods for the preschool child with congenital below-elbow amputation: a comparison of two training programmes. J Bone Joint Surg 1985 67B, 273–277

Hubbard S, Galway R, Urquhardt K ... (et al.) Preschool myoelectric program: a three-year review (abstract). J Assoc Child Prosthet Orthot Clin 1985 20, 38

Hubbard S, Heim W, Giavedoni B. Paediatric prosthetic management. Curr Orthop 1997 11, 114–121*. (2029505)

Hudgins B, Parker P, Scott RN. A new strategy for multifunction myoelectric control. IEEE Trans Biomed Eng 1993 40, 82–94

Humbert SD, Snyder SA, Grill WM. Evaluation of command algorithms for control of upper-extremity neural prostheses. IEEE Trans Neural Syst Rehabil Eng 2002 10, 94–101

Hunter GA, Heger H, Millstein S. A review of the failures in the below elbow myoelectric prosthesis (abstract). Orthop Trans 1982 6, 485

Hunter Peckham P, Keith MW, Kilgore KL ... (et al.) Efficacy of an implanted neuroprosthesis for restoring hand grasp in tetraplegia: a multicenter study. Arch Phys Med Rehabil 2001 82, 1380–1388

Hunter Peckham P, Kilgore KL, Keith MW ... (et al.) An advanced neuroprosthesis for restoration of hand and upper arm control using an implantable controller. J Hand Surg 2002 27A, 265–276*. (2240141)

Hutnick GF, Rothenberg, Ahlert J. Thermoplastic below elbow prostheses (abstract). J Assoc Child Prosthet Orthot Clin 1991 26, 18

Ingvarsson B, Karlsson I, Ottosson L-G ... (et al.) Proposal for test instructions and test report for the technical testing of mono-functional myoelectrically-controlled prosthetic hands. Report 2/80.- Linkoping, Sweden: University Hospital, Department of Rehabilitation Medicine, 1980. 29 pp*. (22151)

Ingvarsson B, Karlsson I, Ottosson L-G ... (et al.) Technical note – test instructions for the technical testing of mono-func-

tional myoelectrically-controlled prosthetic hands: a proposal. Prosthet Orthot Int 1982 6, 41–42

Ingvarsson B, Karlsson I, Ottosson L-G ... (et al.) Test instructions for the technical testing of mono-functional myoelectrically-controlled prosthetic hands: a proposal (technical note). Prosthet Orthot Int 1982 6, 41–42

Jacobsen SC ... (et al.) Development of the Utah artificial arm. IEEE Trans Biomed Eng 1982 29, 249–269*. (01586)

Jacques GE, Ryan S, Naumann S ... (et al.) Application of quality function deployment in rehabilitation engineering. IEEE Trans Rehabil Eng 1994 2, 158–164

James MA. Choosing the right prosthesis for a child with congenital upper extremity absence: an ethical analysis (abstract). Orthop Trans 1998/99 22, 1206

Jerard RB, Jacobsen SC. Laboratory evaluation of a unified theory for simultaneous multiple axis artificial arm control. Trans ASME J Biomech Eng 1980 102, 199–207

Johansen PB, Breitholtz M, Cavrini R ... (et al.) Prosthetic rehabilitation in bilateral high above elbow amputation. Scand J Rehabil Med 1987 19, 85–87

Johnsson U, Korner L, Herberts P. A microprocessor based control system for multifunctional hand prostheses. Int J Rehabil Res 1984 7, 193–195

Jouin E. La pronosupination dans les protheses myoelectriques (pronation/supination with myoelectric prostheses). Rev Readapt 1983 11, 43–45

Kaitan R. Die verwendung von mikrocontrollern in der prothetik (microcontrollers in the field of prosthetics). Med Orthop Tech 1997 117, 26–30

Kampas P. Myoelektroden – optimal eingesetz (the optimal use of myo-electrodes). 2001 121, 21–27

Kato I. Trends in powered upper limb prostheses. Prosthet Orthot Int 1978 2, 64–68

Kato I, Morita H, Onozuka T. Development of myoelectric control system for an above-knee prosthesis. In: Second CISM/IFTOMM International symposium on the theory and practice of robots and manipulators, 1977. p74–78*. (02406)

Kejlaa GH. Consumer concerns and functional value of prostheses to upper limb amputees. Prosthet Orthot Int 1993 17, 157–163

Kelly MF, Parker PA, Scott RN. The application of neural networks to myoelectric signal analysis: a preliminary study. IEEE Trans Biomed Eng 1990 37, 221–230

Kelly MF, Parker PA, Scott RN. Neural network classification of myoelectric signal for prosthesis control. J Electromyogr Kinesiol 1991 1, 229–236

Kirtley C, Andrews BJ. Control of functional electrical stimulation with extended physiological proprioception. J Biomed Eng 1990 12, 183–188

Kiryu T, De Luca CJ, Saitoh Y. AR modeling of myoelectric interference signals during a ramp contraction. IEEE Trans Biomed Eng 1994 41, 1031–1038

Kitzenmaier P, Boenick U. Moglichkeiten der myoelektrischen Ansteuerung von Gliedmaßenprothesen (methods of achieving myoelectrical control of prostheses). Biomed Tech 1992 37, 170–180*. (9307737)

Knowles JB, Stevens BL, Howe L. Myo-electric control of a hand prosthesis. J Bone Joint Surg 1965 47B, 416–417

Kohn JG, Dunbar L, Bolding D … (et al.) Reports of a pilot program: myoelectric prostheses (abstract). Orthop Trans 1998/99 22, 458

Korner L … (et al.) The etiology of amputation stump fatigue in patients controlling myoelectric prostheses. Acta Orthop Scand 1981 52, 693

Kostuik JP. Amputation surgery and rehabilitation: the Toronto experience. - New York: Churchill Livingstone, 1981

Kritter AE. The bilateral upper extremity amputee. Orthop Clin North Am 1972 3, 419–433*. (9513936)

Kritter AE. The Milwaukee experience with myoelectric prostheses (abstract). ICIB 1984 19, 1

Kritter AE. Myoelectric prosthesis. J Bone Joint Surg 1985 67A, 654–657

Kritter AE. Myoelectric prosthesis: current status (abstract). J Assoc Child Prosthet Orthot Clin 1985 20, 36–37

Kruganti U, Hudgins B, Scott RN. Two-channel enhancement of a multifunctional control system. IEEE Trans Biomed Eng 1995 42, 109–111

Kruger LM. A comparison study of the myoelectric and body-powered hand in children (abstract) Orthop Trans 1988 12, 580

Kruger LM, Fishman S. Myoelectric and body-powered prostheses. J Pediatr Orthop 1993 13, 68–75

Kruger L, Skewes E, Haas J. Surlyn socket for below-elbow myoelectric prostheses (abstract). J Assoc Child Prosthet Orthot Clin 1988 23, 34

Kruit J, Cool JC. Body-powered hand prosthesis with low operating power for children. J Med Eng Technol 1989 13, 129–133

Kuiken TA, Popovic M, Taslove A. A 2-D finite element model of myoelectric signals (abstract). Arch Phys Med Rehabil 1999 80, 1122

Kuiken T, Stoykov N, Lowery M … (et al.) The use of nerve-muscle grafts to improve myoelectric prosthesis control. Capabilities 2001 10(3), 1–3, 11*. (2135185)

Kurtz I. The Nintendo Entertainment System – Myoelectric Signal Interface System (NEMESIS) (abstract). J Assoc Child Prosthet Orthot Clin 1993 28, 15

Kurtz I, Mifsud M, Hubbard S … (et al.) Microcomputer-based muscle site identification for electrode placement in myoelectric prostheses (abstract). J Assoc Child Prosthet Orthot Clin 1988 23, 35

Kuruganti U, Hudgins B, Scott RN. Two-channel enhancement of a multifunctional control system. IEEE Trans Biomed Eng 1995 42, 109–111

Kyberd P. The control of artificial hands. Postgrad Doct Middle East 1991 14, 392–398*. (9821565)

Kyberd P. Prosthetics lead the way. Electr Wireless World 1989 95, 176–177*. (21601)

Kyberd PJ. The appropriate control of manipulators for rehabilitation robotics. In: Mechatronics – the integration of engineering design: papers prepared for the University of Dundee and the Solid Mechanics and Machine Systems Group of the Institute of Mechanical Engineers. 1992, p123–130*. (9821569)

Kyberd PJ, Chappell PH. The Southampton Hand: an intelligent myoelectric prosthesis. J Rehabil Res Dev 1994 31, 326–334

Kyberd PJ, Chappell PH, Nightingale JM. Sensory control of a multifunction hand prosthesis. Biosensors 1987/88 3, 347–357*. (22966)

Kyberd PJ, Holland OE, Chappell PH … (et al.) MARCUS: a two degree of freedom hand prosthesis with hierarchical grip control. IEEE Trans Rehabil Eng 1995 3, 70–76

Kyberd PJ, Mustapha N, Carnegie F … (et al.) A clinical experience with a hierarchically controlled myoelectric hand prosthesis with vibro-tactile feedback. Prosthet Orthot Int 1993 17, 56–64

Lamande F. Krankengymnastik zur vorbereitung des patienten fur eine myoelektrische prothesenversorgung (physical therapy for preparation of patients for a myoelectrically controlled prosthesis). Med Orthop Tech 1992 112, 20–24

Lamande F. La reeducation preprothetique: en vue d'un appareillage myoelectrique ou myoelectronique du membre superieur ampute (pre-prosthetic rehabilitation: an aspect of fitting a myoelectric or myoelectronic upper limb amputee). Kinesitherapie Scientifique 1993 329, 10–17

Lamb DW. Upper limb amputations including prosthetic fitting. Curr Opin Orthop 1991 2, 819–823

Lambert CM, Pellicore RJ, Hamilton RC … (et al.) Twenty-three years of clinic experience. ICIB 1976 15(3/4), 15–20, 25

Leblanc MA. Clinical evaluation of externally powered prosthetic elbows. Artificial Limbs 1971 15(1), 70–77

Leblanc MA. Externally powered prosthetic elbows: a clinical evaluation.- Washington, DC: National Research Council. Committee on Prosthetics Research and Development, 1970. 16 pp*. (22669)

Leblanc M. Study of body powered upper limb prostheses in Europe.- Washington, DC: World Rehabilitation Fund, 1986

Leblanc MA. Upper-limb prosthetics current status and future needs. Orthot Prosthet 1977 31(4), 6–9

Lee RE. Reassessing myoelectric control: is it time to look at alternatives. Can Med Assoc J 1987 136, 467–469*. (05551)

Lehmann A, Muller N, Zapfe J. Der nutzen neuer technologie fur trager von myoelektrischen armprothesen (new battery technology now also available for myoelectric arm prostheses). Orthop Tech 1998 49, 192–194

Leite Da Cunha F, Schneebeli H-JA, Dynnikov VI. Development of anthropomorphic upper limb prostheses with human-like interphalangian and interdigital couplings. Artif Organs 2000 24, 193–197*. (2031739)

Light CM, Chappell PH. Development of a lightweight and adaptable multiple-axis hand prosthesis. Med Eng Phys 2000 22, 679–684

Light CM, Chappel PH, Hudgins B ... (et al.) Intelligent multi-functional myoelectric control of hand prostheses. J Med Eng Technol 2002 26, 139–146

Lind K. The electric elbow. ICIB 1969 8(7), 8–9

Lippay AL. Clinical experience with a myoelectric prosthesis. ICIB 1967 6(4), 25–31

Lippay AL. External power and the amputee: an engineer's view. ICIB 1968 7(5), 7–12

Livingstone SM. Some arguments in favour of direct electric drive for an artificial elbow. J Bone Joint Surg 1965 47B, 453–454

Lombardo JR. Myoelectric camp: an innovative interdisciplinary concept for fitting myoelectric prostheses (abstract). J Assoc Child Prosthet Orthot Clin 1991 26, 22

Lopez JMM. Protesis mioelectricas para amputaciones de mano (myoelectric aids for hand-prostheses). Mundo Electronico 1979 82, 41–51*. (23733)

Lovely DF, Buck CS, Scott RN. Improved battery saving device for use with myoelectric control systems. Med Biol Eng Comput 1986 24, 203–205

Lovely DF, Hruczkowski TW, Scott RN. A microprocessor based trainer for both single-site and two-site myoelectric prostheses. J Microcomputer Applications 1988 11, 31–45*. (20936)

Lovely DF, Hudgins B, Stocker DE. A wireless electrode for myoelectric training (abstract). Orthop Trans 1995 19, 122

Lovely DF, Stocker D, Scott RN. A computer-aided myoelectric training system for young upper limb amputees. J Microcomput Appl 1990 13, 245–259*. (9001823)

Lozac'h Y. An improved and more versatile myoelectric control. ICIB 1972 11(8), 13–15

Lucaccini LF, Kaiser PK, Lyman J. The French electric hand: some observations and conclusions. Bull Prosthet Res 1966 10(6), 30–51

Luzzio CC. Controlling an artificial arm with foot movements. Neurorehabil Neural Repair 2000 14, 207–212

Lyttle D, Sweitzer R, Steinke T ... (et al.) Experiences with myoelectric below-elbow fittings in teenagers. ICIB 1974 13(6), 11–20

Malone JH, Childers SJ, Underwood J ... (et al.) Immediate postsurgical management of upper extremity amputation: conventional, electric and myoelectric prosthesis. Orthot Prosthet 1981 35(2), 1–9

Mann RW. Cybernetic limb prosthesis. Ann Biomed Eng 1981 9, 1–43*. (00547)

Mann RW. Tradeoffs at the man-machine interface in cybernetic prostheses/orthoses. In: Perspectives in biomedical engineering: proceedings of a symposium organised in association with the Biological Engineering Society, and held in the University of Strathclyde, Glasgow, Scotland, June./ edited by RM Kenedi.- London: MacMillan Press, 1973. p73–77*. (9207493)

Manneschi V, Palmerio B, Pauluzzi P ... (et al.) Contact Dermatitis from myoelectric prostheses. Contact Dermatitis 1989 21, 116–117*. (23148)

Marquardt E. Prothetische Versorgung nach Amputationen (prosthetic treatment after amputation). Chirurg 1984 55, 311–317*. (10488)

Marquardt E, NEFF G. The angulation osteotomy of above-elbow stumps. Clin Orthop 1974 104, 232–238

Marquardt E, Trauth J. Kriterien fur die Versorgung von Kindern mit Hand und Armprothesen (criteria for the supply of children with hand and arm prostheses). Orthop Tech 1985 36, 524–529

Mason CP. Design of a powered prosthetic arm system for the above-elbow amputee. Bull Prosthet Res 1972 10(18), 10–24

Mason CP. Practical problems in myoelectric control of prostheses. Bull Prosthet Res 1970 10(13), 39–45

Mauriello GE. Some electronic problems of myoelectric control of powered orthotic and prosthetic appliances. J Bone Joint Surg 1968 50A, 524–534

Mayagoita R, Ozuna S. Design and development of a myoelectrically controlled hand prostheses. Proc Int Conf Med Biol Eng 1985 August, 617–618*. (23660)

McCarthy CF, De Luca CJ. A myofeedback instrument for clinical use. J Rehabil Res Dev 1984 21(2), 39–44

McDonnell PM. Developmental response to limb deficiency and limb replacement. Can J Psychol 1988 42, 120–143*. (21165)

McDonnell PM, Scott RN, Dickison J ... (et al.) Do artificial limbs become part of the user? New evidence. J Rehabil Res Dev 1989 26, 17–24

McKenzie DS. The clinical application of externally powered artificial arms. J Bone Joint Surg 1965 47B, 399–410

McKenzie DS. Powered arms. Ann R Coll Surg Engl 1967 40, 279–286*. (9206195)

McKenzie DS. The Russian myo-electric arm. J Bone Joint Surg 1965 47B, 418–420

McLaurin CA. On the use of electricity in upper extremity prostheses. J Bone Joint Surg 1965 47B, 448–452

McLaurin CA. Prosthetic research and training unit. ICIB 1966 6(2), 13–22

McLeod KJ, Lovely DF, Scott RN. A biphasic pulse burst generator for afferent nerve stimulation. Med Biol Eng Comput 1987 25, 77–80

Medical Research Council. Centre for Muscle Substitutes. Group on power and control systems for upper limb prostheses. Progress Report No. 1. / by AB Kinnier Wilson, SR Montgomery, R McWilham. - London: MRC, 1966

Medical Research Council. Powered Limbs Unit. The design and development of an experimental externally powered upper-limb prosthetic system. Progress Report No. 2. / by R McWilham, SR Montgomery, DD Sanderson. - London: MRC, 1970

Meek SG, Fetherston SJ. Comparison of signal-to-noise ratio of myoelectric filters for prosthesis control. J Rehabil Res Dev 1992 29(4), 9–20

Meek SG, Jacobsen SC, Goulding PP. Extended physiologic traction: design and evaluation of a proportional force feedback system. J Rehabil Res Dev 1989 26(3), 53–62

Meghdari A, Arefi M, Mahmoudian M. Geometric adaptability: a novel mechanical design in the Sharif artificial hand. Int J Robotics Autom 1992 7, 80–85*. (9410017)

Mendez MA. Evaluation of a myoelectric hand prosthesis for children with a below-elbow absence. Prosthet Orthot Int 1985 9, 137–140

Mendez MA. Myoelectric hands. Newsletter. Demonstration Centres in Rehabilitation 1984 33, 71–73

Menkveld SR, Novotny MP, Schwartz M. Age-appropriateness of myoelectric prosthetic fitting. J Assoc Child Prosthet Orthot Clin 1987 22, 60–65

Meredith JM. Comparison of three myoelectrically controlled prehensors and the voluntary-opening split hook. Am J Occup Ther 1994 48, 932–937

Meredith JM, Uellendahl JE, Keagy RD. Successful voluntary grasp and release using the Cookie Crusher myoelectric hand in 2-years old. Am J Occup Ther 1993 47, 825–829

Michael JW, Bowker JH. Prosthetics/orthotics research for the twenty-first century: summary of 1992 conference proceedings. J Prosthet Orthot 1994 6, 100–107

Mifsud M, Al-Temen I, Sauter W ... (et al.) Variety village electromechanical hand for amputees under two years of age. J Assoc Child Prosthet Orthot Clin 1987 22, 41–46

Mifsud M, Galway HR, Milner M. Current myoprosthetic developments at the Hugh MacMillan Medical Centre. J Assoc Child Prosthet Orthot Clin 1986 21, 1–7

Mifsud M, Hubbard TS, Verburg G ... (et al.) Microcomputer-based myoelectric assessment system (abstract). J Assoc Child Prosthet Orthot Clin 1989 24(2/3) 36

Mifsud M, Milner M. Two-channel miniature data-acquisition device. Med Biol Eng Comput 1986 24, 199–202

Mifsud M, Naumann S, Milner M. Powered upper extremity prosthetics research and developments. Can J Rehabil 1987 1, 119–122*. (23931)

Miault D, Dechamps E, Lamande F ... (et al.) Erfahrungen mit der "UTAH" – armprothese (experience with the "UTAH" – Arm). Med Orthop Tech 1992 112, 17–19

Miguelez JM. Clinical factors in electrically powered upper-extremity prosthetics. J Prosthet Orthot 2002 14, 36–38

Miguelez JM. High-level bilateral upper extremity amputee patient: a case study (abstract). Arch Phys Med Rehabil 1997 78, 1046

Millstein S, Heger H, Hunter G. A review of the failures in use of the below elbow myoelectric prosthesis. Orthot Prosthet 1982 36(2), 29–34

Millstein SG, Heger H, Hunter GA. Prosthetic use in adult upper limb amputees: a comparison of the body powered and electrically powered prostheses. Prosthet Orthot Int 1986 10, 27–34

Mongeau M. New hope for the patient with severe upper-extremity deficiencies: externally powered prostheses. ICIB 1968 7(5), 1–6

Moradi AA, Fallah A, Mikaili R. Control of the electric motor in a cybernetic arm. Cybernet Syst 1991 22, 119–134*. (9514018)

Morin E, Parker A, Scott RN. Operator error in a level coded myoelectric control channel. IEEE Trans Biomed Eng 1993 40, 558–562

Moscow research team develops 'cybernetic' prosthesis (news item). ICIB 1963 2(6), 8

Moseley M, Baron E. Myoelectric wiring technique for children and young adults. J Prosthet Orthot 1988 1, 41–44

Moss JR, Jackson JA. Myoelectric prosthesis for children. Br J Occup Ther 1979 42, 40

Moss Rehabilitation Hospital. Rehabilitation Engineering Center. Pattern-recognition arm prosthesis: an historical perspective./ by R Wirta, D Taylor, FR Finley. - Philadelphia, PA: Rehabilitation Engineering Hospital, Moss Rehabilitation Hospital, 1977

Muilenburg AL, Leblanc MA. Body-powered upper-limb components. In: Comprehensive management of the upper-limb amputee./ edited by DJ Atkins, RH Meier.- New York: Springer-Verlag, 1988. p28–38*. (9927072)

Munoz R, Leija L, Tovar B ... (et al.) Real-time digital myoelectric pattern detector system. In: Proceedings of the 18th Annual International Conference of the IEEE Engineering in Medicine and Biology Society, 31 October-3 November, 1996, Amsterdam.- Piscataway: IEEE, 1997. p21–23*. (9823659)

Murray D. Problems in prosthetics. Can Fam Physician 1989 35, 309–312*. (21812)

Myers DR, Moskowitz GD. Myoelectric pattern recognition for use in the volitional control of above-knee prostheses. IEEE Trans Syst Man Cybern 1981 11, 296–302*. (02112)

Myoelectric hand – more available for more children. DHSS Press Release 1981, 27 July. 3 pp*. (05519)

Nader M. Industrielle Fertigung und Forschung (industrial production and research). Med Orthop Tech 1987 107, 111–115

Nader M, Ing EH. The artificial substitution of missing hands with myoelectric prostheses. Clin Orthop 1990 258, 9–17

Neal M. Coming to grips with artificial hand design. Design Eng 1993 March, 26–27, 29, 32, 34*. (9410134)

Neff G. Prothetische versorgung nach winkel osteotomie (prosthetic management following angulation osteotomy in above-elbow amputees). Orthop Tech 1979 30, 1–5

Nickel VL, Waring W. Future developments in externally powered orthotic and prosthetic devices. J Bone Joint Surg 1965 47B, 469–471

Nightingale JM. Microprocessor control of an artificial arm. M Microcomputer Applications 1985 8, 167–193*. (9821804)

Norris JF, Lovely DF. Real-time compression of myoelectric data utilising adaptive differential pulse code modulation. Med Biol Eng Comput 1995 33, 629–635

Northmore-Ball MD, Heger H, Hunter GA. The below-elbow myo-electric prostheses: a comparison of the Otto Bock myo-electric prosthesis with the hook and functional hand. J Bone Joint Surg 1980 62B, 363–367

O'Neill PA, Morin EL, Scott RN ... (et al.) Myoelectric signal characteristics from muscles in residual upper limbs. IEEE Trans Rehabil Eng 1994 2, 266–270

O'Shea BJ, Dunfield VA. Myoelectric training for preschool children. Arch Phys Med Rehabil 1983 64, 451–455

Otto EJ, Shannon GF. A microelectronic myofeedback control system. Aust J Biomed Eng 1980 1, 4–9*. (9000486)

Otto J. O & P technology: soaring into the new millenium. O & P Business News 2000 9(3), 40–49

Paciga JE ... (et al.) Clinical evaluation of UNB 3-state myoelectric control for arm prostheses. Bull Prosthet Res 1980 10(34), 21–33

Paciga JE, Richard PD, Scott RN. Error rate in five-state myoelectric control systems. Med Biol Eng Comput 1980 18, 287–290

Paquin JM, Andre JM, Herment JP ... (et al.) Le bras UTAH: Premiere experience a propos de quatre amputes des deux bras appareilles bilateralement (the UTAH arm: first experience with four two arm amputees bilaterally fitted). Probl Med Reed 1989 16, 98–105*. (22584)

Parker P, Korner L, Almstrom C ... (et al.) Skeletal muscle force, pressure and myoelectric signal. Zdrav Vestn 1982 51(Suppl 1), 33–34*. (9207473)

Parker PA, Scott RN. Myoelectric control of prostheses. Crit Rev Biomed Eng 1995 13, 283–310*. (9515086)

Patterson DB, McMillan PM, Rodriguez RP. Acceptance rate of myoelectric prosthesis. J Assoc Child Prosthet Orthot Clin 1989 24(2/3), 37

Patterson DB, McMillan PM, Rodriguez RP. Acceptance rate of myoelectric prosthesis. J Assoc Child Prosthet Orthot Clin 1990/1991 25, 73–76

Patterson PE, Katz JA. Design and evaluation of a sensory feedback system that provides grasping pressure in a myoelectric hand. J Rehabil Res Dev 1992 29(1), 1–8

Patton JG. Upper-limb prosthetic components for children and teenagers. In: Comprehensive management of the upper-limb amputee./ edited by DJ Atkins, RH Meier.- New York: Springer-Verlag, 1988. p99–120*. (9927086)

Patton JG, Shida-Tokeshi J, Setoguchi Y. Prosthetic components for children. Phys Med Rehabil: State Art Rev 1991 5, 245–264

Peizer E. External power in prosthetics, orthotics and orthopaedic aids. Prosthet Int 1971 4(1), 4–60

Peizer E, Pirrello T. Principles and practice in upper extremity prostheses. Orthop Clin North Am 1992 3, 397–417*. (9513937)

Petersen I. Electromyography in cases of congenital and traumatic arm amputations. Acta Orthop Scand 1966 37, 166–176

Philipson L. The electromyographic signal used for control of upper extremity prostheses and for quantification of motor blockade during epidural anaesthesia. Linkoping Studies Sci Technol 1987 172, 8–126*. (20529)

Philipson L, Childress D, Strysik J. Digital approaches to myoelectric state control of prostheses. Bull Prosthet Res 1982 10(36), 3–11

Philipson L, Sorbye R. Control accuracy and response time in multiple-state myoelectric control of upper-limb prostheses: initial results in nondisabled volunteers. Med Biol Eng Comput 1987 25, 289–293

Philipson L, Sorbye R. Myoelectric elbow and hand prosthesis controlled by signals from 2 muscles only, in a 9 year old girl. Prosthet Orthot Int 1981 5, 29–32

Philipe-Auguste JS, Gibbons DT, O'Riain MD. Simulation and modelling of a microcomputer controlled above-elbow prosthesis. Automedica 1989 11, 99–109*. (22605)

Picken R. Myoelectric prosthesis for a partial hand amputee (abstract). J Assoc Child Prosthet Orthot Clin 1986 21, 30

Platt W, Shutty MS, Buckelew SP ... (et al.) Biofeedback-assisted assessment and myoelectric training in an adolescent below elbow amputee (abstract). Arch Phys Med Rehabil 1989 70(11), A99–A100

Plettenburg DH. A myoelectrically controlled pneumatically powered hand prosthesis for children. J Rehabil Sci 1988 1, 135–137

Plettenburg DH. Electric versus pneumatic power in hand prostheses for children. J Med Eng Technol 1989 13, 124–128

Ploger J, Baumgartner R. Die Kineplastik nach Sauerbruch im Zeitalter der Myoelektrik (Sauerbruch's cineplasty versus myoelectric prostheses). Med Orthop Tech 1986 106, 110–113

Popov B. The bio-electrically controlled prosthesis. J Bone Joint Surg 1965 47B, 421–424

Pouthier F, Vincent C, Morissette M-J ... (et al.) Clinical results of an investigation of paediatric upper limb myoelectric prosthesis fitting at the Quebec Rehabilitation Institute. Prosthet Orthot Int 2001 25, 119–131

Prehension assessment: prosthetic therapy for the upper limb child amputee./edited by David Krebs. - Thorofare, NJ: Slack, 1987

Proot W. The New York electric elbow, the New York prehension actuator, and the NU-VA synergetic prehension. In: Comprehensive management of the upper-limb amputee./ edited by DJ Atkins, RH Meier.- New York: Springer-Verlag, 1988. p221–226*. (9927080)

Puchhammer G. Der taktile rutschsensor: integrated miniaturisierter sensorik in einer myo-hand (the tactile sup sensor: integration of a miniaturized sensory device on an myoelectric hand). Orthop Tech 1999 50, 564–569 (E)

Putzi R. Myoelectric partial-hand prosthesis. J Prosthet Orthot 1992 4, 103–108

Radocy R. Willkurlich schlieBende eigen kraftprothesen in den USA (voluntary closing devices for body-powered upper extremity prostheses in the USA). Med Orthop Tech 2001 121, 18–20

Rebuck C, Ciocco R, Harrington SE ... (et al.) The ultimate camp experience (abstract). Orthop Trans 1998/99 22, 1199

Reswick JB. Development of feedback control prosthetic and orthotic devices. Adv Biomed Eng 1972 2, 139–217*. (01866)

Ringaert L, Lyttle D. Wearing patterns and usage of myoelectric prostheses in a population of young amputees (abstract). J Assoc Child Prosthet Orthot Clin 1991 26, 25

Robdeutscher W, Hammerl M, Wen L ... (et al.) Ein myo-trainer mit animierter darstellung – neue moglichkeiten des muskeltrainings fur amputierte (a myoelectric training system with animated presentation – new possibilities of muscle training with amputees). Orthop Tech 1999 50, 560– 562

Robertson E. Rehabilitation of arm amputees and limb deficient children. - London: Bailliere Tindall, 1978

Rodriquez RP. Amputation surgery and prostheses. Orthop Clin North Am 1996 27, 525–539*. (9617644)

Roesler H. Entwicklung, stand und perspektiven kunstlicher hande (development present state and perspectives of artificial hands). Orthop Tech 1982 33, 101–105*. (23741)

Rohland TA. Sensory feedback in upper-limb prosthetic systems. ICIB 1974 13(9), 1–4

Ronald JR, Kingston JE. How early can we start myoelectrics (abstract). BAPO Newsletter 1997 No. 2, 25

Ronald JR, Kingston JE. Myoelektrische prothesen fur kinder mit ellbogen-exartikulationsamputationen (myoelectric prostheses for children with elbow distraction). Orthop Tech 1997 48, 918–924

Rossdeutscher W. Steuerungsmoglichkeiten in der armprothetik (facilities of control of upper limb prosthetics). Orthop Tech 2000 51, 865–868

Rowe J. Record breaking development in artificial limb technology. Within Reach 1999 No. 69, 6

Rubin G, Harris F. An above-elbow electrically controlled prosthesis complicated by the presence of a cardiac pacemaker. Clin Prosthet Orthot 1987 11, 251–253

Sacchetti R, Schmidl H. Les protheses dan le traitement de l'enfant (prostheses used in treatment of children). Techn Orthop Int 1994 No. 25, 4–13*. (9411213)

Salam Y. The use of silicone suspension sleeves with myoelectric fittings. J Prosthet Orthot 1994 6, 119–120

Sanderson ER, Caldwell RR, Wedderburn Z ... (et al.) Myoelectric below-elbow prostheses in the very young child (abstract). ICIB 1984 19, 55

Sauter WF. Application of a three-state myoelectric control system. ICIB 1977 16(1/2), 9–12

Sauter WF. Erfahrungen mit elektrischen Antriebs-und steuersystemen in armprothesen fur kinder und erwachsene (experiences with electrically powered and myoelectric control systems in upper extremity prosthetics for children and adults). Med Orthop Tech 1992 112, 13–16

Sauter WF. Reassessing myoelectric control: is it time to look at alternatives? (letter) Can Med Assoc J 1987 137, 10*. (16944)

Sauter WF, Bush G, Sommerville J. A single case study: myoelectrically controlled exoskeletal mobilizer for amyotrophic lateral sclerosis (ALS) patients. Prosthet Orthot Int 1989 13, 145–148

Sauter WF, Dakpa R, Galway R ... (et al.) Development of layered "Onionized" silicone sockets for juvenile below-elbow amputees. J Assoc Child Prosthet Orthot Clin 1987 22, 57–59

Sauter WF, Dakpa R, Hamilton E ... (et al.) Prosthesis with electric elbow and hand for a three-year-old multiply handicapped child: case note. Prosthet Orthot Int 1985 9, 105–108

Sauter WF, Naumann S, Milner M. A three-quarter type below-elbow socket for myoelectric prostheses. Prosthet Orthot Int 1986 10, 79–82

Schultz CJ, Kritter AE. Myoelectric single-site electrode fitting for a short below-elbow amputee. ICIB 1983 18(3), 1–6

Scotland TR, Galway HR. A long-term review of children with congenital and acquired limb deficiency. J Bone Joint Surg 1983 65B, 346–349

Scott RN. Biomedical engineering in upper-extremity prosthetics. In: Comprehensive management of the upper-limb amputee./ edited by DJ Atkins, RH Meier, - New York: Springer-Verlag, 1988. p9173–189*. (9927084)

Scott RN. Feedback in myoelectric prostheses. Clin Orthop 1990 256, 58–63

Scott RN. Myo-electric control. Science J 1966 March, 8pp*. (17327)

Scott RN. Myo-electric energy spectra (technical note). Med Biol Eng 1967 5, 303–305*. (17326)

Scott RN. Myoelectric control of prostheses. Arch Phys Med Rehabil 1966 47, 174–181*. (17328)

Scott RN. Myoelectric control of prostheses and orthoses. Bull Prosthet Res 1967 10(7), 93–114

Scott RN. Myoelectric control systems. In: Advances in biomedical engineering and medical physics. Vol.2./ edited by SN Levine.- New York, NY: Wiley 1962 p45–72*. (01453)

Scott RN. Myo-electric control systems. Progress report No. 5. University of New Brunswick. Bioengineering Institute, 1965. 25 pp*. (22668)

Scott RN. Myo-electric control systems. Progress report No. 6. University of New Brunswick. Bioengineering Institute, 1967. 41 pp*. (22667)

Scott RN. Myoelectric control systems research at the Bioengineering Institute, University of New Brunswick. Med Prog Technol 1990 16, 5–10*. (9002083)

Scott RN ... (et al.) New myoelectric control system (abstract). J Assoc Child Prosthet Orthot 1986 21, 30

Scott RN. Reassessing myoelectric control: is it time to look at alternatives? (letter). Can Med Assoc J 1987 137, 10*. (16962)

Scott RN. Understanding and using your myoelectric prostheses. / by RN Scott ... (et al.) -New Brunswick: Bioengineering Institute, University of New Brunswick, 1985

Scott RN, Brittain RH, Caldwell PR ... (et al.) Sensory feedback system compatible with myoelectric control. Med Biol Eng Comput 1980 18, 65–69

Scott RN, Dunfield VA, Richard PD ... (et al.) A myoelectric control system for young children (abstract). ICIB 1984 19, 4–5

Scott RN, Lovely DF. Amplifier input impedances for myoelectric control. Med Biol Eng Comput 1986 24, 527–530

Scott RN, O'Shea BJ, Dunfield VA ... (et al.) Myo-electric control systems. Muscle function analysis. Progress report No. 7. University of New Brunswick. Bioengineering Institute, 1968. 30 pp*. (22666)

Scott RN, Parker PA. Myoelectric prostheses: state of the art. J Med Eng Technol 1988 12, 143–151

Scott RN, Parker PA. A review of the criteria for setting switching levels in myoelectric prostheses (abstract). J Assoc Child Prosthet Orthot Clin 1990 25, 46

Scott RN, Parker PA, O'Neill PA ... (et al.) Criteria for setting switched levels in myoelectric prostheses. J Assoc Child Prosthet Orthot Clin 1990 25, 11–14

Scott RN, Sanderson ER. Sensory feedback in prosthetics: where do we go now? (abstract). ICIB 1984 19, 54

Scott RN, Tucker FR. Surgical implications of myoelectric control. Clin Orthop 1968 61, 248–260*. (17300)

Scott TRD, Hunter Peckham P, Kilgore KL. Tri-state myoelectric control of bilateral upper extremity neuroprostheses for tetraplegic individuals. IEEE Trans Rehabil Eng 1996 4, 251–263

Sears HH. Approaches to prescription of body-powered and myoelectric prostheses. Phys Med Rehabil Clin North Am 1991 2, 361–371*. (9104940)

Sears HH, Andrew JT, Jacobsen SC. Experience with the Utah Arm, Hand, and Terminal Device. In: Comprehensive management of the upper-limb amputee./ edited by DJ Atkins, RH Meier.- New York: Springer-Verlag, 1988. p194–210*. (9927082)

Sears H, Rendi J. A look at myoelectric prosthetic technology. O & P Business World 1999 2(1), 48–52

Sears HH, Shaperman J. Proportional myoelectric hand control: an evaluation. Am J Phys Med Rehabil 1991 70, 20–28

Selvarajah K, Datta D. An unusual complication of a myoelectric prosthesis. Prosthet Orthot Int 2001 25, 243–245

Sensky TE. A consumer's guide to "bionic arms". Br Med J 1980 12 July, 126–127*. (00190)

Setoguchi Y. Alternative pediatric prosthetic fittings. Capabilities 1993 3(1), 4–5*. (9308315)

Shannon GF. The case for sensory feedback on artificial limbs. Inst Eng Australia Elect Eng Trans 1975 EE11, 36–38*. (05586)

Shannon GF. A comparison of alternative means of providing sensory feedback on upper limb prostheses. Med Biol Eng 1976 14, 289–294

Shannon GF. A myoelectrically-controlled prosthesis with sensory feedback. Med Biol Eng Comput 1979 17, 73–80

Shannon GF. Characteristics of a transducer for tactile displays. Biomed Eng 1974 9, 247–249

Shannon GF. Sensory feedback for artificial limbs. Med Prog Technol 1979 6, 73–79*. (23739)

Shannon GF. Some experience in fitting a myoelectrically controlled hand which has a sense of touch. J Med Eng Technol 1978 2, 312–314

Shannon GF, Agnew PJ. Fitting below-elbow prostheses which convey a sense of touch. Med J Aust 1979 24 March, 242–244*. (17363)

Sherman ED, Gingras G, Lippay AL ... (et al.) New trends in externally powered upper extremity prostheses. World Med J 1968 15, 121–125*. (9822159)

Sherman ED, Lippman Al, Gingras G. Prosthesis given new perspectives by external power. Hosp Management 1965 100, 44–49*. (17329)

Sherman ED, Lippay AL, Gingras G. Prosthesis given new perspectives by external power (abstract). ICIB 1966 5(10), 10–12

Silcox DH, Rooks MD, Vogel RR ... (et al.) Myoelectric prostheses: a long-term follow-up and a study of the use of alternate prostheses. J Bone Joint Surg 1993 75A, 1781–1789

Skewes E, Haas J, Kruger LM. Surlyn sockets for below-elbow myoelectric prostheses. J Assoc Child Prosthet Orthot Clin 1988 23, 19–23

Solomonow M ... (et al.) The myoelectric signal of electrically stimulated muscle during recruitment: an inherent feedback parameter for a closed-loop control scheme. IEEE Trans Biomed Eng 1986 33, 735–745

Solomonow M, Adair C, Lyman JH. Harnessing technique for myoelectric arm prosthesis – technical note. Bull Prosthet Res 1979 10(32), 208–212

Sorbye R. Myoelectric controlled hand prostheses in children. Int J Rehabil Res 1977 1, 15–25

Sorbye R. Myoelectric prosthetic fitting in young children. Clin Orthop 1980 148, 34–40

Sorbye R. Myoelektrisch gesteuerte handprothese fur kinder – klinische betrachtungen (myoelectrically controlled hand prostheses in children – clinical considerations). Orthop Tech 1980 31(1), 19–22*. (23744)

Sorbye R. Upper-extremity amputees: Swedish experiences concerning children. In: Comprehensive management of the upper-limb amputee./ edited by DJ Atkins, RH Meier.- New York: Springer-Verlag, 1988. p227–239*. (9927085)

Spaeth JP ... (et al.) Handbook of externally powered prostheses for the upper extremity amputation. - Springfield, Ill: CC Thomas, 1981

Spiegler SR. Adult myoelectrical upper-limb prosthetic training. In: Comprehensive management of the upper-limb amputee./ edited by DJ Atkins, RH Meier.- New York: Springer-Verlag, 1988. p60–71*. (9927074)

Spittler AW, Rosen IE. Cineplastic muscle motors for prostheses of arm amputees. J Bone Joint Surg 1951 33A, 601– 611

Stack DM, McDonnell PM. Conditioning 1–6 month old infants by means of myoelectrically controlled reinforcement. Int J Rehabil Res 1995 18, 151–156

Stein RB, Charles D, James KB. Providing motor control for the handicapped: a fusion of modern neurosciences, bioengineering, and rehabilitation. Adv Neurol 1988 47, 565–581*. (19917)

Stein RB, Charles D, Walley M. Bioelectric control of powered limbs for amputees. Adv Neurol 1983 39, 1093–1109*. (05011)

Stein RB, Walley M. Functional comparison of upper extremity amputees using myoelectric and conventional prostheses. Arch Phys Med Rehabil 1983 64, 243–248

Stern PH, Lauko T. A myoelectrically controlled prosthesis using remote muscle sites. ICIB 1973 12(7), 1–4

Stinus H, Baumgartner R, Schuling S. Uber die akzeptanz von armprothesen (on the acceptance of upper extremity prostheses). Med Orthop Tech 1992 112, 7–12

Stocker D, Caldwell R. Pattern of usage of cosmetic gloves for myoelectric prostheses (abstract). J Assoc Child Prosthet Orthot Clin 1993 28, 17

Stocker DE, Lovely DF, McDonnell PM. Children using computer video games in myoelectric training. Rehabil Digest 1991 22, 7–10

Stocker D, McDonnell PM, Lovely DF. Computer aided myoelectric training (abstract). J Assoc Child Prosthet Orthot Clin 1991 26, 17

Thaury MN, Gauquil C, Vergnettes J ... (et al.) Le point sur les protheses myoelectriques (position on myoelectric prosthesis). Probl Med Reed 1989 16, 91–98*. (22585)

Thyberg M, Johansen PB. Prosthetic rehabilitation in unilateral high above-elbow amputation and brachial plexus lesion: case report. Arch Phys Med Rehabil 1987 67, 260–262

Triolo RJ, Moskowitz GD. The experimental demonstration of a multichannel time-series myoprocessor: system testing and evaluation. IEEE Trans Biomed Eng 1989 36, 1018–1027

Trost FJ. A long term follow-up on amputees with myoelectric prostheses (abstract). J Assoc Child Prosthet Orthot Clin 1993 28, 30

Tura A, Lamberti C, Davalli A ... (et al.) Experimental development of a sensory control system for an upper limb myoelectric prosthesis with cosmetic covering. J Rehabil Res Dev 1998 35, 14–26

Uellandahl J. Pediatric myolectric fittings. Capabilities 1993 3(1), 1,4*. (9308313)

Uellandahl JE. Upper extremity myoelectric prosthetics. Phys Med Rehabil Clin North Am 2000 11, 639–652

Uellandahl JE, Heelan JR. Prosthetic management of the upper limb deficient child. Phys Med Rehabil: State Art Rev 2000 14, 221–235

Ulsass W. Les possibilities fonctionnelles pour un ampute des quatre membres (the functional possibilities for a quadrimembral amputee). Ortho-Scop 1980 1, 55–58

Upper-limb electronic technology moves forward. O & P Business News 1999 8(23), 1, 20–23

Van Lunteren A, Van Lunteren-Gerritsen GHM, Stassen HB ... (et al.) A field evaluation of arm prostheses for unilateral amputees. Prosthet Orthot Int 1983 7, 141–151

Vitali M ... (et al.) Amputations and prostheses. – London: Bailliere Tindall, 1978

Wakefield GS, Auty B, Tottle CR. Powered exo-skeleton for the treatment of paralytic upper limb disease. Rehabilitation (Lond) 1975 No. 94, 22–25

Wang G, Zhang X, Zhang J ... (et al.) Gripping force sensory feedback for a myoelectrically controlled forearm prosthesis. In: IEEE International Conference on Systems, Man and Cybernetics; intelligent systems for the 21st century, Vancouver, B.C., October 22–25, 1995. – Piscataway, N.J: IEEE, 1995. p501–504*. (9615942)

Waring W. Spectrum analysis of the myoelectric signal: a bibliography. Bull Prosthet Res 1972 10(18), 5–9

Waring W, Antonelli DJ. Myoelectric control systems. Orthop Prosthet Appl J 1967 21(1), 27–32*. (9308714)

Wasserman WL. Human amplifiers. Int Sci Technol, 1964. 9 pp*. (17301)

Weaver SA, Lange LR, Vogts VM. Comparison of myoelectric and conventional prostheses for adolescent amputees. Am J Occup Ther 1988 42, 87–91

Weaver SA, Lange LR. Myoelectric prostheses versus body powered prostheses with unilateral, congenital, adolescent below elbow amputees (abstract). Orthot Prosthet 1986 39(4), 56

Wedlick LT. External power and recent concepts in control of limb prostheses. Med J Aust 1969 8 February, 278–280*. (16671)

Weir RFF, Grahn EC, Duff SJ. A new externally powered, myoelectrically controlled prosthesis for persons with partial-hand amputations at the metacarpals. J Prosthet Orthot 2001 13, 26–31

Weir RFF, Heckathorne CW, Childress DS. Cineplasty as a control input for externally powered prosthetic components. J Rehabil Res Dev 2001 38, 357–363

Wetz HH, Gisbertz D. Amputation und prothetik: teil 1: amputation und prothesenversorgung der oberen extremitat (amputation and prosthetics: part 1: the upper limb. Orthopade 1998 27, 397–411*. (9824061)

What normality means to a girl called Aasa. New Scientist 1978 9 March, 659*. (23736)

Williams TW. One-muscle infant's myoelectric control. J Assoc Child Prosthet Orthot Clin 1989 24(2/3), 53–56

Williams TW. Practical methods for controlling powered upper-extremity prostheses. Assistive Technol 1990 2, 3–18

Williams TW. The Boston elbow. SOMA 1986 1(2), 29–33

Williams TW. Use of the Boston Elbow for high-level amputees. In: Comprehensive management of the upper-limb amputee./ edited by DJ Atkins, RH Meier.- New York: Springer-Verlag, 1988. p211–220*. (9927081)

Williams TW, Polsky S, Gans B ... (et al.) Hybrid myoelectric prosthesis for congenital elbow disarticulation (abstract). J Assoc Child Prosthet Orthot Clin 1986 21, 53

Winkler W, Bierwirth W, Fitzlaff G. Myoelektrische Prothesen bei Amputationen oberhalb des Ellenbogens (myoelectric prostheses for above-elbow amputations). Med Orthop Tech 1986 106, 114–119

Wirta R, Taylor DR, Finley FR. Pattern-recognition arm prosthesis: a historical perspective – a final report. Bull Prosthet Orthot Res 1978 10(30), 8–35

Withrow CA, Schuck M. Early prosthetic fittings – the Grenville experience (abstract). J Assoc Child Prosthet Orthot Clin 1991 26, 26

Wood JC, Barry DT, Alter B ... (et al.) Myoacoustic control of upper-extremity prostheses (abstract). J Assoc Prosthet Orthot Clin 1989 24(2/3), 37

Wood JE, Meek SG, Jacobsen SC. Quantitation of human shoulder anatomy for prosthetic arm control – 1. Surface modelling. J Biomech 1989 22, 273–292

Wright TW, Hagen AD, Wood MB. Prosthetic usage in upper extremity amputations. J Hand Surg 1995 20A, 619–622*. (9515453)

Yeh EC, Chung WP, Chan RC ... (et al.) Development of neural network controller for below-elbow prosthesis using single-chip mircontroller. Biomed Eng Appl Basis Comm 1993 5, 340–346*. (9411761)

Yu W, Yokoi H, Nishikawa D. Adaptive electromyographic (EMG) prosthetic hand control using Reinforcement Learning. In: Intelligent autonomous systems./ edited by Y Kakuza, M Wada, T Sato.- Amsterdam: ISO Press, 1998. p266–271*. (9924804)

Zhang Y, Gruver WA. Force distribution of power grasps based on the controllability of contact forces. In: IEEE International Conference on Systems, Man and Cybernetics; intelligent systems for the 21st century, Vancouver, B.C., October 22–25, 1995.- Piscataway, N.J: IEEE, 1995. p83–88*. (9615938)

Zhang YT, Parker PA, Scott RN. Control performance characteristics of myoelectric signal with additive interference. Med Biol Eng Comput 1991 29, 84–88

Zwaan A. Der gebrauchswert einer myoelektrischen prothese: eine nachuntersuchung an 12 patienten (utility value of the myoelectric prosthesis – follow-up study on 12 patients). Orthop Tech 1992 43, 727–731

Subject Index